PERSISTENT RENAL-GENITOURINARY DISORDERS

DEVELOPMENTS IN NEPHROLOGY

Gruskin, A.B. and Norman, M.E., eds.: Pediatric Nephrology. 1981. ISBN 90-247-2514-3.

Schück, O., ed.: Examination of the Kidney Function. 1981. ISBN 0-89838-565-2.

Strauss, J., ed.: Hypertension, Fluid-Electrolytes and Tubulopathies in Pediatric Nephrology. 1981. ISBN 90-247-2633-6.

Strauss, J., ed.: Neonatal Kidney and Fluid-Electrolytes. 1983. ISBN 0-89838-575-X.

Strauss, J., ed.: Acute Renal Disorders and Renal Emergencies. 1984. ISBN 0-89838-663-2.

Didio, L.J.A. and Motta, P.M., eds.: Basic, Clinical and Surgical Nephrology. 1985. ISBN 0-89838-698-5.

Friedman, E.A. and Peterson, C.M., eds.: Diabetic Nephropathy: Strategy for Therapy. 1985. ISBN 0-89838-735-3.

Dzurik, R., Lichardus, B. and Guder, W., eds.: Kidney Metabolism and Function. 1985. ISBN 0-89838-749-3.

Strauss, J., ed: Homeostasis, Nephrotoxicity, and Renal Anomalies in the Newborn. 1986. ISBN 0-89838-766-3.

Oreopoulos, D.G., ed: Geriatric Nephrology. 1986. ISBN 0-89838-781-7.

Paganini, E.P., ed: Acute Continuous Renal Replacement Therapy. 1986. ISBN 0-89838-793-0.

Cheigh, J.S., Stenzel, K.H. and Rubin, A.L., eds.: Hypertension in Kidney Disease. 1986. ISBN 0-89838-797-3.

Deane, N., Wineman, R.J. and Bemis, J.A., eds.: Guide to Reprocessing of Hemodialyzers. 1987. ISBN 0-89838-798-1.

Ponticelli, C., Minetti, L. and D'Amico, G., eds.: Antiglobulins, Cryoglobulins and Glomerulonephritis. 1987. ISBN 0-89838-810-4.

Persistent Renal-Genitourinary Disorders

Current Concepts in Dialysis and Management

Proceedings of Pediatric Nephrology Seminar XII
held at Bal Harbour, Florida
February 25–28, 1985

edited by
José Strauss, MD
Division of Pediatric Nephrology
University of Miami
School of Medicine
Miami, Florida, USA

with the assistance of
Louise Strauss, MS, MA

Martinus Nijhoff Publishing
a member of the Kluwer Academic Publishers Group
Boston/Dordrecht/Lancaster

Distributors for North America:
Kluwer Academic Publishers
101 Philip Drive
Assinippi Park
Norwell, MA 02601, USA

Distributors for the UK and Ireland:
Kluwer Academic Publishers
MTP Press Limited
Falcon House, Queen Square
Lancaster LA1 1RN, UNITED KINGDOM

Distributors for all other countries:
Kluwer Academic Publishers Group
Distribution Centre
Post Office Box 322
3300 AH Dordrecht, THE NETHERLANDS

Library of Congress Cataloging-in-Publication Data

Pediatric Nephrology Seminar (12th : 1985 : Bal Harbour, Fla.)
Persistent renal-genitourinary disorders.

(Developments in nephrology ; DIN 17)
Includes indexes.
1. Kidneys—Diseases—Congresses. 2. Genitourinary organs—Diseases—Congresses. 3. Pediatric nephrology—Congresses. 4. Pediatric urology—Congresses. I. Strauss, José. II. Strauss, Louise. III. Series: Developments in nephrology ; 17. [DNLM: 1. Kidney Diseases—in infancy & childhood—congresses. 2. Urologic Diseases—infancy & childhood—congresses. W1 DE998EB v. 17 / WS 320 P373 1985p]
RF466.P3675 1985 618.92′6 86-28465
ISBN 0-89838-845-7

Printed in the United States of America

ERNESTO STRAUSS

my big brother

found his own way to glory

*

living for giving

caring and sharing

1928–1985

CONTENTS

FOREWORD

This Pediatric Nephrology series is a focus on salient points which at the time of each annual seminar are of importance to the practicing pediatrician and nephrologist, the clinical researcher, and basic researcher interested in clinical problems. Hence the format of selected papers and panel discussions to capture the tenor of the times. More thorough coverage of many of the subjects can be found in current journals and textbooks listed in the authors' references. Those searching for the conventional should look there rather than here since our aim is not to cover each subject in its entirety but to secure attention to the controversial aspects of the subjects, dispel the notion that there is one answer to a question, and raise the level of inclination toward dynamic problem solving.

The basic subject chosen this year reflects dominant concerns this year and the participants chosen--speakers and discussants--represent certain views relevant to the subject at this time. To reflect the tempo and flavor produced by this unique blend, the discussions are included almost verbatim. For some this means readability; for others, excess verbiage. The careful reader will notice that I have been the chairman of all sessions and have moderated all discussions. This is in keeping with our aim to ferret out interrelated basic questions and varying answers to the subjects--seen as related in problems and solutions. In the discussions, all names have been deleted. This is in agreement with participants who thus are encouraged to speak with less inhibition and more candor. My point is, this volume must be evaluated on the basis of its aim, not by standard textbook criteria.

I consider most valuable (30 M.D.) my realization that what is considered known--"the facts"--is temporal, still a question in search of a new answer--even what we think of as basic facts. I would consider myself to have made a significant contribution to the field of medicine if I could stimulate preference for a dynamic approach to any problem--no matter how "standard". We too often see what we look for rather than whatever else there might be, and in the very process of educating, dull the inclination to question, consider alternatives. What seems to be "old stuff"/"routine procedures" may not be/should not be. Of course, we cannot face the volume of our responsibility without using routine procedures; we do not have time or energy to question our every step every day, but absolutely essential to the practice of "good medicine" is an attitude of questioning--removal of the film of familiarity covering truly unresolved questions.

Thus, my hope in this volume (as in the eleven preceding it) is to gently disturb the status quo, to challenge the physician/researcher to think as he acts, to see when he looks. Those who have conspired with me in this effort this year include guest faculty Sidney Blumenthal, Joan Chesney, Russell Chesney, Richard Fine, Warren Grupe, Alan Gruskin, Julie Ingelfinger, Abdollah Iravani, Barry Kahan, Peter Kwiterovich, Norman Siegel, Kirsti Thodenius, and local faculty Carolyn Abitbol, Jacques Bourgoignie, Michael Freundlich, George Kyriakides, Jorge Lockhart, Joshua Miller, Victoriano Pardo, Charles Lynne, Catherine Poole, Gwendolyn Scott, George Sfakianakis, Carlos Vaamonde, and Gaston Zilleruelo.

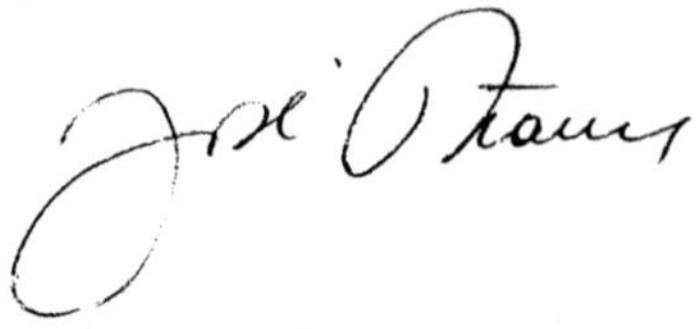

ACKNOWLEDGEMENTS

This volume is made from camera-ready copy prepared by each author which means that each one assumes complete responsibility for the content of his work and each made the effort to prepare his manuscript as required by the publisher. Annual publication would be impossible without the authors' willingness to do this significant part of the job. Even so, more time and effort than an unfamiliar one would imagine go into the final bundle sent to Martinus' Barbara Ward who then carries the copy through to its book form. The one who did the parts that tied everything together is Linda Lane, truly remarkable in her skill, efficiency and perserverance. Also invaluable were Pearl Seidler, Bonnie Ladich and the cooperation of Pediatric Nephrology Division members who tolerated the occasional domination of these efforts.

Those who expressed their support of the Seminar on which this book is based in much more than words include:

American McGaw
Ayerst Laboratories
Beach Pharmaceuticals
Burroughs Wellcome Company
CD Medical, Inc.
Chesebrough Pond's Inc.
Cobe Laboratories
Florida Children's Medical Services
Merck, Sharp & Dohme
National Kidney Foundation
R&D Laboratories
Ross Laboratories
Sandoz Pharmaceuticals
Schering Corporation
Smith, Kline, & French Laboratories
Travenol Laboratories, Inc.
Upjohn Company
Wyeth Laboratories

As in years past, the approval and moral support of the University of Miami School of Medicine's Department of Pediatrics Chairman William Cleveland and Dean Bernard Fogel form the foundation of our contribution to continuing medical education.

José Strauss

I

PRIMARY NEPHROTIC SYNDROME

IDIOPATHIC NEPHROTIC SYNDROME: PROLIFERATIVE NEPHROPATHY AND MEMBRANOUS NEPHROPATHY

Russell W. Chesney, M.D. and Antonia C. Novello, M.D., M.P.H.

In this chapter we shall cover those disorders in children which result in a proliferative and/or membranous renal morphologic appearance. If one considers only the idiopathic nephrotic syndrome and excludes known causes of these disorders such as systemic lupus erythematosus, chronic hepatitis antigenemia, and partial lipodystrophy, three conditions should be considered: membranoproliferative glomerulonephritis (mesangiocapillary glomerulonephritis), mesangial proliferative glomerulonephritis, and membranous nephropathy. These three conditions account for only a small percent of the cases of the idiopathic nephrotic syndrome in childhood, occurring in less than 10% of cases in series from North America, Britain and Western Europe. It is our intention to review each of these three disorders, focusing on the major references and on recent reports which indicate the progress in our understanding of these conditions. At the outset it is essential to remember that the etiology and pathogenesis of each is poorly understood and that effective, clearly established forms of treatment for each are not presently available.

MEMBRANOPROLIFERATIVE GLOMERULONEPHRITIS (MESANGIOCAPILLARY GLOMERULONEPHRITIS)

Membranoproliferative or mesangiocapillary glomerulonephritis (MPGN) is a distinctive form of chronic glomerulonephritis which can cause the primary nephrotic syndrome in children or adults. First described in autopsy lesions and called subacute and chronic lobular glomerulonephritis (1, 2), two groups independently reported in 1965 that certain children with persistence of the nephrotic syndrome and reduction of serum complement concentrations, had the glomerular changes that are now considered characteristic of MPGN (3, 4). In this chapter we hope to summarize what we have learned about this entity in the intervening 20 years.

Although clinically similar, two major and three minor subtypes in terms of <u>morphologic appearance</u> account for most cases. <u>Type I MPGN</u> is characterized by subendothelial deposits, mesangial cell interposition and splitting of the basement membrane (5). <u>Type II MPGN</u> or dense deposit disease (DDD) consists of dense, ribbon-like deposits within the basement membrane. Burkholder et al. (6) have described a type with features common to membranous and MPGN, so called Burkholder, Type III. Davis et al. (7) described patients with the features of type I (splitting and proliferation) and irregular intramembranous dense deposits separated by varying lengths of normal-appearing basement membrane. However, the most common minor variant consists of focal, segmental proliferative lesions and and occasionally with widespread subendothelial and subepithelial deposits (8). This latter variant is now generally called Type III MPGN in most series. Immunofluorescent microscopy reveals granular deposition of C_3 and properdin in the mesangium and along the peripheral glomerular basement membrane in type I and the distinctive lesion of C_3 along the margin but not in the deposits in type II which give the parallel double linear bands called "railroad tracks" (5). In type III MPGN, mesangial fluorescence to C_3 and segmental granular fluorescence to IgG in the focal, segmental lesions is evident (8). Each of these subtypes has distinctive electron microscopic features which aid in the identification: in type I a normal basement membrane with mesangial interposition gives rise to the split basement membrane or "train tracking". Type II has the deeply electron dense intramembranous deposit, easily one of the most distinctive electron microscopic findings in renal biopsies (5). In type III the segmental lesions are characterized by mesangial cellular and matrix proliferation.

Not all authorities agree that MPGN should be broken down into these two major and three minor subtypes. It has recently been proposed that type II MPGN be called "dense deposit disease" and that types I and III be lumped together as "mesangiocapillary glomerulonephritis" (9). The fluorescent dye thioflavin T intensely stains these type II dense deposits and can be used to distinguish it from types I and III, although amyloidosis and light chain disease have similar tinctorial properties. In addition, some histologic properties tend to link the three minor subvariants of MPGN (6-8), particularly urinyl acetate or lead citrate staining.

The pathogenesis of MPGN is unknown but probably involves immune complex induced renal disease (5, 10). Several factors suggest that immune complexes are involved including the fact that patients with type I disease have hypocomplementemia with consumption of components of complement by the classical and alternative pathways, that the disease may represent the consequences of persistent antigenemia, the presence of cryoglobulins and Clq-binding immune complexes in serum and the finding that chronic bacteremia leads to similar lesions. In type II disease, the finding of granular deposition of immunoglobulins and the presence of circulating immune complexes indicate an immune complex pathogenic mechanism (5).

A variety of complement system abnormalities are apparent. The serum complement values are variable in type I and may be reduced at the time of diagnosis in only 25 to 33% of the patients (5, 10, 11). Hypocomplementemia occurs sometime during the course of the disease in patients with type I disease, although recent series of patients in whom serial serum complement values were measured indicate that this is not always correct. Types I and III have similar patterns of complement abnormalities. The complement abnormalities in type II disease are different in that persistent hypocomplementemia is frequent (5, 12, 13), the concentrations of the early (classical pathway) components such as Clq and C_4 are normal, and the components of the alternative pathway, such as factor B and properdin, are reduced (5, 12-14). The autoantibody, C_3 nephritic factor (C_3NeF), which appears to be directed against the alternative pathway C_3 convertase is far more common in patients with type II MPGN than in

Table I. Clinical Features of MPGN in Children

Series	Habib (12)	Davis (14)	McEnery (20)	Cameron (11)	Together
Year	1973	1978	1980	1983	
Patients	105	27	27	45	204
Males	45	14	18	17	94(46%)
Females	60	13	9	28	110(54%)
Female/Male Ratio	1.33	0.93	0.5	1.65	1.17
TYPE of MPGN					
I	76	13	15	23	127(62%)
II	29	14	5	22	70(34%)
III	--	--	7	--	7 (3%)
Age of Onset	10yr.	9.5yr.	9.5yr.	11.5yr.	10yr.
Azotemia %	31%	22%	30%	51%	33%
Hypertension	25%	41%	41%	20%	32%
ONSET Acute glomerulonephritis	88%	78%	93%	47%	77%
Nephrotic Syndrome	67%	56%	52%	33%	52%
Proteinuria	--	--	--	20%	20%
Hypocomplementemia	--	78%	74%	43%	65%
Extensive Crescents	15%	15%	15%	17%	16%
Years of follow-up	1-16yr.	1-8yr.	1-18yr.	2-21yr.	
Persistent Remissions	6%	--	37%	56%	
Development of ESRD	40%	67%	15%	36%	
Actuarial ESRD	50% by 11th yr.	67% by 6th yr.	11% by 12th yr.	61% by 16th yr.	

type I disease (5, 11, 15, 16).

Put together, the immunofluorescence studies, the presence of immune complexes and the serum complement abnormalities indicate an immunologic etiology. Certain features also suggest that chronic antigenemia may be an important factor since a clinical and morphologic picture resembling MPGN can be seen in bacteremia with visceral abscesses, subacute endocarditis, shunt nephritis and chronic active hepatitis (10). Other less common disorders, such as chronic mucocutaneous candidiasis, may also be associated with MPGN (17). Studies on the composition of glomerulosclerosis indicate that mesangial sclerosis in MPGN consists of the glycoprotein laminin, and collagen type IV, components usually present within the glomerulus, but that crescentic lesions usually contain type III collagen, not normally found in the glomerulus (18). Alpha-1-antitrypsin can be used as a marker for infiltrating monocytes and indicates that monocytic infiltration is marked in severe MPGN (19). Finally, it should be emphasized that the pathogenesis of MPGN is not well understood, that evidence for chronic antigenemia is rarely found and that the cause of complement consumption is uncertain. As well C_3NeF, although common in MPGN, may circulate in the serum of patients with other glomerular disorders.

The clinical course of MPGN has considerable heterogeneity (Table I). Patients may present with a picture suggesting acute post-infectious glomerulonephritis, with the nephrotic syndrome, with isolated proteinuria, with hematuria and proteinuria or with hematuria, either macroscopic or microscopic, alone (3-14). Children appear to have MPGN type II more commonly and hypertension and a reduced GFR less frequently than adults (11), but the breakdown into type I or type II disease is quite variable. Table I consists of a review of 4 large series (11, 12, 14, 20) and examines children with both types I and II lumped together. Although such a comparison can be criticized on the basis that different criteria are established for each center - Paris, Boston, Cincinnati and London - these results are of interest. A total of 204 patients are analyzed in whom 46% are males and 54% females. Of these, 62% had type I MPGN, 34% type II disease and only 3% had type III. This latter figure may be somewhat misleading, since Cameron et al. (11) have lumped types I and III together and Habib et al. (12) did not consider this entity. Davis et al. (7) have elsewhere indicated that perhaps as many as 10% of patients have type III disease. The mean age of onset is approximately 10 years of age and approximately one-third of patients appear to be azotemic at the onset. A mean of 77% have hematuria, over half (52%) have the nephrotic syndrome and hypocomplementemia is found at some time in two-thirds of the patients. The length of follow-up ranged from 1-21 years and anywhere from 6 to 56% had persistent remission of their disease with 15 to 67% developing end stage renal disease or death.

Additional features that may sometimes be apparent are the association of MPGN type II (and rarely type I) with partial lipodystrophy (5), an anemia that is unexplained by the degree of azotemia and a mild hyperchloremic metabolic acidosis (5).

In Table II is listed the major differences between type I and II MPGN, but it should be appreciated that these differences are of little help in assessing the morphologic form of the disease that a given patient may have.

Table II. Differences Between Types I and II MPGN in a Group of Patients*

Feature	Type I	Type II
Renal Biopsy		
Subendothelial Deposits	Present	Absent
Intramembranous dense deposits	Absent	Present
Thioflavin T Staining	Absent	Present
C_3 Mesangial rings	Absent	Present
C_4 immunofluorescence	Present	Absent
Complement (serum)		
C_3	Normal or Reduced	Reduced
C_1 and C_4	Reduced	Normal
C_3 NeF	Uncommon	Common
Clinical Course		
Acute Nephritis	Uncommon	Common
Nephrotic Syndrome	Common	Common
Hematuria	Common	Common
Hypertension	Common	Common
Progression to Renal Failure if Nephrosis present	Common	Common
Progression to Renal Failure if Nephrosis absent	Less Common	Less Common
Recurrence in Transplants	Rare	Common

* Adapted from References 5, 11, 14 and 21

It is notable that the features and findings presented in tables I and II are similar to two other large series of patients (21, 22). The first is a series of patients from Minnesota reported in 1970 indicating how the clinical features have remained constant since the recognition of this disorder (2-4, 21) and how they are similar to recent reports (11). However, it is remarkable that a series of patients from Hacettepe Children's Hospital in Ankara, Turkey who have MPGN due to secondary causes have clinical features quite similar to the large western series we have reviewed (11, 12, 14, 20-22). These 21 patients have the morphologic features of the MPGN in association with systemic lupus erythematosus, Hodgkin's disease, shunt infections, osteomyelitis, endocarditis, chronic active hepatitis, cirrhosis and rheumatic fever. In this series the mean age of onset is 8.6 years, 52% are males, azotemia was present in 53%, hypertension in 21%, a nephritic picture in 57%, nephrotic syndrome in 19% and asymptomatic proteinuria in 24%. In this Turkish series, secondary MPGN represented 9% of all cases of MPGN (22). Thus the only remarkable difference from this series in Asia Minor is that fewer patients had the nephrotic syndrome.

The well known association of MPGN type II with partial lipodystrophy (10, 22) will not be further discussed.

The treatment of MPGN is not entirely satisfactory and several therapeutic approaches have been employed with varying degrees of success (Table III). Currently three approaches are available. West and his group (20, 23) have uncontrolled data suggesting that alternate day prednisone is of benefit with improvement in both the clinical features, such as hematuria and proteinuria, and in the histologic appearance on serial renal biopsy specimens. These results have met with some skepticism and the International Study for Kidney Disease in Children report indicated no clear benefit of prednisone treatment and that patients receiving oral glucocorticoids in this prospective trial experienced considerable morbidity in the form of glucocorticoid side effects (24). The reasons for these differences are not immediately apparent, but it is noteworthy that the Cincinnati series includes patients from a single center in whom therapy was initiated within 1.5 years of the discovery of MPGN. McEnery et al. (20) compared the patient survival in their series to the published series of Habib et al. (12) and Davis et al. (14) and using the actuarial method, found an 89% survival versus a 50% survival. These differences could not be accounted for by readily obvious factors such as type of MPGN, mean age of disease onset, presence of the nephrotic syndrome, hypertension, crescents, hematuria or azotemia. Two additional factors are of importance. First, in all the series discussed, patients do undergo spontaneous prolonged remissions of their disease (5, 11, 12, 14, 20, 21). Secondly, in all series employing steroids some patients appear to improve.

Hasegawa et al. (25) used pulse intravenous methylprednisolone therapy (30 mg/kg) followed by alternate-day prednisone (1mg/kg/48h) for 2 years in 15 children with MPGN and compared their course to 18 untreated age-matched controls. Creatinine clearance increased from 46 to 68 ml/min and two-thirds of the patients showed a clinical improvement. The renal biopsy showed a decrease in mesangial hypercellularity not seen in controls. Global sclerosis was not altered. Unfortunately a full report of this trial has not appeared.

Table III. Therapy of Mesangiocapillary Glomerulonephritis

A. Alternate Day Prednisone		
1. McAdams (J Pediatr 86:23, 1975)	Retrospective	Benefit
2. McEnery (Clin Nephrol 13:117, 1980)	Retrospective	Benefit
3. ISKDC (Kidney Int 21:150A, 1982)	Prospective	No Benefit High Morbidity
4. Hasegawa (Proc 8th Int Congress Nephrol) (1981)	Controlled + IV Methylprednisolone	Benefit
B. Immunosuppressive Agents		
1. Cameron (Br Med J 4:7, 1970)	Retrospective	No Benefit
2. Herdman (Medicine 49:207, 1970)	Retrospective	No Benefit
3. Holland (Am J Dis Child 123:439, 1972)	Retrospective	No Benefit
4. Davis (Clin Nephrol 8:184, 1978)	Retrospective	No Benefit
5. Donadio (Mayo Clin Proc 54:141, 1979)	Retrospective Pred + Cyclo	No Benefit
C. Indomethacin		
1. Michielsen (Glomerulonephritis 1973)	Not Controlled	Benefit
2. Vanrenterghem (Clin Neph 4:218, 1975)	Plus Cyclophos-phamide	Benefit
3. Ponticelli (Contrib Nephrol 34:33, 1982)	Plus Cyclophos-phamide	No Benefit
D. Anticoagulant Therapy		
1. Kincaid-Smith (Med J Aust 2:587, 1975)	Cyclo + Dipyr Retrospective	Benefit
2. Tiller (Eighth Int Congress Nephrol 1981)	Cyclo + Dipyr + Warf controlled	High Dropout rate
3. Cattaran (Eighth Int Congress Nephrol 1981)	Cyclo + Dipyr + Warf Prospective Randomized	No Benefit
4. Donadio (Seminars Nephrol 2:214, 1982)	ASA + Dipyr Prospective, Controlled	Benefit Iothalamate Clearance
5. Zimmerman (Am J Med 75:920, 1983)	Dipyr + Warf Controlled, Crossover	? Benefit in Treatment year

As noted in Table III, five series have not found any benefit from the use of a variety of immunosuppressive agents used under the conditions of an uncontrolled, non-randomly selected retrospective study. These references will not be given in the reference list aside from 2 that are presently there (14, 21). Although it has never been shown in an appropriate controlled, randomized trial that the use of azathioprine or cyclophosphamide in conjunction with prednisone may be of benefit, these 5 reports are so negative that such a controlled trial seems completely unwarranted.

A third form of treatment that has been employed is indomethacin, usually in conjunction with cyclophosphamide (26, 27). Indomethacin at a dose of 1.5mg/kg/day was employed for 1 year alone or with cyclophosphamide (50mg/day) in 33 adults with MPGN I and II (26). At 10 years the actuarial survival of these patients was improved and after prolonged therapy, proteinuria seemed to be less. This latter statement is not surprising since powerful cyclo-oxygenase inhibitors are known to reduce GFR. Another study in 7 treated patients and 8 controls employing the same dosage schedule of these agents showed no difference in the degree of proteinuria or in GFR after 2 years (27). Thus the benefits of indomethacin are uncertain and no studies in children are available.

The most gratifying response to treatment has occurred in trials in adults employing various anticoagulants. Because fibrin deposition is sometimes present in glomerular vessels, Kincaid-Smith (28) used "triple therapy" consisting of cyclophosphamide, dipyridamole and warfarin in doses which would double prothrombin time in 16 patients and compared results in 13 untreated patients. Ten treated patients showed clinical improvement, but no improvement was found in the control subjects or in 6 treated patients. Two further trials from Australia and Toronto, demonstrated no benefit and indicated the high dropout rate using this type of therapy (Table III). Donadio et al. (29) reported stabilization of iothalamate clearances after using 925 mg of aspirin and 225 mg of dipyridamole. Zimmerman et al. (30) examined warfarin and dipyridamole in 18 patients with MPGN using a control or treatment crossover trial. Unpaired analysis showed stable renal function in the treated as compared to non-treated subjects. The slope of the regression lines for reciprocal serum creatinine values was significantly different between groups. In patients undergoing both phases, renal function improved and urine protein decreased in the treatment year. Bleeding was a frequent complication. These studies suggest that anticoagulants may have a beneficial effect in MPGN, but further trials are required.

The ultimate prognosis of MPGN is shown in Table II, where it is apparent that 15 to 50 percent of patients develop end stage renal failure in 10 years (5, 11, 12, 14, 20, 21). Hence any effective therapy would be of benefit in patients with this disorder. An important characteristic of patients with MPGN who require kidney transplantation because of end stage renal failure is that MPGN may recur in the transplanted kidney (31, 32). In general, this complication occurs in patients with type II disease and complement is consumed by the alternative pathway. Recurrence of dense deposits is typical and immunofluorescent microscopy often reveals C_3, IgG and properdin (31, 32). Most authorities agree that this disease is milder than recurrent focal sclerosing glomerulonephritis following kidney transplant (5, 11, 32).

To summarize, much has been learned concerning MPGN since its initial description in 1965 (3, 4). However, its relentless nature and chronic course indicate that an effective form of therapy is badly needed.

MESANGIAL PROLIFERATIVE GLOMERULONEPHRITIS

Diffuse proliferation of mesangial cells has been seen in a small number of children with the nephrotic syndrome who undergo a renal biopsy (33-35). This association was clearly appreciated in the initial clinicopathological studies of White et al (33). Several recent series of this morphologic entity have been reported with various clinicopathological analyses being made (36-42). However, it is not clearly established that this disorder is distinct from either minimal lesion nephrotic syndrome or focal sclerosing glomerulonephritis (35, 36, 39, 41, 42) in terms of its steroid responsivity, clinical progression and ultimate prognosis.

This disorder is characterized morphologically by diffuse mesangial hypercellularity and by mesangial matrix expansion, but the basement membrane is spared (33-36). Although the immunofluorescent stains are often negative, mesangial deposits of IgM and C_3 may be found, giving rise to the term IgM nephropathy (42). Garin et al. (41) make the point that depending on the degree of mesangial hypercellularity that is included in this designation, the ultimate clinical status will be influenced. Investigators who have included pure mesangial hypercellularity without other features tend to report a favorable response to glucocorticoid therapy and a good prognosis (36, 37), while other studies where more severe mesangial lesions were encountered reported a high frequency of steroid resistance and even a progression to renal failure (35, 39-41). Garin et al.(41) showed that patients with greater degrees of mesangial proliferation had more serious disease. Although patients appear to have a poorer initial response to glucocorticoid therapy, it is still likely that mesangial proliferative glomerulonephritis is closely related to minimal lesion disease (41, 42). It is also important to appreciate that some patients with minimal lesion disease may develop mesangial proliferative disease and visa versa. Nevertheless, mesangial proliferation may be complicated by focal sclerosis and focal sclerosis appears to be much more common in mesangial proliferative than in minimal lesion disease (43). Finally, those patients with nephrotic syndrome who experience a recurrence post transplant are more likely to have been one of the 2-5% of patients with mesangial proliferation (42-44).

Finally, it appears very unlikely that IgM deposition has any pathogenic or prognostic significance in this disorder.

MEMBRANOUS NEPHROPATHY

Idopathic membranous nephropathy (MGN), also known as epimembranous, is a chronic glomerular disease that is unusual in children and adolescents. Most patients are older than 35 years and the peak incidence occurs in the fifth decade (45). Membranous nephropathy and membranous glomerulonephropathy (MGN) are today the most accepted terms for the disease. The term membranous nephropathy describes a distinctive clinicopathological entity, with absence of inflammation and/or proliferation, that usually is associated with the nephrotic syndrome, and appears in the absence of systemic disease or known precipitating factors. In some instances it may represent an underlying disease which has not yet expressed itself (46).

Membranous nephropathy is characterized by the presence of granular deposits of immunoreactants along the glomerular capillary wall and pathologically by thickening of glomerular capillary basement membrane. Primary or Idiopathic, and Secondary membranous nephropathy, seen in association with a known cause, are the two main categories. Secondary disease has been associated with infections (hepatitis B, syphilis, leprosy, filariasis, malaria); multisystem diseases (SLE, rheumatoid arthritis, sarcoidosis, diabetes mellitus); neoplasms (carcinoma of lung, colon, breast, stomach); lymphoma (Hodgkins); medications (organic gold, elemental mercury, d-penicillamine, captopril); heredofamilial and metabolic diseases (sickle cell, thyroiditis) and miscellaneous disorders (Fanconi, chronic allograft rejection, bullous pemphigoid) (46).

In children, the association with malignancy is rare, and only a single case with Wilms' tumor has been reported (47). Libit has stated that SLE is the main cause of MGN in children (48), emphasizing that the nephropathy may precede serologic evidence of SLE by several years. Renal vein thrombosis has often been reported with MGN, but this might be a consequence of the glomerulopathy, rather than its cause (46). Hepatitis B, SLE, carcinoma, organic gold, elemental mercury, and D penicillamine, account for about 75 percent of the secondary forms of membranous glomerulopathy (46).

Incidence

Actual incidence in childhood is difficult to assess. The overall prevalence in earlier studies, which relied heavily on light microscopy, may have been underestimated. The International Study of Kidney Disease in children reported that 2 of 127 nephrotic children had membranous nephropathy (49). In a more selected group Habib found 37 children with MGN among 406 nephrotics. Analyzing all available data, Pollak concluded that MGN occurs in 6 percent of nephrotic children and 19 percent of nephrotic adults. Row, however found an incidence of 2.7 percent in children and of 20 percent in adults (47). The percentage of nephrotic children with MGN has varied from 2.7 percent to 6 percent in all children with nephrotic syndrome (50).

The prognosis is variable. In adults, Cameron estimated that 75 - 80 percent of patients will be alive five years after the diagnosis, and 50 percent after ten years (51). In children, however, Habib has reported progression to renal failure in only 10 percent, over 5 years, suggesting a better prognosis in children than in adults (52). The histologic stage of glomerular lesion appears to correlate with ultimate prognosis in adults. The same correlation has not been well studied in pediatric patients. The prognosis in children appears to be not as good if the clinical course is characterized by unremitting nephrotic proteinuria, severe hypertension, and renal vein thrombosis. The age at presentation is also considered a prognostic feature in children. Obing indicates that patients whose disease onset occurs before 10 years of age have a better prognosis than patients with onset after that (53). No correlation between age at onset and outcome, however, was found in other series (50, 54).

Clinical Features

Membranous nephropathy is known for its well defined clinical expression. The onset is usually insidious and the disease occurs at all ages, including infancy, and as in adult series, males are more affected than females. Proteinuria is always present and often is associated with the nephrotic syndrome. Proteinuria is usually non-selective, but highly selective proteinuria can occur in up to 20 percent of patients (50). Microscopic hematuria is common, and gross hematuria is rare, but hematuria usually disappears during the course of the disease (50).

The C_3 complement in plasma and other complement components are nearly always normal. If abnormal, they point to a multisystem involvement. HLA-DRW-3 is found in 65-75 percent of cases (46). Hypertension and azotemia are encountered less often in children than in adults. Signs of proximal tubular dysfunction, however, have been described in children, as have polyarthralgias, rash, purpura and thrombocytopenia (50).

Splenic reticuloendothelial function in MGN is defective, as evidenced by delayed clearance of IgG. This defect does not correlate with disease activity and is associated with HLA-B8 and DR3 (55). During the nephrotic stage of MGN the proportion of T lymphocytes decreases with simultaneous increase in the proportion of B lymphocytes. Similarly, in nephrotic MGN patients' impaired lymphocyte reactivity with lower Con A and PHA responses as compared to controls, is evident. However, the mean mitogenic responses to the antigens in patients with MGN in remission were similar to those of the control subjects (56). The frequency of HLA-B8 antigen in MGN is 57 percent, the frequency of HLA-DR3 antigen is 65 percent. Of further interest, the half life of sensitized erythrocytes is 67 minutes; this prolongation appears to correlate with exacerbations of the disease while normal values are obtained with remission. During exacerbations the T-lymphocyte subset fractions are normal, whereas OKT3 and OKT4 are decreased during remission. These studies indicate that MGN is a strongly HLA-linked disease (57). A strong association of MGN with HLA-DR2 and MT1 in Japanese patients has also recently been reported; these findings suggest that an immunological disturbance under the influence of genetic factors may confer a susceptibility to membranous nephropathy (58).

Pathologic Features

The typical light microscopic lesion in MGN is a diffuse and uniform thickening of the capillary wall, usually without proliferation of endothelial, mesangial or epithelial cells. Spiky argyrophilic projections, arising from the glomerular basement membrane, can be demonstrated using silver stains. These spikes give the typical comb-like appearance to the capillary wall (46). Four patterns are distinguished by electron microscopy representing histologic evolution of the disease. Stage I: BM (basement membrane) is normal but small, discrete electron-dense subepithelial deposits, under the foot processes of epithelial cells, are evident. Stage II: Projections of variable shape arise from the BM between adjacent deposits. Many of these spikes encircle the deposit, giving a dome-like appearance. Stage III: Foot processes are greatly distorted. Stage IV: Deposits are progressively incorporated into the BM, where they lose their density and become difficult to distinguish from the basement membrane itself. By immunofluorescence, IgG is nearly always present in a uniform granular distribution, outlining the capillary loop, but sparing the mesangium. IgM and IgA are scanty, and C3 is present in a pattern similar to IgG. Deposits of other endogenous antigens may be found when secondary illnesses are present. Certain IgG subclasses are found in glomerular deposits with IgG4 predominating. This IgG4 may play an important role in the pathogenesis of MGN (59). C3d deposits are also evident in membranous nephropathy and patients found to have glomerular C3 deposits excrete more protein then those without C3 deposits (60).

The histological stage of the lesion correlates with the duration of the illness. The lesions may remain stable over long periods or may progress with little change in the clinical course. Although remission of proteinuria may be accompanied by some resolution of findings, the relationship between the extent of proteinuria and the severity of glomerular lesion is not reliable (46). Some investigators have described no modifications of histologic lesions in repeat biopsies in patients in remission. Others have observed disappearance of deposits in patients free of proteinuria, while others have reported no remissions in patients with Stage III or higher (61). Recently, Ramirez et al found less progression to renal insufficiency in patients with Stage I and Stage II assessed by electron microscopy examination of renal tissue, suggesting that the stage of the lesion on the initial biopsy may be a good predictor of the course of the disease in children (62). This finding was not found by Lantham et al (54) whose study suggested that it was not possible to predict the outcome of patients from the pathologic stage of the disease.

Course and Therapy

The outcome is much more favorable in children than in adults. The overall prognosis in children is excellent with less than 5 percent progressing to renal failure within the first five years and 90 percent surviving for more than ten years (52). The majority of children will experience a complete remission of proteinuria within five years of diagnosis; those with asymptomatic proteinuria carry a better prognosis. In adults, Cameron has estimated that 75-80 percent of patients will be alive without renal failure five years after the diagnosis, but only 50 percent at the end of ten years (51). Spontaneous remission of proteinuria occurs in 25 percent of adult patients, with an additional 25 percent sustaining a spontaneous partial remission. A relapsing and remitting course, similar to the one observed in minimal change nephrotic syndrome, may also be seen in adults. Remission of proteinuria is most likely to occur in the early stages of the disease. Renal failure seldom occurs in patients sustaining a partial remission (46). The persistence of the nephrotic syndrome, in children and in adults, is an ominous sign (46, 50), as is the presence of the nephrotic syndrome at the onset of the nephropathy (62). Hypertension is another clinical finding that correlated with the clinical outcome. Fewer patients who are hypertensive at onset of the disease, go into remission (54). A recent study, in membranous nephropathy utilizing multivariate life table analysis, was able to predict the risk of developing renal failure in patients with membranous nephropathy. The risk was found to be higher in men, lower in those treated with prednisone, and inversely related to serum albumin. Except in those cases where there were electron dense deposits, the electron microscopic findings had no predictive value (63).

It is known that membranous glomerulopathy develops in renal allografts, but it has a low recurrence rate in renal transplants. Similarly, MGN has developed "de novo" in renal transplants. A survey of the clinical and morphological features of both "de novo" and "recurrent" disease failed to find a specific cause of the MGN. The authors speculate that immunosupression in transplanted patients may lower the antibody response to levels that favor the development of MGN (64). Despite the presence of "de novo" MGN in renal allografts, it generally does not appear deleterious for the graft function (65).

Because of the indolent nature of this disease, the tendency for spontaneous remissions, and the varied clinical course, evaluation of appropriate treatment has been difficult. In the opinion of Habib, the low mortality of MGN does not justify the use of drugs with potential side effects, unless the patients at risk for renal failure can be identified (50). Most investigators consider that none of the treatment modalities currently available affect the course of the disease. In the past, retrospective studies have found no differences in steroid-treated vs steroid-untreated groups. In a recent study, the natural history of renal function in 64 untreated MGN in adults, was reported with a mean follow-up ranging from two to fifteen years (66). During the follow-up, no deterioration in renal function was found in 30 patients, steady deterioration in 27 patients, a slow deterioration in 5 patients, and change in deterioration away from the mode in 2 patients (cause identified as RVT and interstitial nephritis respectively). In the 27 patients that showed a steady deterioration, it took, on the average, 30 months for the serum creatinine to double, and 32 months to reach 400 µmoles/l. The reciprocal of the sequential serum creatinine with time indicated that the rate of deterioration was essentially constant in all patients. Poor indicators of prognosis were as previously reported, nephrotic syndrome at presentation, impaired function at time of diagnosis, male patients and older age (66). In the collaborative study of the adult idiopathic nephrotic syndrome, a significant reduction in proteinuria, and the prevalence of complete or partial remissions of proteinuria in treated vs placebo groups, was achieved when higher doses of prednisone (120 to 150 mg - QOD x 8 weeks or more) were employed (67). Although at the end of three years, no differences in the patients remaining in remission was noted, there was a significant reduction in the occurrence of renal failure in the steroid treated group (67). Although further randomized trials are needed to confirm these observations, considering the potential benefits and the relative safety of the program, investigators feel that a course of alternate day steroids to patients with uncomplicated MGN should be offered (46). If progression of renal failure has already occurred, Hopper has suggested that high dose alternate day steroid will often stabilize or improve renal function (46).

Recently, the use of steroids has been advocated in order to improve the long term prognosis in children (68). In children remissions have occurred more frequently during or after the administration of steroids or immunosuppressants (alone or in combination). Remissions, however, have been reported more frequently in untreated patients or in those without therapy for more than a year (50). Kincaid Smith has reported a high remission rate using a combination of anticoagulants and immunosuppressants (69). The frequency of remission, however, was not higher than in some untreated series.

The role of cytotoxic agents in the management of MGN is uncertain. No beneficial effect has been demonstrated with azathioprine or cyclophosphamide although chlorambucil has reduced proteinuria when used for prolonged periods (46). Occasionally, the simultaneous administration of cyclophosphamide or azathioprine along with alternate daily steroids has been associated with a reduction in proteinuria or reversal of progression into renal failure (70).

Recently, a controlled treatment trial of methylprednisolone and chlorambucil was conducted for a period of one to seven years in 67 adults with MGN. At the end of the follow-up, 23 of the 32 treated patients were in complete or partial remission, as compared with 9 of 30 control patients. Renal function did not change in the treated group, while renal function worsened in the control group. The results showed that steroid alternated with chlorambucil treatment every other month for a total of six months induced remission in the nephrotic syndrome in adults with MGN, and could potentially preserve renal function for at least several years (71).

In another recent study, beneficial effects of steroids in the treatment of membranous nephropathy and the use of cyclophosphamide in patients not responding to steroids alone has been advocated (72). Therapy may have to be prolonged before a remission can be observed. It is apparent that further studies under controlled circumstances are needed before treatment modalities for membranous nephropathy in both children and adults are widely and globally accepted.

References

1. Allen, A.C.: The clinicopathological meaning of the nephrotic syndrome. Am J Med 18:277-314, 1955.

2. Ellis, A.: Natural history of Bright's disease: Clinical histological and experimental observations. Lancet 1:1-7, 1942.

3. West, C.D., McAdams, A.J., McConville, J.M., Davis, N.C. and Holland, N.H.: Hypocomplementemic and normocomplementemic persistent (chronic) glomerulonephritis; clinical and pathological characteristics. J Pediatr 67:1089-1112, 1965.

4. Gotoff, S.P., Fellers, F.X., Vawter, G.F., Janeway, C.A. and Rosen, F.S.: The beta$_{1C}$globulin in childhood nephrotic syndrome. Laboratory diagnosis of progressive glomerulonephritis. N Engl J Med 273:524-529, 1965.

5. Kim, Y. and Michael, A.F.: Idiopathic membranoproliferative glomerulonephritis. Ann Rev Med 31:273-288, 1980.

6. Burkholder, P.M., Marchand, A., Krueger, R.P.: Mixed membranous and proliferative glomerulonephritis. A Correlative light, immunofluorescence and electron microscopic study. Lab Invest 23:459-479, 1970.

7. Davis, A.E., Schneeberger, E.E., McCluskey, R.T. and Grupe, W.E.: Mesangial proliferative glomerulonephritis with irregular intramembranous deposits. Another variant of hypocomplemententemic nephritis. Am J Med 63:481-486, 1977.

8. Strife, C.F., McAdams, A.J. and West, C.D.: Membranoproliferative glomerulonephritis characterized by focal, segmental proliferative lesions. Clinical Nephrology 18:9-16, 1982.

9. Churg, J., Duffy, J.L. and Bernstein, J.: Identification of dense deposit disease. Arch Pathol Lab Med 103:67-72, 1979.

10. Jones, D.B.: Membranoproliferative glomerulonephritis. One or many diseases? Arch Pathol Lab Med 101:457-461, 1977.

11. Cameron, J.S., Turner, D.R., Heaton, J., Williams, D.G., Ogg, C.S., Chantler, C., Haycock, G.B., and Hicks, J.: Idiopathic mesangiocapillary glomerulonephritis. Comparison of types I and II in children and adults and long term prognosis. Am J Med 74:175-192, 1983.

12. Habib, R., Kleinknecht, C., Gubler, M.C. and Levy, M.: Idiopathic membranoproliferative glomerulonephritis in children. Report of 105 cases. Clin Nephrol 1:194-214, 1973.

13. Kim, Y., Vernier, R.L., Fish, A.J. and Michael, A.F.: Immunofluorescence studies of dense deposit disease. The presence of railroad tracks and mesangial rings. Lab Invest 40:474-480, 1979.

14. Davis, A.E. III, Schneeberger, E.E., Grupe, W.E. and McCluskey, R.T.: Membranoproliferative glomerulonephritis (MPGN type I) and dense deposit disease (DDD) in children. Clin Nephrol 9:184-193, 1978.

15. Spitzer, R.E., Vallota, E.H., Forristal, J., Sudora, E., Stitzel, A., Davis, N.C. and West, C.D.: Serum C'3 lytic system in patients with glomerulonephritis. Science 164:436-437, 1969.

16. Davis, A.E. III, Ziegler, J.B., Gelfand, E.W., Rosen, F.S. and Alper, C.A.: Heterogeneity of nephritic factor and its identification as an immunoglobulin. Proc Natl Acad Sci USA 74:3980-3983, 1977.

17. Chesney, R.W., O'Regan, S., Guyda, J.H. and Drummond, K.N.: Candida endocrinopathy syndrome with membranoproliferative glomerulonephritis: demonstration of glomerular candida antigen. Clin Nephrol 5:232-237, 1976.

18. Morel-Maroger, L., Killen, P.D., Chi, E. and Striker, G.E.: The composition of glomerulosclerosis. I Studies in focal sclerosis, crescentic glomerulonephritis and membranoproliferative glomerulonephritis. Lab Invest 51:181-192, 1984.

19. Leohapand, T., Cattell, V. and Gabriel, J.R.T.: Monocyte infiltration in human glomerulonephritis: Alpha-1-antitrypsin as a marker for mononuclear phagocytes in renal biopsies. Clin Nephrol 19:309-316, 1983.

20. McEnery, P.T., McAdams, A.J. and West, C.D.: Membranoproliferative glomerulonephritis: improved survival with alternate day prednisone therapy. Clin Nephrol 13:117-124, 1980.

21. Herdman, R.C., Pickering, R.J., Michael, A.F., Vernier, R.L., Fish, A.J., Gewurz, H. and Good, R.A.: Chronic glomerulonephritis associated with low serum complement activity (chronic hypocomplementemic glomerulonephritis). Medicine 49:207-226, 1970.

22. Ormeci, A.R., Tinaztepe, B. and Tinaztepe, K.: Associated conditions in childhood membranoproliferative glomerulonephritis during 15 years of experience at the Hacettepe Children's Hospital. Turkish J Pediatr 24:211-225, 1982.

23. McAdams, A.J., McEnery, P.T. and West, C.D.: Mesangiocapillary glomerulonephritis: Changes in glomerular morphology with long term alternate day prednisone therapy. J Pediatr 86:23-31, 1975.

24. International study of kidney disease in children: Alternate-day steroid therapy in membranoproliferative glomerulonephritis: a randomized controlled clinical trial (abstr). Kidney Int. 21:150, 1982.

25. Hasegawa, O., Honda, M., Nakakara, T., Hazekano, H., Ito, H., Sakaguki, H.: Methylprednisolone pulse therapy for membranoproliferative glomerulonephritis (MPGN) in children. Proc 8th Int Congr Nephrol, Athens, 1981.

26. Vanrenterghem, Y., Roels, L., Verbeckmoes, R. and Michielsen, P.: Treatment of chronic glomerulonephritis with a combination of indomethacin and cyclophosphamide. Clinical Nephrol 4:218-222, 1975.

27. Ponticelli, C., Banfi, G., Imbascanti, E. and Tarantino, A.: Immunosuppressive therapy in primary glomerulonephritis (Pros). Contr Nephrol 34:33-54, 1982.

28. Kincaid-Smith, P.: The treatment of chronic mesangiocapillary (membranoproliferative) glomerulonephritis with impaired renal function. Med J Aust 2:587-592, 1972.

29. Donadio, J. and Holley, K.: Membranoproliferative glomerulonephritis. Seminars in Nephrol 2:214-227, 1982.

30. Zimmerman, S.W., Moorthy, A.V., Dreher, W.H., Friedman, A. and Varanasi, V.: Prospective trial of warfarin and dipyridamole in patients with membranoproliferative glomerulonephritis. Am J Med 75:920-927, 1983.

31. Zimmerman, S.W., Hyman, R., Uehling, D.T. and Burkholder, P.M.: Recurrent membranoproliferative glomerulonephritis with glomerular properdin deposition in allografts. Ann Intern Med 80:169-172, 1974.

32. McLean, R.H., Geiger, H., Burke, B., Simmons, R., Najarian, J., Vernier, R.L. and Michael, A.F.: Recurrence of membranoproliferative glomerulonephritis following kidney transplantation. Serum complement component studies. Am J Med 60:60-72, 1976.

33. White, R.H.R., Glasgow, E.F., Mills, R.J.: Clinicopathological study of nephrotic syndrome in childhood. Lancet 1:1353, 1970.

34. International study of kidney disease in children: The nephrotic syndrome in children: Prediction of histopathology from clinical and laboratory characteristics at time of diagnosis. Kidney Int 13:159-165, 1978.

35. Waldherr, R., Gubler, M.C., Levy, M., Broyer, M. and Habib, R.: The significance of pure diffuse mesangial proliferation in idiopathic nephrotic syndrome. Clin Nephrol 10:171, 1978.

36. Brown, E.A., Upadhyaya, K., Hayslett, J.P., Kashgarian, M. and Siegel, N.J.: The clinical course of mesangial proliferative glomerulonephritis. Medicine 58:219, 1980.

37. Murphy, W.M., Jukkola, A.F. and Roy, S. III: Nephrotic syndrome with mesangial-cell proliferation in children - a distinct entity? Am J Clin Path 72:42-47, 1979.

38. Pascal, J.F., Molina, M. and Lopez, J.: Long-term assessment of chlorambucil in children with nephrotic syndrome who fail to respond adequately to corticosteroids. Contr Nephrol 27:65-74, 1981.

39. Allen, W.R., Travis, L.B., Cavallo, T., Brouhard, B.H. and Cunningham, R.J.: Immune deposits and mesangial hypercellularity in minimal change nephrotic syndrome: clinical relevance. J Pediatr 100:188-191, 1982.

40. Koskimies, O., Vilska, J., Rapola, J. and Hallman, N.: Long-term outcome of primary nephrotic syndrome. Archiv Dis Child 57:544-548, 1982.

41. Garin, E.H., Donnelly, W.H., Geary, D. and Richard, G.A.: Nephrotic syndrome and diffuse mesangial proliferative glomerulonephritis in children. Am J Dis Child 137:109-113, 1983.

42. Habib, R., Churg, J., Bernstein, J., Cameron, J.S., Cohen, A.H., Gagnadoux, M.F. and Lewis, E.J.: Minimal change disease, mesangial proliferative glomerulonephritis and focal sclerosis: Individual entities or a spectrum of disease. In Robinson, R.R. (ed.): Nephrology. New York: Springer Verlag, 1984, pp 634-644.

43. Scheoneman, M.J., Bennett, G. and Greifer, I.: The natural history of focal segmental glomerulosclerosis with and without mesangial hypercellularity in children. Clin Nephrol 9:45-54, 1978.

44. A report of The Southwest Pediatric Nephrology Study Group: Childhood nephrotic syndrome associated with diffuse mesangial hypercellularity. Kidney Int 24:87-94, 1983.

45. Ehrenreich, J. and Churg, J: Pathology of membranous nephropathy. Pathol Annu 3:45, 1968.

46. Glassock, R.J., Cohen, A.H., Bennett, C.M. and Martinez-Maldonado, M: Primary glomerular diseases. In Brenner, B.M., and Rector, F.C., Jr., (eds.): The Kidney Vol. II. Philadelphia: W.B. Saunders Co., 1981, pp 1351-1492.

47. Row, P.G., Cameron, J.S., Turner, D.R., Evans, D.J., White, R.H.R., Ogg, C.S., Chantler, C.B. and Brown, C.B.: Membranous nephropathy. Long term follow-up and association with neoplasia BJ Med 44:207, 1975.

48. Libit, S.A., Burke, B., Michael, A.F. and Vernier, R.L.: Extramembranous glomerulonephritis in childhood: Relationship to systemic lupus erythematosus. J Pediatr 88:394, 1976.

49. Churg, J., Habib, R. and White, R.H.R.: Pathology of the nephrotic syndrome in children. Lancet 1:1299, 1970.

50. Habib, R., Kleinknecht, C., Gubler, M.D., Levy, M.: Membranous glomerulonephropathy in children. In Edelmann, C.M. Jr., (ed.): Pediatric Kidney Disease, Vol. 2. Boston: Little, Brown and Company, 1978, pp 646-660.

51. Cameron, J.S.: Pathogenesis and treatment of membranous nephropathy, Kidney Int 15:88, 1979.

52. Habib, R. and Kleinknecht, C.: Idiopathic extramembranous glomerulonephritis in children. In Kincaid-Smith, P., Mathew, R.H. and Becker, E.L. (eds.): Glomerulonephritis. Morphology, Natural History and Treatment, Part I. New York: John Wiley and Sons, 1973, p 461.

53. Olbing, H., Greifer, I., Bennett, B.P., Berstein, J. and Spitzer, A.: Idiopathic membranous nephropathy in children. Kidney Int 3:381, 1973.

54. Latham, P., Poucell, S., Koresaar, A., Arbus, G. and Baumal, R.: Idiopathic membranous glomerulopathy in Canadian children: A clinicopathologic study. J Pediatr 101:682-685, 1982.

55. McGinley, E., Martin, W., Henerson, N., Boulton-Johnes, J.M.: Defective splenic reticuloendothelial function in idiopathic membranous nephropathy. Clin Exp Immunol 56:295, 1984.

56. Matsumoto, K., Osakabe, K., Katayama, H., Moshizawa, N., Harada, M., Hatano, M.: Cell mediated immunity in idiopathic membranous nephropathy. Int Arch Allergy Appl Immunol 66:310, 1981.

57. Berthoux, F.C., Laurent, B., Le Petit, J-C., Cenin, C., Broutin, F., Touraine, F., Hassan, A.A., Champailler, A.: Immunogenetics and immunopathology of human primary membranous glomerulonephritis: HLA-A, B, DR antigens; functional activity of splenic macrophage Fc-receptors and peripheral blood T-lymphocyte subpopulations. Clin Nephrol 22:15-20, 1984.

58. Tomura, S., Kashiwahara, H., Tuchida, H., Shishido, H.L., Sakurai, S., Miyajima, T., Tsuji, K., Takeuchi, J.: Strong association of idiopathic membranous nephropathy with HLA-DR2 and MT1 in Japanese Nephron 36:242, 1984.

59. Doi, T., Mayumim, Kanatsu, K., Suehiro, F., Hamashima, Y.: Distribution of IgG subclasses in membranous nephropathy. Clin Exp Immunol 58:57, 1984.

60. Doi, T., Kanatsu, K., Nagai, H., Suehiro, F., Kuwahara, T., Hamashima, Y.: Demonstration of C3d deposits in membranous nephropathy. Nephron 37:232, 1984.

61. Habib, R., Kleinknecht, C. and Gubler, M.C.: Extramembranous glomerulonephritis in children: Report of 50 cases. J Pediatr 82:754, 1973.

62. Ramirez, F., Brouhard, B.H., Travis, L.B. and Ellis, E.N.: Idiopathic membranous nephropathy in children. J Pediatr 101:677-681. 1982.

63. Tu, W.H., Pettitti, D.B., Biava, C.G., Tulunay, O., Hopper, J.Jr.: Membranous nephropathy: predictions of terminal renal failure. Nephron 36:118, 1984.

64. Verani, R., Dan, M.: Membranous glomerulonephritis in renal transplant. A case report and review of the literature. Am J Nephrol 2:316, 1982.

65. Charpentier, B., Levy, M.: Cooperative study of de novo extramembranous glomerulonephritis in renal allografts in humans. Nephrologie 3:1158, 1982.

66. Davison, A.M., Cameron, J.S., Kerr, D.N., Ogg, C.S. and Wilkinson, R.W.: The natural history of renal function in untreated idiopathic membranous glomerulonephritis in adults. Clin Nephrol 22:61, 1984.

67. Collaborative study of the adult idiopathic nephrotic syndrome. A controlled study of short-term prednisone treatment in adults with membranous nephropathy. N Engl J Med 301:1301, 1979.

68. Ehrenreich, T., Porush, J.G., Churg, J., Garfinkel, L., Glabman, S., Goldstein, M.H., Grishman, E. and Munis, S.L.: Treatment of idiopathic membranous nephropathy. N Engl J Med 295:741, 1976.

69. Laver, M.D. and Kincaid-Smith, P.: The natural history and treatment of membranous glomerulonephritis. In P. Kincaid-Smith, T. H. Mathew and E. L. Becker (eds). Glomerulonephritis, Vol. 1. New York: Wiley, 1973, pp 441.

70. Randall, R.E., Treng, M.G., Abukurah, A.R., Still, W.J.S., Brackett, N.C. and Setter, J.G.: Responsiveness of adult idiopathic membranous nephropathy to cyclophosphamide. Am Soc Nephrol 4:65, 1970.

71. Ponticelli, C., Zucchelli, P., Imbasciati, E., Cagnoli, L., Pozzi, C., et al. Controlled trial of methyl prednisolone and chlorambucil in idiopathic membranous nephropathy. N Engl J Med 310:946, 1984.

72. Suki, W.N., Chavez, A.: Membranous nephropathy: response to steroids and immunosuppression. AM J Nephrol 1:11, 1981.

FOCAL AND SEGMENTAL GLOMERULOSCLEROSIS

Karen M. Gaudio, M.D. and Norman J. Siegel, M.D.

Fahr (1) and Rich (2) described children who had lipoid nephrosis but demonstrated glomerular sclerosis on examination of renal specimens at autopsy. It was not until the early 1970's that this lesion began to attract considerable attention based on reports by Hayslett (3) and others (4,5,6). Today, there is general agreement concerning the histologic appearance of this lesion but the clinical correlates remain controversial. This chapter will address four clinical issues regarding focal and segmental glomerulosclerosis:

1. Does this lesion define a distinct disease?
2. What is the clinical course of this lesion in children with idiopathic nephrotic syndrome?
3. What is the relationship of focal and segmental glomerulosclerosis (FSGS) to other lesions in children with lipoid nephrosis?
4. What are the implications of this lesion with respect to renal transplantation?

HISTOPATHOLOGY

The morphologic criteria to establish a diagnosis of focal and segmental glomerulosclerosis (FSGS) were defined by the ISKDC (6) and more recently refined by the World Health Organization (7). By light microscopy, hylanosis and sclerosis of glomerular capillaries are the essential feature of this lesion. Moreover, the obliteration, scarring and adhesion of glomerular capillaries must be focal in that they affect some but not all glomeruli and segmental in that these changes occur only in a portion of the glomerular capillary tufts of the affected glomeruli. Condensation and scarring of the entire glomerulus is termed focal global obsolescence and is felt to have different clinical implications (5). The other characteristic feature of this lesion is focal tubular atrophy and interstitial fibrosis. In some cases, these interstitial lesions may be more evident than the glomerular changes on an early biopsy specimen and these lesions have been associated with tubular defects such as glycosuria. Electron microscopy generally reveals an increase in matrix material and may have effacement of epithelial cell foot processes in those patients with proteinuria. Immunofluorescence microscopy is usually non-specific with occasional staining with IgM and C_3 in sclerotic areas of the mesangium. Several investigators have attempted to determine specific histopathologic changes which would predict the clinical outcome for patients with this lesion (5,8,9). In large part, such studies have been retrospective and require the presence of large numbers of glomeruli in tissue specimens for accurate prognostication. Because the sclerotic lesions are focal, careful examinations of the non-affected glomeruli may be more helpful in this regard. For example, patients with FSGS and minimal change lesions in the non-sclerotic glomeruli have a better clinical course than similar patients with FSGS and mesangial proliferative lesions (10).

DOES THIS LESION DEFINE A DISTINCT DISEASE?

It is evident from Figure 1 that histomorphologic changes which meet the criteria for FSGS can be observed in a number of different clinical settings. The clinical course of these patients is generally more related to their underlying condition. The broad spectrum of diseases in which this lesion can be found and the observation that it generally becomes clinically apparent late in the

FIGURE 1

CLINICAL CONDITIONS ASSOCIATED WITH FOCAL AND SEGMENTAL GLOMERULOSCLEROSIS

Idiopathic Nephrotic Syndrome

Infantile Nephrotic Syndrome

Asymptomatic Proteinuria

Drug-Abuse Nephropathy

Hereditary Nephritis

Hypertension

Pyelonephritis

Reflux Nephropathy

IgA Nephropathy

Sickle Cell Disease

Oligomeganephronia

Acquired Immune Deficiency Syndrome

Massive Obesity

Aging

FIGURE 2

PROGNOSIS FOR CHILDREN WITH FOCAL AND SEGMENTAL GLOMERULOSCLEROSIS AND NEPHROTIC SYNDROME

		RELATIONSHIP OF LESION TO CLINICAL COURSE	
		AT ONSET	LATER IN DISEASE
RELATIONSHIP TO TREATMENT	RESPONSIVE	GUARDED	EXCELLENT
	RESISTANT	POOR	GUARDED

clinical course would suggest that the glomerular alterations, i.e., sclerosis, adhesions, and obliteration, represent a final common pathway of glomerular injury rather than a specific entity.

In the mid-1970's, the question arose as to whether or not FSGS represented a distinct entity in children with idiopathic nephrotic syndrome (11-14). The observation that the presence of focal sclerotic lesions early in the course of nephrosis is associated with a) a high degree of resistance to steroid therapy, b) significant progression to renal failure, and c) recurrence following transplantation, led some investigators to propose that this lesion represented a distinct nosologic entity (11,14). Other investigators who noted that a) there is a transition from minimal change disease to FSGS in serial biopsy specimens, b) FSGS could be found in children with a steroid responsive course, and c) some patients with steroid resistant disease had only minimal change lesions, proposed that FSGS and minimal change disease were part of a disease spectrum (12,13). Lacking a specific pathogenetic factor or cellular mechanism which could distinguish between these entities, this question remains unresolved and moot.

WHAT IS THE CLINICAL COURSE OF THIS LESION IN CHILDREN WITH IDIOPATHIC NEPHROTIC SYNDROME?

The clinical course of children with idiopathic nephrotic syndrome and FSGS is dependent on two factors: a) the relationship of the lesion to the onset of the disease and b) the responsiveness to treatment with steroids or cytotoxic agents (Figure 2). Unfortunately, it is not possible to determine the interval from the onset of disease to the appearance of FSGS in many reports. Yet, this relationship may have importance with respect to the likelihood of response to treatment and ultimate prognosis. Children who have FSGS early in the course of nephrotic syndrome tend to be a) older at the onset of the disease, b) more likely to have microscopic hematuria, c) equally distributed between males and female, d) more refractory to therapy and have persistent proteinuria or nephrotic syndrome, e) more likely to develop renal failure, and f) at risk for recurrence of FSGS in a transplanted kidney (4,5,13). Although early reports suggested that children with FSGS were quite unlikely to respond to initial corticosteroid therapy, more recent data indicate that 25-35% of such patients will achieve a complete remission of their nephrotic syndrome (15-17). Mongeau (15) found that 27% of his patients responded to corticosteroids while Arbus reported a 33% response (17) and the ISKDC (16) noted that 29.7% of patients had cleared their proteinuria within 8 weeks of initiation of steroid therapy. Unfortunately, this initial response to therapy may not predict a favorable outcome for all children with early onset FSGS. Despite an initial response to corticosteroids, children with an early onset of FSGS tend to have a refractory clinical course which may include a) a short initial response lasting only a few weeks, b) frequent relapses after either steroids or cytotoxic drugs, and c) development of resistance to conventional therapy within 12-18 months after onset of nephrotic syndrome (17,18). The guarded prognosis for children with early onset FSGS despite treatment responsiveness was documented by Arbus and associates (17). These investigators described seven children with FSGS which was documented within 6-8 months of onset of nephrotic syndrome and which initially responded to steroids but became resistant to treatment within 18 months. Five of these seven patients have developed end stage renal disease (17). In contrast, none of 19 patients with FSGS who remained responsive to treatment have progressive renal failure. Unfortunately, the relationship of FSGS to onset of disease is not clear in this latter group (17).

For children with early onset FSGS which is unresponsive to treatment, the prognosis is quite poor. These patients frequently experience a clinical course which includes persistence of nephrotic syndrome with severe edema formation, early appearance of hypertension, tubular defects and progressive loss of renal function. Halevy and Hayslett (19) have analyzed the rate of development of end stage renal disease in five studies of FSGS. These authors note that 20-40% of patients have end stage renal disease within five years, 35-50% within 10 years and 40-75% within 15 years of onset of nephrotic syndrome with FSGS (19).

Children in whom FSGS has been reported to occur later in the course of nephrotic syndrome are characterized by a) young age at onset of nephrosis, b) a steroid responsive although frequently relapsing clinical course, c) male predominance, d) good response to cytotoxic therapy, and e) relatively lower incidence of progression to renal failure (12,18,20). We have observed 18 patients who had steroid responsive idiopathic nephrotic syndrome and were found to have FSGS on renal biopsies performed 3-5 years after onset. After an extensive period of follow-up which was more than 10 years after the appearance of FSGS in all patients, only three have developed end stage renal disease. The importance of treatment responsiveness in children with late onset FSGS is illustrated by comparing our experience with that reported by Tejani and associates (20). These investigators reported 10 patients with FSGS 1.5 to 11 years after onset of corticosteroid responsive nephrotic syndrome. Only one of seven patients achieved a remission when treated with cytoxan and five patients have renal failure or died. All 18 of our patients

FIGURE 3

HISTOLOGIC SPECTRUM IN LIPOID NEPHROSIS

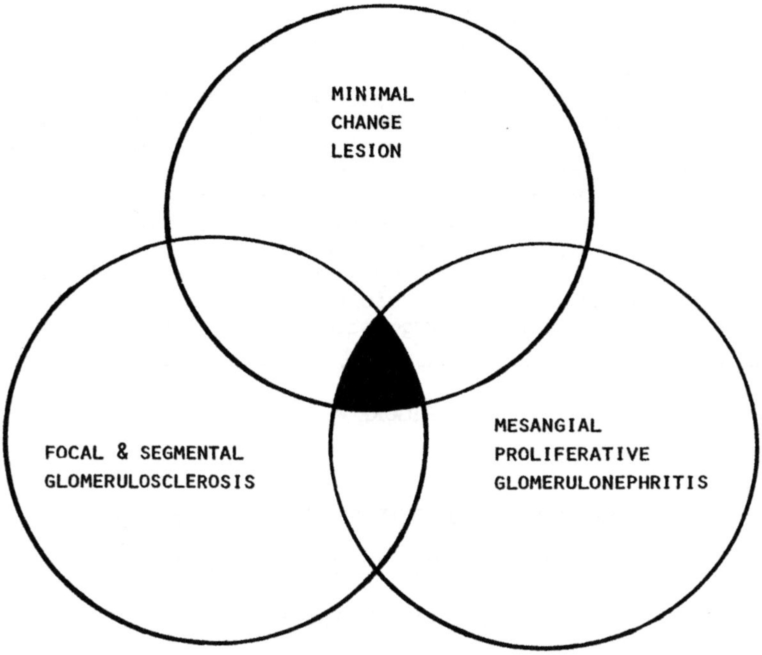

were treated with cyclophosphamide; 15 responded to this therapy and only three patients have developed renal insufficiency. Although multiple differences between the patient populations may have contributed to the respective outcomes, treatment responsiveness appears to be a critical factor with regard to prognosis for children with late onset FSGS.

WHAT IS THE RELATIONSHIP OF FSGS TO OTHER LESIONS IN CHILDREN WITH LIPOID NEPHROSIS?

The complex interaction of FSGS and the other lesions which are commonly found in children with lipoid nephrosis, defined as steroid responsive nephrotic syndrome, is shown in Figure 3. The areas of overlap between FSGS, Minimal Change Lesion (MCL) and Mesangial

Proliferative Changes (MPC) occur in regard to both the interpretation of renal biopsy specimens and the clinical course associated with these lesions. Certainly, there is a fine line which separates the degree of increase in mesangial matrix material which is acceptable as part of the spectrum of MCL and that which requires classification as MPC. Likewise, the number of glomeruli which demonstrate FSGS may be quite small, since this is a focal lesion, in comparison to the other glomeruli which may have minimal or mesangial changes and, in some instances, such specimens may be classified according to the more dominant lesions. In several early reports children with FSGS or MPC were called minimal change disease because their nephrosis had remitted with steroids and it was presumed that only patients with minimal change lesions would respond to steroid therapy (21,22).

The intimate relationship between these three lesions is also evident clinically. Figure 4 compares the relative distribution of these lesions in children with steroid responsive disease. When a renal biopsy is carried out at the onset of disease, the dominant histology is MCL. However, when evaluated after 3-5 years of steroid responsive disease, there is a considerable redistribution of these lesions such that FSGS and MPC comprise over 50% of the group. These differences can be accounted for by several factors. First, there is a transition from MCL to other lesions during the course of childhood nephrotic syndrome. This was suggested by early reports from our

FIGURE 4

DISTRIBUTION OF HISTOPATHOLOGIC LESIONS

IN CHILDHOOD LIPOID NEPHROSIS

(PERCENT OF PATIENTS)

	Biopsy At Onset Initial Steroid Response*	Biopsy After 3-5 Years Steroid Dependent - Frequent Relapse**
Minimal Change Lesion	90	45
Mesangial Proliferative Lesion	5	25
Focal and Segmental Glomerulosclerosis	5	30

*Based on Data from ISKDC, Reference #16

**Based on Data from Siegel and Gaudio, Reference #18

FIGURE 5

FSGS FOLLOWING RENAL TRANSPLANTATION

1. RISK OF RECURRENCE 6 - 30%

2. ALMOST ALWAYS ASSOCIATED WITH RECURRENCE OF NEPHROTIC SYNDROME.

3. FACTORS FAVORING RECURRENCE:

   PRIMARY NEPHROTIC SYNDROME
   EARLY ONSET/STEROID RESISTANT DISEASE
   YOUNG PATIENTS

4. FACTORS REDUCING RISK:

   SECONDARY CAUSES OF LESION
   OLDER PATIENTS
   SLOWLY PROGRESSIVE CLINICAL COURSE

5. LESION MAY OCCUR AS PART OF SPECTRUM OF GLOMERULOPATHY OF CHRONIC REJECTION.

---

group (3,12,18) and has been directly observed on sequential renal biopsy specimens by several investigators (17,19,20). Although the possibility of sampling error can always be evoked to explain the absence of MPC or FSGS on the initial biopsy specimens, the combination of reports based on clinical observation and biopsy documentation from several centers makes it likely that a transition in histopathology occurs and is not an artefact. Secondly, it can be argued that many patients with MCL have a short-term steroid responsive course followed by cessation of their nephrosis and, therefore, they are not included in patients biopsied later in the course of disease. Based on our current understanding of the natural history of minimal change disease, this explanation seems quite probable because a) 15-20% of minimal change lesion patients have only one episode of nephrosis, b) only 30% of such patients follow a frequently relapsing course, c) non-minimal change lesions seem to have a more prolonged clinical course characterized by multiple relapses, and d) patients selected for biopsy several years after onset have had a complicated clinical course and are generally being considered for cytotoxic therapy (18,23). Thus, a number of children, who would be expected to have MCL lesion at onset because of young age and steroid responsive disease, will actually be found to have either FSGS or MPC if biopsied 3-5 years after onset (18). Based on these pathologic and clinical studies, it becomes clear that FSGS, MCL and MPC must be considered part of the spectrum of lipoid nephrosis.

WHAT ARE THE IMPLICATIONS OF THIS LESION WITH RESPECT TO RENAL TRANSPLANTATION?

Because of the poor outcome for patients with FSGS which is unresponsive to treatment, this question has received considerable attention. Hoyer (24) first reported the recurrence of this lesion following transplantation. Subsequently, similar reports have come from a number of transplant centers (25-29). Figure 5 summarizes the salient and clinically relevant information from several of these reports. Although the risk of recurrent FSGS is reported from 6-30%, most reports suggest a recurrence rate of 20-25%. Interestingly, recurrences have been reported almost exclusively in patients who had idiopathic nephrotic syndrome but not in children with FSGS associated with other diseases. Unfortunately, those patients at greatest risk for recurrences of the lesion are also those at greatest risk for steroid resistant disease. Thus, those patients with the more severe clinical course are also at highest risk for recurrence of the lesion. Lastly, FSGS has been described as part of the spectrum of histopathologic changes associated with chronic rejection. Therefore, in some patients, the appearance of FSGS in a transplanted kidney may represent chronic rejection rather than recurrence of the original entity. Paradoxically, although FSGS may recur in a transplanted kidney, the reappearance of this lesion may not adversely affect graft survival (20).

REFERENCES

1. Fahr, T.: Pathologische Anatomie des Morbus Brightii. In: Hencke and Lubarsch, Handbuch der speziellen pathologischen anatomie. Springer, Berlin, 1925.

2. Rich, A.R.: A hitherto undescribed vulnerability of the juxtamedullary glomeruli in lipoid nephrosis. Bulletin of Johns Hopkins Hospital, 100:173, 1957.

3. Hayslett, J.P., Krassner, L.S., Bensch, K.G., Kashgarian, M. and Epstein, F.H.: Progression of "lipoid nephrosis" to renal insufficiency. N. Engl. J. Med., 281:181, 1969.

4. White, R.H.R., Glasgow, E.F. and Mills, R.J.: Clinicopathological study of nephrotic syndrome in childhood. Lancet, 1:1353, 1970.

5. Habib, R.: Focal glomerular sclerosis. Kidney Inter., 4:355, 1973.

6. Churg, J., Habib, R. and White, R.H.R.: Pathology of the nephrotic syndrome in children. A report of the International Study of Kidney disease in children. Lancet, 1:1299, 1970.

7. Churg, J. and Sobin, L.H.: Focal and segmental glomerulosclerosis. In: Churg, J. et al. (eds.): Renal Disease-Classification and Atlas of Glomerular Diseases. Igaku-Shoin, Tokyo, New York, p. 37, 1982.

8. Ellis, D., Kapur, S., Antonovych, T.T., Salcedo, J.R. and Yunis, E.J.: Focal glomerulosclerosis in children: Correlation of histology with prognosis. J. Pediat., 93:762, 1978.

9. Kohaut, E.C., Singer, D.B. and Hill, L.L.: The significance of focal glomerular sclerosis in children who have nephrotic syndrome. Am. J. Clin. Pathol., 66:545, 1976.

10. Schoenemann, M.J., Bennett, B. and Greifer, T.: The natural history of focal segmental glomerulosclerosis with and without mesangial hypercellularity in children. Clin. Nephrol., 9:45, 1978.

11. Glasgow, E.F. and White, R.H.R.: "Not so minimal". Nephron, 8:403, 1971.

12. Siegel, N.J., Kashgarian, M., Spargo, B.H. and Hayslett, J.P.: Minimal change and focal sclerotic lesions in lipoid nephrosis. Nephron, 13:125, 1974.

13. Kashgarian, M., Hayslett, J.P. and Siegel, N.J.: Lipoid nephrosis and focal sclerosis distinct entities or spectrum of disease. Nephron, 13:105, 1974.

14. Unsigned Editorial: Focal glomerulosclerosis. Lancet, 2:367, 1972.

15. Mongeau, J.G., Corneille, L., Robitaille, P., O'Regan, S. and Pelletier, M.: Primary nephrosis in childhood associated with focal glomerular sclerosis: Is long-term prognosis that severe? Kidney Inter., 20:743, 1981.

16. ISKDC: The primary nephrotic syndrome in children: Identification of children with minimal change nephrotic syndrome from initial response to prednisone. J. Pediat., 98:561, 1981.

17. Arbus, G.S., Poucell, S., Bachevyie, G.S. and Baumal, R.: Focal segmental glomerulosclerosis with idiopathic nephrotic syndrome: Three types of clinical response. J. Pediat., 101:40, 1982.

18. Siegel, N.J., Gaudio, K.M., Krassner, L.S., McDonald, B.M., Anderson, F.P. and Kashgarian, M.: Steroid-dependent nephrotic sydnrome in children: Histopathology and relapses after cyclophosphamide treatment. Kidney Inter., 19:454, 1981.

19. Halevy, J. and Hayslett, J.P.: Clinical features and course of focal glomerulosclerosis. In: Brenner, B.M. and Stein, J.H. (eds). Contemporary Issues in Nephrology, Churchill-Livingston, New York, 1985.

20. Tejani, A., Nicastri, A.D., Sen, D., Chen, C.K., Phadke, K., Adamson, O. and Butt, K.M.H.: Long term evaluation of children with nephrotic syndrome and focal segmental glomerular sclerosis. Nephron, 35:225, 1983.

21. Cameron, J.S., Turner, D.R., Ogg, C.S., Sharpstone, P. and Brown, C.B.: The nephrotic syndrome in adults with "minimal change" glomerular lesions. Quart. J. Med., N.S., XLIII, 171:461, 1974.

22. Jao, W., Pollak, V.E., Norris, S.N., et al.: Lipoid nephrosis: An approach to the clinicopathologic analysis and dismemberment of idiopathic nephrotic syndrome with minimal glomerular change. Medicine, 52:445, 1973.

23. Siegel, N.J., Goldberg, B., Krassner, L.S. and Hayslett, J.P.: Long-term follow-up of children with steroid responsive nephrotic syndrome. J. Pediat., 81:251, 1972.

24. Hoyer, J.R., Vernier, R.L., Najarian, J.S., Raij, L., Simmons, R.L. and Michael, A.F.: Recurrence of idiopathic nephrotic syndrome after renal transplantation. Lancet, 2:343, 1972.

25. Malekzadeh, M.J., Heuser, E.T., Ettenger, R.B., Pennisi, A.J., Uittenbogaart, C.H., Warshaw, B.L. and Fine, R.N.: Focal glomerulosclerosis and renal transplantation. J. Pediat., 95:249, 1979.

26. Leumann, E.P., Briner, J., Donckerwolcke, R.A.M., Kuijten, R. and Largiader, F.: Recurrence of focal segmental glomerulosclerosis in the transplanted kidney. Nephron, 25:65, 1980.

27. Pinto, J., Lacerda, G., Cameron, J.S., Turner, D.R., Bewick, M. and Ogg, C.S.: Recurrence of focal segmental glomerulosclerosis in renal allografts. Transplantation, 32:83, 1981.

28. Hamburger, J., Crosnier, J. and Noel, L.H.: Recurrent glomerulonephritis after renal transplantation. A. Rev. Med., 29:67, 1978.

29. Zimmerman, C.E.: Renal transplantation for focal segmental glomerulosclerosis. Transplantation, 29:172, 1980.

ABNORMAL LIPID METABOLISM IN PRIMARY NEPHROTIC SYNDROME

Gaston Zilleruelo, M.D., S. L. Hsia, M.D., Michael Freundlich, M.D., Carolyn Abitbol, M.D., Milan Novak, Ph.D., Marianne Fordyce, M.D. and Jose Strauss, M.D.

The idiopathic nephrotic syndrome (NS) in children is usually defined by the presence of heavy proteinuria, hypoalbuminemia, edema and moderate to severe hyperlipidemia (1). Hyperlipidemia Type 2B with increase in serum cholesterol and triglycerides is the most common and recognized metabolic complication in patients with NS. However, the precise mechanisms involved in its pathogenesis, the associated clinical complications of hyperlipidemia and the best approach for its management are not well established.

In this review we will address four basic questions: 1) What are the common findings in nephrotic hyperlipidemia? 2) What are the mechanisms of hyperlipidemia? 3) What are the possible clinical complications associated with hyperlipidemia? 4) How can we control better the hyperlipidemia in NS?

1. Common Findings in Nephrotic Hyperlipidemia

The term hyperlipidemia has been used interchangeably with hyperlipoproteinemia and reflects an increase in total cholesterol (TC), triglycerides (TG) or both, over the normal fasting levels for age, sex and race. The degree of hyperlipidemia in NS is quite variable from one patient to another and several factors may influence it, including severity and duration of NS, age, diet, corticosteroids, diuretics, beta blockers, nutritional state, and renal function (2). In general, serum cholesterol, phospholipids and free (unbound) fatty acids (FFA) are elevated more consistently than TG (3). Increased levels of very low and low density lipoproteins (VLDL, LDL) are observed early in the course of NS, but VLDL rise at a faster rate than LDL. High density lipoproteins (HDL) have been reported as being low, normal or elevated in NS (4, 5). In a recent study in 59 children with NS, serum TC and TG were found to be over the 95th percentile for age and sex in all patients with minimal change NS in relapse (mean value of 354 mg/dl and 249 mg/dl, respectively) and in those with non-minimal change nephrotic syndrome and persistent proteinuria (mean value of 557 mg/dl and 620 mg/dl, respectively) (6) (Figure 1). Over 40 percent of patients with MCNS in remission,and most of them off corticosteroids, had some lipids

---

This study was funded in part under an agreement with the Department of Health and Rehabilitative Services, State of Florida Children's Medical Services.

abnormally high including either LDL or VLDL. HDL level was found significantly increased during relapse only in children with MCNS; it was decreased in patients with non-MCNS and persistent proteinuria (Figure 2).

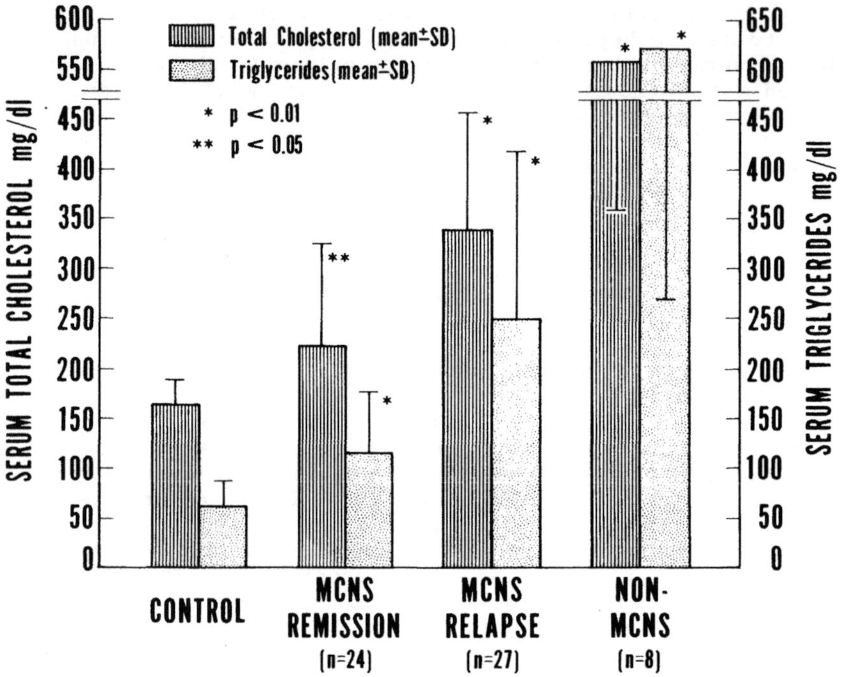

Figure 1: Mean values and standard deviations for serum cholesterol and triglycerides in different subgroups of children with nephrosis according to activity of disease.

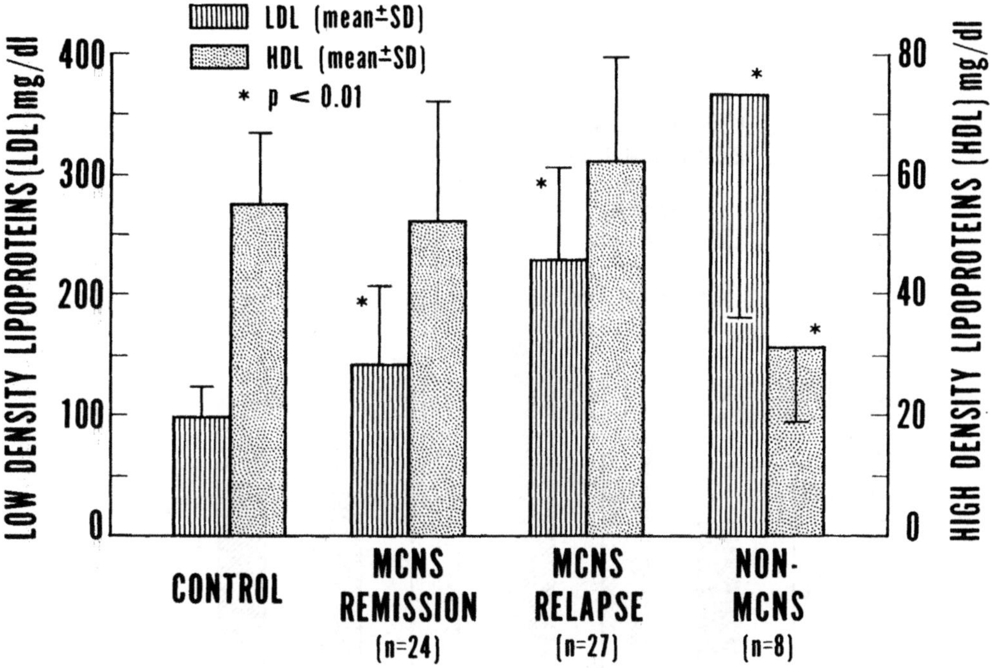

Figure 2: Mean values and standard deviations for low and high density lipoproteins in different subgroups of children with nephrosis according to activity of disease.

Severity and persistence of lipid changes correlated well with duration of disease and frequency of relapses (Figure 2) (6). Many patients had transient hyperlipidemia and this correlated well with activity of the disease; in others, however, hyperlipidemia persisted for prolonged periods of time with elevated cholesterol and LDL levels even months or years after remission. Patients with history of frequent relapses or corticosteroid dependency had significantly elevated TC levels during relapse and remission as compared with controls. Highest values of serum TC were observed in patients with non-MCNS and persistent proteinuria (Figure 3). In this group of patients, no clear correlation between HL and urinary protein excretion was observed.

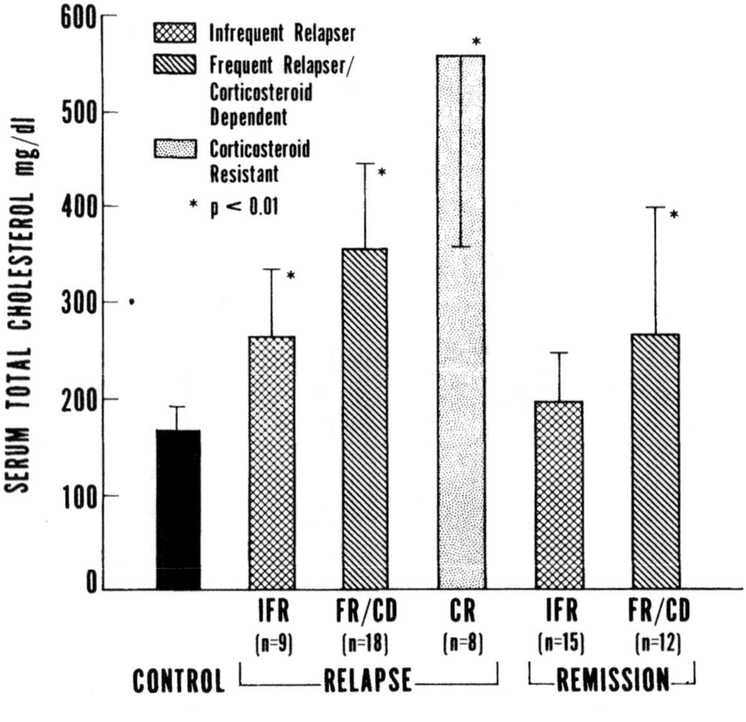

Figure 3: Mean values and standard deviations for serum cholesterol in different subgroups of children with nephrosis according to activity of disease and frequency of relapses. From: Zilleruelo, G., Hsia, S.L., Freundlich, et al.: Persistence of serum lipid abnormalities in children with idiopathic nephrotic syndrome. J. Pediatr 104:61, 1984 (with permission).

In order to obtain further insight into the lipid metabolism in children with NS, we conducted a study of the fatty acid composition in adipose tissue in 13 children with primary NS and normal glomerular filtration rate (7). All had a history of frequent relapses or corticosteroid resistance, but four were studied during remission and off steroids for several months or years. These children were found to have abnormal composition of adipose tissue fatty acids with a significant elevation of linoleic acid (20% versus 14% in healthy controls) and concomitant reduction of palmitic acid (16% versus 19% in healthy controls). In addition, these children had an abnormal fatty acid composition of plasma phospholipids with a significant increase in arachidonic acid (25% versus 10% in healthy controls). These changes were present in children even after years in remission of their NS. The abnormal fatty acid distribution of adipose tissue and plasma phospholipids possibly reflect an abnormal fatty acid transport or metabolism in NS which needs further clarification. It is worthwhile to mention that linoleic acid is a natural precursor of arachidonic acid and the latter is the principal precursor of the prostaglandin cascade. The significance of our findings and their relationship with the demonstrated increased plasma and urinary concentration of prostaglandins in children with NS deserve further study (8, 9).

2. Mechanisms of Hyperlipidemia

The causes of hyperlipidemia in NS are probably multifactorial. Numerous studies in humans and in animal models have shown a marked increase in the rate of hepatic synthesis of both lipid and protein moieties of the lipoprotein fraction (10, 11). The increased liver synthesis seems to result from the non-specific stimulation by the decreased oncotic pressure (hypoalbuminemia) or increased plasma viscosity (12, 13). Other studies have shown a decrease in the removal rate of lipoproteins from the circulation. This decrease in the catabolism of lipoproteins apparently is due to a decrease in lipoprotein lipase with slower removal of VLDL or a decrease in Lecithin Cholesterol Acyl Transferase (LCAT) with the resulting reduced HDL production (14, 15). Finally, there seems to be an intravascular trapping of TC and TG because of increased mobilization from fat tissue stores, increased lipolysis and reabsorption of fats from the gastrointestinal tract.

Although hypoalbuminemia probably plays a major role in the pathogenesis of lipid abnormalities in NS (16), it should be emphasized that the correlation between serum albumin and cholesterol is not always linear (6). In fact, we have found that serum albumin has no correlation with cholesterol during remission and only a poor, though significant, linear inverse correlation with serum cholesterol during relapse (Figure 4). Many patients in either relapse or remission had elevated serum cholesterol despite serum albumin greater than 3.5 g/dl. In addition, patients with similar serum albumin levels may have markedly different degrees of hyperlipidemia and patterns of hyperlipoproteinemia.

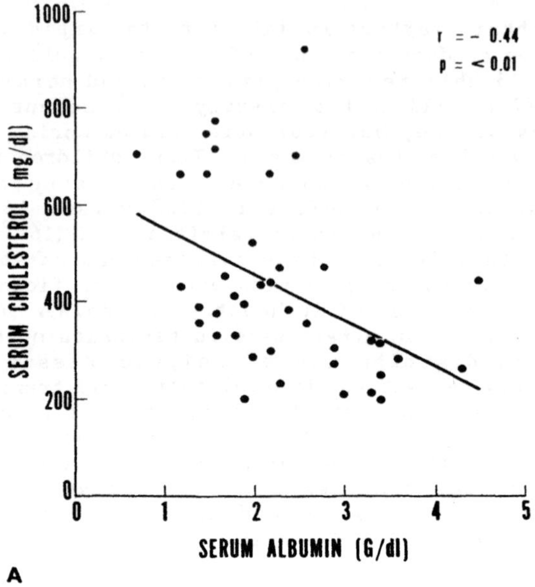

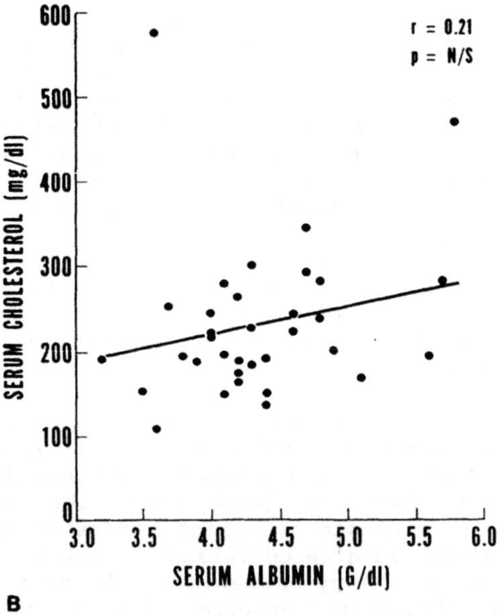

Figure 4: Correlation between serum albumin and serum cholesterol concentrations in 35 children with idiopathic nephrotic syndrome during relapse (A) (more than one determination in some children at different times), and remission (B). From: Zilleruelo, G., Hsia, S.L., Freundlich, et al.: Persistence of serum lipid abnormalities in children with idiopathic nephrotic syndrome. J. Pediatr 104:61, 1984 (with permission).

Important losses of apolipoprotein A during episodes of massive proteinuria have been shown to contribute to the decrease in serum levels of HDL (17). The role played in the pathogenesis of hyperlipidemia by various hormones (including thyroid hormone, androgens and insulin), and by several drugs, should all be considered when evaluating a patient with nephrotic syndrome and hyperlipidemia.

3. Clinical Complications Associated with Hyperlipidemia

The hyperlipidemia of NS has been associated with several clinical complications, although the precise cause/effect relationship is not well established. Table 1 summarizes the possible clinical and laboratory consequences of hyperlipidemia in patients with NS.

TABLE 1

POSSIBLE COMPLICATIONS ASSOCIATED WITH NEPHROTIC HYPERLIPIDEMIA

Premature atherosclerosis
Thromboembolism
Hyperchylomicronemia syndrome
Immune deficiency
Pseudohyponatremia
Progression of renal disease ("nephrotoxicity")
Carnitine and Vitamin E deficiency

A. Premature atherosclerosis. In view of the epidemiologic information obtained on the relationship of elevated serum cholesterol and coronary heart disease, a large number of nephrotic children would be at increased risk of premature atherosclerosis (18, 19). In particular, the group of patients with persistent proteinuria, decrease in HDL and HDL/LDL ratio should be at an increased risk of premature atherosclerosis and coronary heart disease. Still, the possible association between hyperlipidemia and premature atherosclerosis in nephrotic children has received little attention and long range follow-up studies with periodic lipid profile evaluations will be needed before further conclusions about this association can be reached.

B. Thromboembolism. Hyperlipoproteinemia, increased platelet aggregation, hyperviscosity and abnormal coagulation factors may all play a role in the increased incidence of thromboembolic accidents observed in nephrotic patients (20). The thromboembolism may affect different veins (renal vein being the most frequent) and arteries.

C. Immunologic effects. Serum inhibitory factors of lymphocyte blastogenesis may be related to lipoprotein bound substances. "Functional hyposplenia" reported in children with NS (21) may be related to the hyperlipidemia inducing blockage of the reticular endothelium system.

D. Pseudohyponatremia. Any patient with active nephrosis and decreased serum sodium should have simultaneous serum osmolality to document the presence of true hyponatremia (in this case, serum osmolality will be low). It should be remembered that lipids are solids with high molecular weight; therefore, their elevation may reduce the percentage of water contained in plasma and induce a low concentration of sodium with normal serum osmolality ("pseudohyponatremia"). Multiplication of the plasma lipid concentration in mg/dl by 0.002 gives the reduction of serum sodium caused by the accumulation of these solids. However, as it has been reported recently (22), true hyponatremia due to continuous activation of the antidiuretic hormone, could also be present in hypovolemic patients.

E. Progression of renal disease (lipid "nephrotoxicity"). There is some circumstantial evidence suggesting that hyperlipoproteinemia in nephrosis or in other chronic renal diseases may induce changes in glomerular structure, mainly mesangial cells, leading to further nephron loss and glomerulosclerosis (23).

F. Various nutrients deficiency. Finally, the excess of circulating plasma lipids including fatty acids may induce a relative deficiency of certain substances needed in lipid metabolism such as carnitine or vitamin E. Frequently, the plasma levels of carnitine and vitamin E are within normal limits, but there might be a relative deficiency due to the high levels of circulating lipids. Carnitine plays an important role in energy production for the transport of fatty acids inside the mitochondrial membrane. On the other hand, Vitamin E is a potent antioxidant substance which prevents lipid peroxidation. Therefore, deficit of both substances may have chemical and/or clinical relevance in the nephrotic syndrome.

4. <u>Management of Hyperlipidemia in NS</u>

There is no agreement on the best approach and how aggressive the clinician should be in the correction of hyperlipidemia accompanying NS. Various steps should be undertaken in order to clarify the type of problem and plan for its management: a) confirm and quantify the degree of hyperlipidemia; b) rule out secondary dyslipidemias associated with diseases such as hypothyroidism, diabetes mellitus, familial hypercholesterolemia, etc; c) rule out the possible adverse effects of certain drugs (such as diuretics, propranolol, corticosteroids, etc.) on lipoprotein metabolism and consider their discontinuation if possible; d) attempt identification and treatment of the cause of the nephrotic syndrome; e) achieve and maintain ideal weight for height; f) practice regular aerobic physical exercises; g) consume only a moderate amount of saturated fats (increase the ratio of polyunsaturated to saturated fatty acids to at least 1:1) and no more than 30 to 35% of calories as fat; h) administer hypolipidemic drugs/substances if there is persistent and severe hyperlipidemia after all the above measures have been instituted.

There is no consensus in terms of the ideal hypolipidemic drug/substance and its dose in this situation. Because of binding to albumin, hypoalbuminemia may cause increase in free drug levels; therefore, the patient should be carefully titrated to determine the best dose. The safety and efficiency of newer antilipidemic drugs, such as Cholestipol, Gemfibrozil and Probucol in nephrotic hyperlipidemia has not been established. From preliminary experience in hyperlipidemia not associated with nephrotic syndrome in children, cholestyramine may be useful. We have recently conducted a preliminary trial using Omega-3 fatty acids supplementation in children with nephrotic syndrome. Since Omega-3 fatty acids have been reported to have unique hypolipidemic effects, we used oral eicosapentanoic acid supplementation (MaxEPA, Thompson Co.) in eight children with nephrotic syndrome and severe hyperlipidemia. Preliminary results are very encouraging since we observed a trend toward a significant reduction in both TC and TG after several weeks of MaxEPA at a dose of 4 g/m^2/day (24).

In conclusion, we believe that nephrotic hyperlipidemia should be evaluated in all children with nephrotic syndrome. These patients should have serum lipid profile evaluations done at regular intervals, with follow-up even during remission. Lipid profiles should include at least levels of HDL and total cholesterol. All identifiable pathogenetic factors should be corrected if possible. Finally, diet, physical activity and even lipid lowering drugs seem beneficial and deserve further evaluation in nephrotic patients with persistent and severe hyperlipidemia.

REFERENCES

1. Rothenberg, M. and Heyman, W.: The incidence of the nephrotic syndrome in children. Pediatrics 19:446, 1957.

2. Zilleruelo, G. and Strauss, J.: Evaluation and management of nephrotic hyperlipidemia. Resident and Staff Physician (in press).

3. Baxter, J.H., Goodman, H.C. and Havel, R.J.: Serum lipid and lipoprotein alterations in nephrosis. J Clin Invest 39:455, 1960.

4. Gherardi, E., Rota, E., Calandra, S. et al.: A Relationship among the concentrations of serum lipoproteins and changes in their chemical composition in patients with untreated nephrotic syndrome. Eur J Clin Invest 7:563, 1977.

5. Vass, V.J., Chilvers, C., Jarrett, R. et al.: Does the nephrotic syndrome increase the risk of cardiovascular disease? Lancet 2:664, 1979.

6. Zilleruelo, G., Hsia, S.L., Freundlich, M. et al.: Persistence of serum lipid abnormalities in children with idiopathic nephrotic syndrome. J Pediatr 104:61, 1984.

7. Zilleruelo, G., Fordyce, M., Christakis, G. et al.: Abnormal adipose tissue fatty acid composition in children with idiopathic nephrotic syndrome. Pediatr Res 17:354A, 1983.

8. Januszewicz, P., Ignatowska-Switalska, H. and Wyszynska, T.: Abnormal prostaglandin excretion in children with minimal change nephrotic syndrome. Prostaglandins Med 7:149, 1981.

9. Garin, E., Sausville, P.J. and Richard, G.: Plasma prostaglandin E_2 concentration in nephrotic syndrome. J Pediatr 103:253, 1983.

10. Oetliker, O.H., Merdasini, R., Lutchg, J. et al.: Lipoprotein metabolism in nephrotic syndrome in childhood. Pediatr Res 14:64, 1980.

11. Michaeli, J., Bar-On, H. and Sharfir, E.: Lipoprotein profiles in a heterogeneous group of patients with nephrotic syndrome. Isr J Med Sci 17:1001, 1981.

12. Baxter, J.H.: Hyperlipoproteinemia in nephrosis. Arch Intern Med 109:742, 1962.

13. Yedgar, S., Weinstein, D.B., Patsch, W. et al.: Viscosity of culture medium as a regulator of synthesis and secretion of very low density lipoproteins by cultured hepatocytes. J Biol Chem 257:2188, 1982.

14. Hyman, L.R., Wong, P.W.K. and Grossman, A.: Plasma lipoprotein lipase in children with idiopathic nephrotic syndrome. Pediatrics 44:1021, 1969.

15. Dixit, V.M. and Hettiaratchi, E.S.G.: The mechanism of hyperlipidemia in nephrotic syndrome. Med Hypoth 5:1327, 1979.

16. Appel, G.B., Blum, C.B., Chien, S. et al.: The hyperlipidemia of the nephrotic syndrome: Relation to plasma albumin concentration, oncotic pressure, and viscosity. N Eng J Med 312:1544, 1985.

17. Lopes-Virella, M., Virella, G., Debeukelear, M. et al.: Urinary high density lipoprotein in minimal change glomerular disease and chronic glomerulopathies. Clin Chim Acta 94:73, 1979.

18. Gordon, T., Kannel, W.B., Casteli, W.P. et al.: Lipoproteins, cardiovascular disease and death: The Framingham Study. Arch Intern Med 141:1128, 1981.

19. Goldburt, U. and Medali, J.H.: High-density lipoprotein cholesterol and incidence of coronary heart disease: The Israeli ischemic heart disease study. Am J Epidemiol 109:296, 1979.

20. Llach, F.: Hypercoagulability, renal vein thrombosis, and other thrombotic complications of nephrotic syndrome. Kidney Int 28:429, 1985.

21. McVicar, M., Chandra, M., Margouleff, D. et al.: Splenic hypofunction in children with nephrotic syndrome. Pediatr Res 17:354A, 1983.

22. Schrier, R.W.: Treatment of hyponatremia. N Engl J Med 312:1121, 1985.

23. Moorhead, J.F., Chan, M.K., El-Nohas, M. et al.: Lipid nephrotoxicity in chronic progressive glomerular and tubulo-interstitial disease. Lancet 2:1309, 1982.

24. Zilleruelo, G., Novak, M., Freundlich, M. et al.: Dietary fish oil supplementation ameliorates hyperlipidemia in nephrotic children. Pediatr Res 20(4):460A, 1986.

MINERAL METABOLISM IN NEPHROTIC SYNDROME

Michael Freundlich, M.D., Gaston Zilleruelo, M.D., Carolyn Abitbol, M.D. and Jose Strauss, M.D.

Although hypocalcemia has been recognized for decades in patients with nephrotic syndrome (NS), it was initially simply related to the reduction in the protein-bound calcium fraction as a result of the heavy proteinuria (1, 2). Thus, true hypocalcemia (low ionized calcium) was assumed to be absent in NS and the observed low serum total calcium concentration was not considered as having clinical significance. However, with the advent of calcium specific electrodes, direct measurements of serum ionized calcium became available in patients with NS.

Lim et al. first showed systematically that the reduction in total serum calcium reflects a decrease in serum ionized calcium in a group of nephrotic adults in which total and ionized calcium were determined simultaneously (3). Furthermore, it was demonstrated that in patients with NS the total serum calcium concentration does not reflect accurately concentration of the ionized fraction, even after correction of total calcium concentration for the hypoproteinemia (4). In the majority of patients, serum protein-bound calcium per gram of serum albumin appeared excessively high. It was suggested that in the nephrotic state, there is increased binding of calcium by macromolecules other than albumin (3). Thus, direct measurements of ionized calcium are needed to determine the true concentration of this ion in patients with NS.

Subsequently, another study mostly in adults (5) confirmed that the reduction in total serum calcium is accompanied by a decrease in serum ionized calcium. More recently, two independent groups of investigators made similar observations in children with NS (6-8). Although tetany is a rare occurrence in children with NS, paresthesias and ill-defined muscle aches during nephrotic relapse could be caused by true hypocalcemia; however, carefully designed studies addressing this issue are lacking.

In addition to hypocalcemia, excessive fecal calcium losses have been described in patients with NS even when glomerular filtration rate (GFR) was normal. Several investigators using metabolic balance techniques (9-11) found that intestinal absorption of calcium may be impaired in some of those patients. However, in many studies the levels of renal function were not stated; since patients with NS,

This project was funded in part under an agreement with the Department of Health and Rehabilitative Services, State of Florida Children's Medical Services.

particularly adults, may have renal failure, the latter may have caused the defective intestinal calcium absorption (13). In contrast, others have found normal intestinal calcium absorption when measured by radiocalcium (14); nevertheless, when corrected to habitual dietary calcium intake, defective intestinal calcium absorption was demonstrated employing similar methodology (3).

A greater understanding of derangements in mineral metabolism in NS coincided with a better knowledge of the role played by vitamin D, its metabolites, and circulating parathyroid hormone (PTH). Availability of new techniques for determination of those compounds made possible their accurate measurement in the various states of relapse, remission, corticosteroid therapy, etc. High serum PTH concentration often accompanied hypocalcemia, even with a normal GFR; occasionally there were radiologic (11) and histologic (10) evidences of decalcification and enhanced bone resorption.

Low circulating levels of 25-hydroxyvitamin D [25(OH)D] were first noted in a group of adults with NS (15-18); the decreased levels presumably were a result of urinary losses (18, 19). More recently, strikingly low plasma 25(OH)D levels were found in a group of children with NS and normal GFR (8). The direct correlation between plasma 25(OH)D and serum albumin (8) and inverse correlation between proteinuria and plasma 25(OH)D (20) support the concept that the low levels of this vitamin D metabolite are due mainly to excessive urinary losses during active NS. Administration of ^{3}H-labelled cholecalciferol in NS patients (18) resulted in rapid appearance of labelled vitamin in the urine, mainly as the 25-hydroxylated metabolite bound to vitamin D-binding globulin (VDBG). The latter, with a MW of 59.000 daltons (smaller than the 69.000 daltons of albumin), constitutes the serum transporting protein for vitamin D metabolites. Diminished serum and elevated urinary concentrations of VDBG have been consistently found in patients with NS (17-19). Current understanding, therefore, supports the concept that urinary losses of 25(OH)D attached to VDBG during the stage of active (proteinuric) NS, lead to decreased plasma levels of this form of vitamin D (21).

In contrast, data on circulating levels of 1,25-dihydroxyvitamin D [$1,25(OH)_2D$] remain controversial and have been reported to be low by some (5, 19) and normal by most (8, 22, 23). The precise nature of these discrepancies is not clear, but several factors may determine the levels of circulating $1,25(OH)_2D$: duration of illness, concurrent administration of corticosteroids, and concentration of serum calcium, phosphorus, magnesium, and PTH (24).

We studied these factors in a group of children with NS and normal GFR during periods of active NS and during periods of remission, with longitudinal observations in some (20). Similar to our initial cross-sectional observations (8), plasma $1,25(OH)_2D$ concentrations were normal during active NS as well as in remission. As expected, hypocalcemia, modest hyperparathyroidism and strikingly low 25(OH)D levels were identified during relapsing periods. Of particular relevance was that most alterations were transient and normalized upon remission (Table). Of further interest was the finding that concurrent administration of glucocorticoid therapy at conventional low dose and short-term (< three months) schedules did not affect results. However, glucocorticoid administration for more than one year, has been associated with diminished circulating levels of $1,25(OH)_2D$ as well as with bone undermineralization (25).

TABLE

LABORATORY DATA DURING RELAPSE AND REMISSION IN 20 CHILDREN WITH NEPHROTIC SYNDROME

	CALCIUM (mg/dl)	PHOSPHORUS (mg/dl)	PARATHORMONE (ulEq/ml)	CALCIDIOL (ng/ml)	CALCITRIOL (pg/ml)
RELAPSE	8.2±0.17	5.1±0.18	123±14	9.0±6.7	44±5.0
REMISSION	9.7±0.08*	4.8±0.12	94±10	26±14*	51±5.0

Values represent mean ± SEM of 43 episodes of relapse and 47 remissions. $^*p < 0.0001$.

Reproduced from Freundlich, M., Bourgoignie, J.J., Zilleruelo, G., et al: Calcium and vitamin D metabolism in children with nephrotic syndrome. J Pediatr 108:383-386, 1986, with permission.

Since the onset and subsequent relapses of NS occur in children during periods of active bone formation and mineral deposition (26), alterations in bone modulating factors could eventually result in altered bone mineralization and structure. While evidence of metabolic bone disease by bone biopsy has been described in adults with NS and normal GFR (16), similar data are lacking in children. We reported diminished bone mineral content when assessed by photon absorptiometry in a group of nephrotic children (8). These and other observations suggest that children (and adults) with NS, particularly those with a protracted or frequently relapsing course, appear to be at risk of developing bone disease even though they have a normal GFR.

A corollary of the above considerations is that prevention of hypovitaminosis D, hypocalcemia, and hyperparathyroidism should be considered in patients with an active NS. Whether this can be achieved and, thereby, prevent undermineralization of bone by administration of a vitamin D metabolite and/or exogenous calcium supplementation, remains to be demonstrated.

REFERENCES

1. Salvesen, H.A., Limder, C.C.: Observations on the inorganic bases and phosphates in relation to the protein of blood and other body fluids in Bright's disease and in heart failure. J Biol Chem, 58:617-634, 1923.

2. Drummond, K.N.: The nephrotic syndrome. In Vaughan, V.C. and Behrman, R.E., (eds.): Nelson Textbook of Pediatrics. Philadelphia:Saunders Co., 1983, pp 1322-1330.

3. Lim, P., Jacob, E., Tock, E.P.C., et al.: Calcium and phosphorus metabolism in nephrotic syndrome. Quart J Med, 46:327-338, 1977.

4. Payne, R.B., Little, A.J., Williams, R.B., et al.: Interpretation of serum calcium in patients with abnormal serum proteins. Br Med J IV, 643-646, 1973.

5. Goldstein, D.A., Haldimann, E., Sherman, D., et al.: Vitamin D metabolites and calcium metabolism in patients with nephrotic syndrome and normal renal function. J Clin Endocrinol Metab, 52:116-121, 1981.

6. Alon, U. and Chan, J.C.M.: Calcium and vitamin-D metabolism in nephrotic syndrome. Int J Pediatr Nephrol, 4:115, 1983.

7. Freundlich, M., Cassady, J.C., Zilleruelo, G., et al.: Altered mineral metabolism in children with nephrotic syndrome and normal renal function. Pediatr Res 17:349A, 1983 (Abst.).

8. Freundlich, M., Bourgoignie, J.J., Zilleruelo, G., et al.: Bone modulating factors in nephrotic children with normal glomerular filtration rate. Pediatrics 76:280-285, 1985.

9. Boyd, G.L., Courtney, A.M. and MacLachlan, I.F.: The metabolism of salts in nephritis. Am J Dis Child 32:29-39, 1926.

10. Scriver, W. de M.: Observations on the excretion of calcium in two cases of nephrosis treated with parathyroid extract. J Clin Invest 6:115-125, 1928.

11. Emerson, K. and Beckman, W.W.: Calcium metabolism in nephrosis. I. A description of an abnormality in calcium metabolism in children with nephrosis. J Clin Invest 24:564-572, 1945.

12. Jones J.H., Peters, D.K., Morgan D.B., et al.: Observations of calcium metabolism in the nephrotic syndrome. Quart J Med. 36:301-320, 1967.

13. Coburn, J.W., Koppel, M.H., Brickman, A.S., et al.: Study of intestinal absorption of calcium in patients with renal failure. Kidney Int 3:264-272, 1973.

14. Mountokalkin, T., Virvidakis, C., Singhellakis, P., et al.: Intestinal calcium absorption in the nephrotic syndrome. Ann Intern Med 86:746-747, 1977.

15. Goldstein, D.A., Oda, Y., Kurokawa, K., et al.: Blood levels of 25-hydroxyvitamin D in nephrotic syndrome. Studies in 26 patients. Ann Intern Med 87:664, 1977.

16. Malluche, H.H., Goldstein, D.A. and Massry, S.G.: Osteomalacia and hyperparathyroid bone disease in patients with nephrotic syndrome. J Clin Invest 63:494-500, 1979.

17. Schmidt-Gayk, H., Grawunder, C., Tschope, W., etal.: 25-hydroxyvitamin D in nephrotic syndrome. Lancet 2:105-108, 1977.

18. Barragry, J.M., Carter, N.D., Beer, M., et al.: Vitamin-D metabolism in nephrotic syndrome. Lancet 2:629-632, 1977.

19. Lambert P.W., De Oreo, P.B., Fu, I.Y., et al.: Urinary and plasma vitamin D3 metabolites in the nephrotic syndrome. Metab Bone Dis Relat Res 4:7-15, 1982.

20. Freundlich, M., Bourgoignie, J.J., Zilleruelo, G., et al.: Calcium and vitamin D metabolism in children with nephrotic syndrome. J Pediatr 108:383-387, 1986.

21. Alon, V. and Chan, J.C.M.: Calcium and vitamin D homeostasis in the nephrotic syndrome. Current status. Nephron 36:1-4, 1984.

22. Korkor, A., Schwartz, J., Bergfeld, M., et al.: Absence of metabolic bone disease in adult patients with the nephrotic syndrome and normal renal function. J Clin Endocrinol Metab 46:496-500, 1983.

23. Tessitore, N., Bonucci, E., D'Angelo, A., et al.: Bone histology and calcium metabolism in patients with nephrotic syndrome and normal or reduced renal function. Nephron 37:153-159, 1984.

24. Rosen, J.F. and Chesney, R.W.: Circulating calcitriol concentrations in health and disease. J Pediatr 103:1, 1983.

25. Chesney, R.W., Hamstra, A.J., Mazess, R.B., et al.: Reduction of serum 1,25-dihydroxyvitamin D3 in children receiving glucocorticoids. Lancet 2:1123-1125, 1978.

26. Barnett, H.L., Schoeneman, M., Bernstein, J., et al.: The nephrotic syndrome. In: Edelmann C.M., Jr., (ed.). Pediatric Kidney Disease, Boston:Little Brown Co., 1978, pp 679-695.

DISCUSSION: PRIMARY NEPHROTIC SYNDROME

PANELISTS: Russell Chesney, M.D., Michael Freundlich, M.D., Warren Grupe, M.D., Norman Siegel, M.D. and Gaston Zilleruelo, M.D.

MODERATOR: Jose Strauss, M.D.

COMMENT: Related to the problem of recurrence in transplants, we talked about recurrence of disease in FSS versus membranous proliferative. The recurrences in focal sclerosing are very complicated recurrences; they look a bit like chronic rejection. It is very difficult to tell whether one has late chronic rejection or true recurrence of focal sclerosis, unless one has the type of situation where proteinuria appears within a day or two. In two of our patients we have even seen actual proteinuria on the operating table at the time of the transplant, proteinuria in the first urine that comes out of the new kidney. In type II membrano-proliferative, where there is said to be a lot of recurrences, the recurrences consist of the presence of intra-membranous ribbon-like material within the basement membrane (tubular and glomerular). However, the clinical implication of this is not so severe; many of these patients do not have evidence of progressive renal disease, and in fact, do quite well. We have had the opportunity to do repeat biopsies in two patients who have recurrent type II MPGN; they have not had any decline in renal function. That is an important distinction. The fact that we get these intra-membranous deposits is an interesting observation but they may not mean that much in terms of the actual clinical course of the patient, at least over the four or five years of follow-up that we and other people have documented.

QUESTION: Not much was said about the juxtaglomerular apparatus as a cause of hypertension. Would you comment on that?

RESPONSE: In other words, you are saying that the hypertension seen in nephrotics may be related to abnormalities of the juxtaglomerular apparatus as reflected by the nephrotic syndrome. I think that the hypertension in nephrotic syndrome is multifactorial. That is one of the things we need to think about but there are other things.

COMMENT: I agree that the hypertension seen in patients with nephrotic syndrome is pretty clearly multifactorial. Certainly some of it is related to the treatment we all dispense in various ways. Depending upon the blood volume status, it is possible to implicate the renin-angiotensin system, and to suggest that in a situation where there is hypovolemia, there may be stimulation of the JG apparatus. At a point where some youngsters have scarring and progression of the disease, as is seen frequently in various glomerulopathies, there is almost certainly renin mediated hypertension.

MODERATOR: What percentage of the nephrotics (minimal change or however we define the various entities that were touched upon today) have hypertension? One of the panelists wrote a review on the subject and gave some figures that to us seemed high--some 20% or so of nephrotics under certain conditions. Could you clarify that question for us?

RESPONSE: About 25-30% of minimal lesion nephrotic children will have blood pressures that are above normal for their size. A good number of those are before the institution of prednisone therapy. One would suspect that in at least some of them this might be related to hypovolemia and the renin-angiotensin system, but I do not know data that clearly show that. Most of these children are not hypertensive to the point that they are having encephalopathy or problems with the hypertension. It is just that their blood pressures are higher than in controls.

COMMENT: Although I am not familiar with available data, conceivably something similar to what happens in adults might happen with children. The opposite is true; the normovolemic or hypervolemic nephrotic patients might be those who are hypertensive with suppression of the renin-aldosterone system. That would be similar to what Laragh and others have found: roughly half of the nephrotic patients are euvolemic or even hypervolemic.

QUESTION: I would like to bring up the whole question of the hyperfiltration syndrome and the role of hyperfiltration. What do you think about the hyperfiltration syndrome as perhaps a central way of explaining focal sclerosis? Maybe several different diseases will manifest themselves in such a way that you would say, "Well, there is an increased GFR per functioning nephron and that is why you see focal sclerosis". I wonder what you think about that.

RESPONSE: The observation that animals who have a significant reduction in renal mass will develop proteinuria and focal segmental glomerulosclerosis if one looks at their kidneys long term, has raised questions about the relationship of this lesion to continued proteinuria and the possibility that this particular type of histologic change is just one that is reflective of continued proteinuria. That is a very difficult question to answer because we do not have a good experimental situation in which to look at this problem. The animal models in which focal and segmental glomerulosclerosis develop, have largely been dependent upon removing one kidney and reducing the renal mass to less than 10% of normal, then watching that animal develop over a period of time. That certainly is not the situation we see either in the patient with early onset or late onset focal segmental glomerulosclerosis. One could argue that the appearance of focal and segmental lesions in children with corticosteroid dependent nephrotic syndrome is derived from the fact that they are having frequent relapses of their disease, have continued proteinuria and are therefore susceptible to the development of this lesion. The appearance of the lesion in reflux nephropathy where it does occur almost exclusively after the reduction in glomerular filtration rate occurs and proteinuria appears suggests that there may be a link to the experimental model. If we take purely the nephrotic syndrome, it is difficult to take that experimental model and move it across to the child with nephrosis or relapsing nephrosis. In some of the other diseases it is a little bit easier to construct a relationship with the experimental model. We do know that in the aging rat, one can find the lesion of focal and segmental glomerulosclerosis developing; we know, at least in human renal biopsy material, that over the age of 50 or 60, it is not unusual to see global sclerosis; totally sclerosed glomeruli even appear in younger patients. But I am not aware of a good study that has shown that classical segmental lesions develop with aging. I think that there is some dropout of glomeruli with time. I am not sure that the hyperfiltration syndrome concept, because it is based largely on a massive reduction in renal mass, is applicable to the child with nephrosis. I guess what I am saying is that I am not in the school that feels that you need to treat asymptomatic proteinuria in the child with nephrotic syndrome. Some people have proposed, based on the hyperfiltration concept, that one should try to reduce the period of proteinuria which these children have. For a period of time after their proteinuria recurs, before putting them back on corticosteroid therapy, we routinely watch children whom we know have corticosteroid responsive disease because some will develop a spontaneous remission of their nephrotic syndrome. We do this particularly if they develop the relapse in relationship to a viral infection or intercurrent viral type of syndrome which so commonly sets off a relapse. I am concerned that we not over-interpret the proteinuria-hyperfiltration concept, and apply it to the child with relapsing nephrotic syndrome.

MODERATOR: Some pediatric nephrologists have accepted the hyperfiltration-hyperperfusion hypothesis as fact, and have started implementing therapeutic changes to fit that hypothesis. For instance, some have started restricting protein intake in patients with nephrotic syndrome. How do you react to that approach?

RESPONSE: My view is that the current concept that restriction of protein intake can diminish the load presented to the glomeruli, and therefore prevent the overworking of the remaining glomeruli after a renal injury has occurred, is exciting; there are lots of experimental data, and the concept has been supported by a number of animal models. I do not think we are ready yet—at least I am not—to implement that. The clinical studies which have been done have relied almost exclusively on the concept that if one looks at the natural history of a renal disease and plots 1/serum creatinine to gauge or to estimate the rate of decline in renal function or the rate of loss of renal mass, the 1/serum creatinine should make a linear plot over time. In many of the renal diseases which we deal with in pediatrics, that clearly is not the case. A classical example is obstructive nephropathy. We all have had the experience of following a child whose creatinine will jump to two and stay there for many months or years, and his renal function will decline in a stepwise fashion, not in a fashion which could be described as linear. I think we have to wait until the concept is proven in the adult who can much more readily sustain protein deprivation, who does not need to grow in height. If that cannot be done, we will have to wait for better measurements or parameters of the effectiveness of that therapy. Also, it will have to be shown that pediatric renal disease follows clinical parameters which are the same as those suggested for adult patients. In sum, I am not quite ready to apply that concept to pediatric patients because of concern about growth and because of concern about the data base upon which the clinical studies have been carried out.

MODERATOR: I agree that those concerns are very important and need to be resolved before acting on the concept. I would like to ask the question, "What is important—the proteinuria or the load of protein to the kidneys?" In studies carried out in the Clinical Research Center here in Miami, we assessed patients who were receiving only water and electrolytes and some continued having up to 10 or more grams of protein in the urine. Those were patients who did not respond to food manipulation; those who did respond had a diuresis and decrease in their proteinuria. We did not specifically try to decrease protein intake but noticed little effect on serum protein after four to five days; in some patients it even increased. We seem to have had patients with plenty of protein production despite the lack of protein intake!

RESPONSE:. One of the important things to recognize about the high protein-hyperfiltration hypothesis is that, in effect, it is a rediscovery of an observation that dates back a long time. There were some observations in the 20's and a resurgence of this in the early 60's, in animal studies and in some human studies, in the so-called Bull diet which was supposed to slow the progression of renal failure. There are several things that we should keep in mind. The first is that a lot of these studies were carried out in the rat. The rat is a peculiar animal; unlike other animals, it actually dies of renal failure. It develops a progressive renal disease and dies between about 20 and 24 months of life with a large heart and often with a proteinuria and glomerular sclerosis of some sort. If one limits the intake of protein in these rats, one can alter this course. When I was working at the NIH, I had the opportunity to become acquainted with a colony of aged rats in which studies could be done. It was very simple to produce these aged rats; one would simply limit the intake of protein to perhaps as low as 13-14% instead of the usual 20-24% found in ordinary rat chow. This observation has been known for a very long time. The idea of hyperfiltration is now, of course, a very appealing one to us, particularly since it fits with diabetic data. But there are two other components of which we must not lose sight: one is that we as pediatricians do not really know how much protein is necessary if we are going to prevent progression of renal failure and yet allow growth; if we limit protein intake by too much, then we potentially are going to limit growth. This is a very crucial and very critical point to be determined. I cannot underscore enough what the other panelist said: the study should be done in adults first and then we should address these questions in children. The second point is, by limiting protein we are also limiting phosphate; this, of course, also has to be recognized. Finally, the point mentioned earlier, the increased synthetic rate of albumin and of other proteins, probably accounts for the finding that there really is little relationship between dietary protein intake and proteinuria in patients with nephrotic syndrome. I would agree 100% on that. The only way that you are going to manipulate protein and account for urinary losses is by the actual infusion of albumin. If you are relying on the diet, you are not really going to change proteinuria very much.

MODERATOR: Conceptually we are all, as pediatricians, in agreement that we should not jump into food, protein, calorie restriction, whatever seems important (their ratios, and so on) until we have solid data. As you know, the NIH is funding a Multi-Center Study on this subject in adults. Some already have stated here that it is not time yet to study this problem in children. But it has been suggested to me that the situation is so entirely different in the adult than in the child that we may end up being strapped by conclusions that an irrelevant-to-children study arrives at in adults. The thought is that we should have a valid parallel study in pediatrics with the growth parameters in mind and the minimal requirements (whatever they are) for proteins and calories. Some of the people at NIH endorse the concept that we should wait for the adult study, but others do not. Again, I think that we are in agreement that we should not take the human adult or rat (not animal but just rat, since that is what seems to be the model) studies as an indication of what we should be doing in children, but how should we proceed at this very crucial point?

COMMENT: I want to comment about that. First of all, yes, it is focused predominantly on rat data, predominantly ablation data, but I think Michel Broyer has come up with some data which are important for us as pediatricians. In ablation data, in rats, the only way he could prolong survival of the rats was by limiting protein intake in the young rats to the point where they did not grow. As soon as he got growth, he got shortening of the life span. That to me is very compelling data relative to us as pediatricians. Even in the model system where it is supposed to work, it works at the expense of growth of the young rat.

MODERATOR: Some people are saying, "Why should pediatricians be so worried and concerned about growth?" It is being said by some adult nephrologists that we are paranoid about growth. They are implying that we should protect the kidneys and let the body and the brain and the rest go to pot. In jest, as nephrologists we might agree, but not as pediatricians.

COMMENT: There is a statement that can be made here. That is, it would be fine if we were able to be assured that the only trade off we would make would be somebody short and not on dialysis. We do not have that kind of data. It has not been proven that you can prevent need for dialysis with low protein diet; you may be able to shift it to the right a little but if you are shifting to the right at the expense of muscle mass and growth and bone and brain development, you are going to end up with something much less than a short person not on dialysis.

COMMENT: I would raise another warning statement. If one looks closely at the experimental data in the ablation model, one can see that it is possible to normalize single nephron GFR; however, there have not been data presented in terms of whole animal GFR. In fact, it may be possible to stabilize single nephron GFR at a relatively normal level; but in a massively reduced number of nephrons, then one would have, by preventing hyperfiltration, an animal which would essentially be uremic. Until we know what the entire GFR is (which may be related to the point just made about the total animal survival), I am not sure that we should jump into this. It is very fashionable, and because we all would like to prevent end stage renal disease, it is very appealing. I would like to see it proven in the adult population that, in fact, protein restriction prevents end stage renal disease; that is, that it allows the stabilization of serum creatinine at 2 or 2.4 mg/dl for a GFR of 25 or 30 cc/min, at a level which we think the patient is medically manageable for a prolonged period of time. Otherwise, our gain may be very small at the expense of growth, intellectual development, and much more. I would not even attempt to design a study that would be applicable to children until we know more about the total therapy.

MODERATOR: All this is terribly important because it has implications for all types of clinical, epidemiological, and, among others, governmental decisions on research support. To feed or not to feed: governments may decide to save money by restricting protein intake because it is good for the people; that brings up the question of national example. When I was in Medellin, Colombia, a few years ago, some people thought at the time that the hyperperfusion hypothesis had been proven. I presented our data about lipid changes which we thought were to a certain extent independent of some of the protein changes. Some of the local people were saying that they have the natural experiment already. They have lots of protein and calorie malnutrition, and they do not see any difference in the progression rate of renal diseases, either acquired or congenital, between Colombia and other countries. We have here physicians from Colombia, Venezuela, Chile, Argentina, Mexico, etc. Would any of you like to comment on that point? What are your thoughts about this problem? Do you see a difference in the progression rate in the population you serve versus the population that we see in Miami or the United States in general?

RESPONSE: Essentially the rate of progression in chronic renal failure which we see is the same as in the United States. However, in Venezuela about 25-27% of the nephrotic population have focal segmental sclerosis, a higher percentage than in other areas of the world. We have only one to two cases per year of mesangial proliferation and membranoproliferative glomerulonephritis but our patients are essentially younger that 18 years of age.

MODERATOR: Would anyone like to comment on that? How does that compare with the figures you would expect in the U.S.?

COMMENT: In general that is a high rate for idiopathic nephrotic syndrome. If you compare this number to the International Study data or most U.S. individual centers, that is a considerably increased rate for that particular lesion.

COMMENT: I would like to offer two comments about the hyperfiltration business. One is the results reported in an abstract which the Einstein group published in the mid-60's: a high protein diet in infants increases the rate of increase in GFR over those given a "normal" diet. The question is, is this some evidence in support of the fact that a high protein diet in someone who intrinsically has a low GFR might just lead to more hyperfiltration? Not that I of necessity am a believer in the theory. The second comment is about the causes of focal segmental glomerulosclerosis. This pertains to the case reports (diffuse and scattered) of children with cyanotic congenital heart disease who have very large glomeruli and perhaps constitute a hyperperfusion model. There are some who have transient proteinuria, and the proteinuria can be reversed by phlebotomy. The other thing in that particular situation, though, is that the effective renal plasma flow or the renal blood flow to the outer cortical glomeruli, is reduced. So, you have perhaps an intrinsic reduction in GFR, and an anatomy that would suggest hyperfiltration. There are a few reports from Japan suggesting that there is an increased incidence of sclerotic glomeruli and hypertension in adult populations. I am not sure where these items stand, but they are interesting observations. In infants at least, they seem to support the hyperperfusion business.

MODERATOR: The population in that abstract from Einstein, were they neonates?

RESPONSE: Yes, they were.

MODERATOR: Did the same thing happen in the work that Edelmann and Barnett published in the JCI in 1959, when protein intake was increased up to about 9 g/kg/day?

RESPONSE: That was looking at the concentrating defect or capacity.

MODERATOR: Yes. But, was there an increase in GFR? I do not believe that the data on GFR were in the paper.

RESPONSE: Neither do I. Also, the time interval may not have been the same. In the paper in the JCI on concentration, I believe that they looked at two - three week intervals, while the GFR and Renal Plasma Flow data were at 8-10 week intervals.

MODERATOR: Going on at Babies' Hospital in New York now is a study about the impact of different protein intakes on GFR in the neonate. The nutrition people there have been testing the effect of different protein intakes on various body functions and they were able to collect blood and urines in premature babies fed about 2 g/kg/day and 4 g/kg/day. So far, there is no difference in GFR in a matter of days, but there are many variables. Again, what we like to emphasize in our group is the relationship of protein intake to total calorie intake. That may be the key to some of the discrepancies of opinions and results.

COMMENT: Another point I want to make about all these data, is the role of phosphate just now mentioned in all these changes in protein intake. Also, what about sodium? You go up and down in the protein content of diets and with that you affect many things.

MODERATOR: Yes. You also might change arterial blood pressure.

COMMENT: Published in the JCI a couple of years ago were some studies which demonstrated the role of fatty acid manipulation in the diet of NZB mice in slowing the progression to end stage renal disease or the prevention of proteinuria with increased survival by the reduction in saturated fatty acids and their replacement with certain polyunsaturated fatty acids. I agree that this is another aspect that needs to be carefully looked into when we assess the effect of certain diets. Everybody is looking at what the protein content is, but not at what is remaining in those diets.

COMMENT: Two things about what has just now been talked about: one, I am not sure that calorie malnutrition is an appropriate control for protein overload so I am not sure that we can make a case out of that. The other point pertains to children who have congenital heart disease and large, congested glomeruli. I am not sure that that is evidence for increased inflow as much as it might be evidence for decreased (due to constriction) outflow from the glomeruli. So it may not be hyperperfusion; it may not be high pressure; it may not be all the things that have been put together as possible contributors. I would like to suggest that oligomeganephronia is a natural human model which I do not think has been looked at appropriately, with this sort of thing in mind. Those patients develop focal and segmental disease as their glomeruli die.

MODERATOR: It is very important that we talk about these things and look at them with as broad a view as possible even though it is becoming unpopular to question some of those items. We have discussed this subject enough. Let us move on to other topics.

QUESTION: There is a study in progress in the Boston area with the use of meclofenamate in the treatment of adults with focal segmental glomerulosclerosis, with the idea of a non-steroidal agent decreasing glomerular filtration and the effect that this would have on decreasing proteinuria and progression of renal disease. Does anyone here know how the results of that study are progressing?

RESPONSE: I do not know about Boston but in Rochester, Minnesota meclofenamate studies in adults with idiopathic nephrotic syndrome have been going on for over a year. I am not fully familiar with all the details of the studies but I do have some generalizations. About 50% of the patients treated who had heavy proteinuria, had a significant reduction in their protein excretion rates. The follow-up time still is too short to make any meaningful interpretation about progression of disease. Since indomethacin was discussed earlier in relation to decrease in GFR with non-steroidal anti-inflammatory agents, I want to comment on that. Although all those agents have in common a decrease in the GFR, at least in the meclofenamate model, when renal functions are evaluated carefully, in almost all patients there will be an initial drop in GFR and a drop in protein excretion rate, but in many, the GFR will return to normal levels while the protein excretion rate remains low. Probably there is a more involved mechanism than a simple decrease in GFR.

MODERATOR: The question in general is throwing all of us off balance in terms of what's good and what's bad when we do something to those patients. At the International Congress of Nephrology in Los Angeles someone brought up the question of antihypertensive medications which we regard as not desirable because they reduce the GFR. He was saying that maybe that is good. So we come back to the question of what is the main determinant if, indeed, the hypothesis works: is the change in load to glomeruli most important, or the basic problem which allows the proteinuria to occur? Should we aim at reducing, increasing or leaving the GFR unchanged?

QUESTION: On the same subject but regarding the treatment of nephrotic syndrome, does anyone have the experience of using pulses of corticosteroids in nephrotic syndrome or in membranoproliferative glomerulonephritis type I, or with the use of immunosuppressors like Cyclophosphamide orally or in pulses?

RESPONSE: The initial evidence in terms of pulse therapy using various medications is that it really is not terribly different from using oral medication provided there is compliance and absorption. You certainly can induce a remission but I do not know that the induction of remission with a pulsed medication is any better or any more sustained than one would get with the same sort of absorption and doses from oral medication. One little caveat in that is some work from Stanford in which patients with frequently relapsing nephrotic syndrome were given pulses almost as if they were on chemotherapy for a tumor. Pulses were given initially over a period of, I think, five days, and then following with almost monthly pulses. They have the feeling that they have been able to keep some patients in remission who otherwise might not have stayed in remission, with a total overall dose lower than "usual". Interestingly enough, they have been keeping these patients on every other day prednisone between these maintenance pulses and there are a large number of nephrotics who have been kept in remission with very low doses of every other day medication. That is one problem. The other is that this has not been done long enough to know what price one might be paying in terms of bone disease. The prevalence of aseptic necrosis seems to be related not just to the total dose of corticosteroids but somewhat to the number of pulses that have been given. So there may be some results to this that are good, but I have not seen any results clearly demonstrating that it is better than the way we have been doing for the last 20 years.

COMMENTS: I would like to touch on the bone disease issue. It is one of the complications of corticosteroids that was just emphasized. We measured bone mineral content in more than 300 children with a variety of renal disorders. We discovered not only that the bone mineral content is somewhat low in children with nephrotic syndrome, but also that this can be enhanced greatly by the use of corticosteroids, and furthermore, that there is a progressive decline in bone mineral content as one uses corticosteroids chronically. We are in the process of analyzing data on children who now have been followed up to 10 years with multiple measurements of bone mineral content. Our impression from the data so far fits the conclusion that we came to a few years ago, that there is a progression in the decline in bone mineral content. There is no question that one has to try to get away with as low a dose of corticosteroids as possible. If it turns out that pulsing ends up using a lower total dose of corticosteroids, there may be some value in it. This has not been looked at in a scientific fashion, however, and thus I would caution against embracing that hypothesis or that philosophy. We also tend to use pulse therapy for a variety of conditions when we are frustrated but our experience is very limited, and I think we may not know what we are doing when we use pulse therapy.

QUESTION: To shift to another area, what is the main reason for doing a biopsy before starting cytotoxic therapy in patients with nephrotic syndrome? Is not the underlying reason basically to determine whether the cytotoxin is going to work or not? Can you actually do that with any of the histologic findings short of actually using the drug?

MODERATOR: A related question is what role does age play as a factor in deciding when to do a renal biopsy before initiating treatment? Some people refer to 7 or 8 or 10 years as the time beyond which all patients should be biopsied. Did the International Study of Kidney Disease in Children recommend an age after which all patients should be biopsied?

COMMENT: My understanding is that the ISKDC really has no specific recommendations as to when to do a renal biopsy. I do not think they have said that children above 10 should have a biopsy with any kind of nephrotic syndrome. On a more personal level, in talking with most of the original ISKDC participants, most of them tend to treat all new nephrotics for four to eight weeks and see if they respond; of course, there may be some exception if a child happens to have low complement or changes in renal function and so on. People tend to individualize but treat most with corticosteroids first and use non-responsiveness as the major indication for biopsy.

MODERATOR: Regarding treatment, when do you treat, when do you not treat, when do you biopsy, and what do you do with the results of the biopsy?

COMMENT: I would like to break my comments into two parts: first, in trying to decide whether or not to biopsy, what factors do you assess when a child presents with a nephrotic syndrome? Based on the most recent publications of the ISKDC which up to age 18 show a continued high incidence or prevalence rate of minimal change disease and a very good rate of response to corticosteroid therapy, one can argue that it is reasonable not to biopsy children but to treat them with a course of corticosteroid therapy and see whether or not they are responders. In fact, that argument was applied to the whole population of patients with nephrotic syndrome, including adults, in a decision analysis published in Kidney International. I do not agree with all the assumptions they made in their profiling. They agreed that one could take the same course in patients from ages 16 to 60 and from ages one to 16. It is fair to say, as it was shown earlier, that the proportion of patients with minimal change disease declines. At least as you begin to look at the adolescent population you go from about an 80% to a 50% prevalence rate for that lesion. On the other hand, there is an interplay between at least two or three different lesions with the nephrotic syndrome, all of which will respond to corticosteroid therapy, including some patients with mild mesangial changes. So one could argue that not only the minimal change patient should be selected for initiating a course of corticosteroid therapy. In that respect, one could go anywhere from saying, "We should biopsy patients who are adolescents or older because there is only a 50% chance of their having minimal change disease", to following the other rationale which, in fact, endorses treating all patients as long as for the course of corticosteroids they do not have high risk factors. That is, they are not diabetic, they do not have hypertension, etc. which obviously would be more applicable to the adult population.

Regarding the other question, "Why do the biopsy before initiating cytotoxic therapy?" Assuming that the question pertains to the patient who has frequently relapsing disease, it is a very valid question. I am asked this question almost every time I admit a patient for that procedure. Analysis of our own data showed that about 50% of the patients would have minimal change disease, 25% would have mild mesangial changes, and 25% would have focal segmental sclerosis; all of those patients responded to Cyclophosphamide. The biopsy would not have helped me select which of those patients should have been treated with Cyclophosphamide. What the biopsy did was identify the patient which is more likely to relapse after the course of Cyclophosphamide. In this population of frequently relapsing nephrotics, the rate of relapse after treatment with Cyclophosphamide was 20% with minimal change disease, 50% with mesangial changes, and 75% with focal segmental sclerosis. So while they all respond to the Cyclophosphamide, for patients who have significant questions about the probability of a relapse of their disease after undertaking therapy with one of the cytotoxic agents which have a number of side effects one can provide additional information at that point. All of the children who relapsed in each of those categories had a very good response to corticosteroids after their course of Cyclophosphamide. If the decision about whether or not the child is at substantial risk for a relapse after the course of Cyclophosphamide is not a pertinent question clinically, you could go ahead and treat him with a course of Cyclophosphamide and see whether or not he responds to that therapy as well.

MODERATOR: Would you now biopsy a patient who comes with what looks like plain nephrotic syndrome who is 10 or older or any other age? Do you yourself use a certain age right now as a cut-off point to perform or not to perform a biopsy?

RESPONSE: At the onset of disease we biopsy patients who are post-pubertal and would have been considered adults if they had not come to us. My own feeling is, in that particular population we begin to see emergence of the various lesions together, and sometimes it is important to have the biopsy information for counseling the patient. We do not biopsy the young patient with "pure nephrosis". Obviously, the other things that were mentioned earlier today, a low complement, gross hematuria, etc., would change that in the younger patient. We do not routinely biopsy patients in the age of 12 or 13 by those criteria.

COMMENT: We tend to believe a fair amount in the selectivity index for proteinuria. So if we have a patient over 10 years of age who is in all other respects minimal lesion but has a low selective protein index, we probably would biopsy him before treatment. The only other thing that would fit against that would be membranous, but it really has not yet reached a high prevalence in the early teens. The selective protein index which we consider low is 0.2 or under. In terms of the specific question you asked, whether or not there is any value in biopsing somebody who seems to have minimal lesions and be corticosteroid responsive but is being treated with a cytoxic drug, don't you think that is where the crux is? I feel strongly that the biopsy ought to be done for three reasons: first of all, we need to be honest with the parents and the child about using a drug that has considerably more toxicity and with which we have considerably less experience than with corticosteroids; they need a maximum amount of information. Second, from our own point of view, we still need information, the kind of information which we've just now talked about. We need to know about the predictive value of these things. And third, there is always that outside chance that you are fooled. How many times have we thought that somebody had minimal lesion by all criteria yet he did not quite follow the usual clinical course and on biopsy turned up with more than that? We are talking about children who are not following the usual clinical course when we pick up a cytotoxic drug; these are children who are having major problems. They may be having problems with their corticosteroids; otherwise, I do not think they should be considered for cytotoxic drugs in the first place.

QUESTION: I want to ask a question regarding biopsy in nephrotic syndrome patients. I am an adult nephrologist trained by some of the Boston people who were participants in the decision analysis referred to earlier. Even though they gave good reasons for not biopsing everybody with nephrotic syndrome, we biopsied everybody. I spent the last eight months in pediatric nephrology and am not sure that we need to look at the pediatric patient so much differently. We can get away with not biopsing anybody, from my little experience, but I do not see why we necessarily should. The cytotoxic agents are very toxic but you would treat the patient using clinical criteria. I would like to ask, what about the patient who has membranoproliferative disease or membranous glomerulonephritis? Is that where the biopsy would change your therapeutic decision?

RESPONSE: Yes. That is what I was talking about, particularly in terms of the older child or the child who is not following the usual course. That is why I feel compelled to do the biopsy before the initiation of cytotoxic therapy. I cannot on clinical grounds absolutely differentiate between membranous and minimal lesion. In terms of membranoproliferative, by and large from the clinical complex we have a pretty good idea that the child has that particularly if you throw in the low complement, but we do not know enough about the various types yet. In terms of directing the therapy, I think whether or not the therapy does anything in membranoproliferative is more dependent on whether you come from Cincinnati or from elsewhere.

MODERATOR: Since one of the panelists is an expert on that last subject, could we hear his response to that? What does the latest published material say in that regard?

COMMENT: To try to say something original at this time is difficult. Obviously, the therapy of membranoproliferative is controversial; a consensus is difficult to achieve. If we did biopsy an individual and discovered membranoproliferative--although I tend to agree with what was just said, that we recognize those people pretty much ahead of time--that would certainly be one compelling reason not to use standard cytotoxic therapy. The other potential therapies you might use, such as aspirin and dipyridamole or alternate day steroids, that would be a compelling reason for doing the biopsy. But on the question, "Should you do a biopsy in everyone?", I have to agree with what was said earlier. In the back of my mind, I was a lot surer 10 years ago than I am today about that very point.

QUESTION: I have a little bit of difficulty in understanding why the arbitrary age of 10 was chosen as a cut off with regards to biopsy. Having biopsied a few children in the last few months, I must say that the three- year-old may be a bit difficult but I am not clear on that. Could somebody clarify the point for me?

RESPONSE: That was an arbitrary decision. They just said that any child above 10 needed to be biopsied. But I think that what my fellow panelists have said is true: they do not really do that in their own personal practice. That was something that was set up at a meeting, is it not so? It was very arbitrary.

QUESTION: In regard to cytotoxic therapy, I noticed in one of the slides shown that nitrogen mustard was listed as the first agent, followed by Cyclophosphamide and Chlorambucil. Would there be a reason to shy away from Cyclophosphamide in the pre-pubertal or pubertal group because of the fertility problem, and use nitrogen mustard. Does anybody know if there is enough information on that?

RESPONSE: I can tell you that the reason it was in the slide first was because it was tried first.

QUESTION: Is there anybody in here who knows if there is any evidence in the literature that nitrogen mustard would be as effective as the other two agents and if there is any evidence that the incidence of side effects is different?

MODERATOR: Didn't Shoeneman present some material on that during one of the ISKDC meetings?

RESPONSE: There has been a recent interest in that by Dr. Shoeneman in New York, and he published an abstract about three or four years ago in the Society for Pediatric Research Meeting. I do not remember that nitrogen mustard was impressively effective in the same way as Chlorambucil and Cyclophosphamide have been. I might comment about the gonadal toxicity of Cyclophosphamide. With the much more cautious use of that medication in the variety of studies which have looked at the dose response type relationship with regard to inducing a remission in the nephrotic syndrome, it has become clear that the gonadal toxicity is also a dose response phenomenon. It is the relationship to the total dose to which the patient has been exposed as well as the period of time that the patient has been off of the Cyclophosphamide for the return of sperm counts or cycling ovulatory periods for the female. The only good evidence that I am aware of which addresses this in some detail is by the group in Toronto. They started using massive doses of Cyclophosphamide for very long periods of time. The only patients that they have reported with permanent oligo- or anespheremia are those who were exposed to huge doses. So that issue, assuming that these children do not require second and third courses, is not now a long term major complication of Cyclophosphamide. This would apply to patients who can be off of the drug for five years or more before they need to be fertile.

COMMENT: Let me make a similar comment regarding chlorambucil. The permanent azoospermia occurs above 25 mg/kg and most of the protocols are talking about 10, 11, 12 mg/kg. So we are well within a good range.

I would like to share an anecdote with you. There was a young gentleman who came to me at about age 25-26 because he had been previously treated with Cyclophosphamide (not by me but by someone else) and had been found to be sterile. He had just married a woman who had four or five children so that he would have a family. He just decided he would drop by and check with me, since I had replaced my predecessor at that point. He seemed to be perfectly healthy to me. I asked him if they were using any kind of contraception and he said, "Oh, no", because this doctor had told him that he was sterile. I said that I thought it might not be a bad idea for him to have a sperm count. He got a sperm count which had this stupendously high count; we repeated it to be absolutely sure. I informed him that in fact he was not sterile, that he was quite okay, at which point he paled a bit and said, "Doc, I am glad that you told me that, now that I am married". That was the best line I had ever had prior to that.

MODERATOR: Any further comments or questions on treatment?

QUESTION: I was a fellow at a New York institution where we used nitrogen mustard basically in children whom we felt were going to be totally non-compliant to a long term or to an eight to ten weeks course of Cyclophosphamide (the only alternative treatment at that time). One of the basic reasons for using nitrogen mustard was that it was given in three or four days to a child who was relatively incarcerated in the hospital so we were sure that the child would get the drug. The major drug that we would go to would be Cyclophosphamide if we got a compliant child.

QUESTION: I have a question relative to treatment. Mesangioproliferative nephrotic syndrome is something of an orphan and may or may not exist as an independent and distinct diagnostic entity. I would like to ask the members of the panel how they would clinically manage a child who is nephrotic, steroid resistant, and who has histological features which clearly show mesangial proliferation but no focal sclerosis or hyalinosis. Should that child be considered for cytotoxic therapy with Chlorambucil or Cyclophosphamide?

RESPONSE: I can give a one word answer: yes. We would treat the child, not because there is a controlled trial but because in our own experience with the group of patients I described to you with relapsing nephrotic syndrome, children with that lesion have responded to that treatment. The fact that the patient you are describing is corticosteroid resistant, does not necessarily make certain that he would not respond to treatment with Cyclophosphamide. Corticosteroid resistant patients with Minimal Change Disease do frequently have a remission of their nephrotic syndrome in association with treatment with Chlorambucil or Cyclophosphamide. So, using that analogy, I would treat the child.

MODERATOR: What about membranous GN? Are we settled on what to do in those patients? Would you like to go back to membranoproliferative?

COMMENT: In terms of mesangioproliferative steroid resistant, we have seen eight children like this in the last ten years and in each of those we were able to induce a prolonged remission using either Chlorambucil or Cyclophosphamide. What that means I am not sure, but that is our experience.

COMMENT: We have had somewhat the same experience in seeing children respond. What disturbs me about that is that in some of the reported series in which people have not been treated, a good number of them lost their proteinuria by the end of the first year, whether they were treated or not. So I am not always certain--even though we have seen responses with both steroids and/or cytotoxic agents--that in fact the treatment has made any difference in the course of the child's disease.

MODERATOR: We are beginning to run out of time but what about membranous GN in pediatrics? Do you treat membranous nephropathy?

COMMENT: I would like to make a delightful comment about that because I agreed so much with what was said today. As the speaker was talking, I turned to my colleague next to me and said "How many kids with primary membranous GN have you really seen (those in which you were certain it was primary)?" And the answer was "two". We now have some 430 nephrotics whom we are following or have followed. We have only one. I think that primary membranous disease in children has come to be a rarity. Unfortunately, with our one, she did not do too well with anything.

MODERATOR: We have had a number of patients here in Miami throughout the years, about 10-12, and we have not treated any of them. Two were transplanted, another one did perfectly well and has been completely asymptomatic for the past five years of so, the others have been in between. Now we have another one who has a positive Australia antigen, is hypertensive and is coming to dialysis. It is such an heterogeneous group that it is hard to predict a given patient's outcome. At one of the past Seminars, Renee Habib was saying that to assess the impact of treatment of these patients is very hard because they are not a uniform population. What one may think one is doing in an uncontrolled population or in a non-blind study, may not be valid, maybe it was a spontaneous (natural) evolution of the disorder. But taking the position of the adult nephrologists, that you should treat those patients, it has come up for discussion even within our group.

COMMENT: The problem I find with membranous is the same problem that was brought out relative to mesangial proliferation and focal and segmental glomerulosclerosis. We have gotten caught with the idea that a morphologic entity is a single disease, and in none of these is it really true.

MODERATOR: Yes, that is so important. We need to clarify how we define an entity and what we understand by a histological finding. That is a very important point: we need to separate the histological picture from the clinical and etiopathogenic ones.

QUESTION-COMMENT: I would like to make a comment and to know the opinion of the Panel. This is in regard to a subject touched upon during one of the presentations today. It was mentioned that vitamin D preparations may need to be used in patients with nephrotic syndrome. Since patients with this syndrome present with a variety of immunological abnormalities, mainly an abnormal blastogenesis, it has been speculated that different mechanisms, like spleen hypofunction or a serum factor, could be responsible. Recent reports have indicated that 1,25 dihydroxy vitamin D is a potent immunosuppressor. One of those reports show that this metabolite of vitamin D causes an important immune suppression and markedly decreases the production of antibodies in vitro. I would like to know if the risk of bone disease outweighs the risk of infection in a patient who is already immunosuppressed because of his primary disease and the use of steroids.

RESPONSE: That is a very good question and it is a very pertinent aspect to deal with when we are faced with a patient who has established bone disease. It is too early in the game to answer that question in a precise manner. There is a recent explosion of literature on the link between vitamin D and the lymphoproliferative and the hematopoietic system. As you pointed out, is bone disease more important than immunosuppression? If we are able to improve bone disease, could we achieve better growth in patients with relapsing nephrotic syndrome? It makes sense but the data are not in yet. We have to look very carefully, and then weigh the risks versus benefits. It is my gut feeling that probably the risks of overwhelming infection in a nephrotic patient following the administration of vitamin D are probably not high, and in a very controlled fashion, that could be a very well-designed study. I would be willing to explore the wisdom of giving vitamin D to a selected group of patients.

RESPONSE: There are two major points that have to be distinguished here. The classical observations in man and in experimental animals are that the primary role of vitamin D is as a modulator of calcium and phosphorus blood level and bone mineralization. This goes back to the discovery of rickets in the mid 16th century onward. A more recent discovery is the in vitro phenomenon that 1,25 dihydroxy vitamin D (not other D metabolites), can serve to modulate the function of a variety of cell lines of lymphocytes, t cells, etc. grown in tissue culture for many generations. This is an in vitro phenomenon; it is not an in vivo phenomenon. These are fascinating observations. The fact that 1,25 DHT can influence certain oncogens of established tumor cell lines, is an absolutely fascinating observation. But thus far there has never been a patient with a malignancy who has been cured by giving 1,25 DHT in any dosage. Certain aspects relating to certain of these tumor cell lines, in terms of the effect of 1,25 DHT, do not have a parallel in vivo. So, I do not think that we should hesitate, if we have a patient with clearly established bone disease, to treat him with D metabolites. The one final thing I would say is that we did try to look at this and we were not able to do so in a fashion that I felt warranted publication. We did take a group of six or seven nephrotics who had a reduction in 1,25 DHT which I felt was in relationship to prolonged use of corticosteroids. We treated them with conventional doses of 1,25 DHT, and in some of them we saw an increase in bone mineral content; in others we saw no change, and in two patients we saw a decline. So, we really saw a mixed pattern; therefore, we did not publish those observations. I am telling this to you now; I have never mentioned it to anybody. I think that if you have clear cut evidence of bone disease, you should go ahead and treat it effectively, because you are dealing with an in vivo phenomenon with vitamin D which has been known for several centuries versus an in vitro phenomenon which has never been shown really to have clinical relevance.

MODERATOR: I have enjoyed tremendously this session and its discussion. Thanks very much to a very effective Panel and an excellent audience.

II

THE KIDNEY IN SYSTEMIC DISEASES

RENAL INVOLVEMENT IN VASCULITIC SYNDROMES IN CHILDREN

Norman J. Siegel, M.D. and Karen M. Gaudio, M.D.

The nomenclature and classification of the vasculitic syndromes are bewildering. The term, vasculitis, is used to describe a wide variety of clinical disorders of diverse presentations and differing etiology (Figure 1). The common denominator for each of these entities is inflammation and necrosis of blood vessels. Although the kidney may be involved in disorders of larger blood vessels, such as polyarteritis, renal involvement is much more of a clinical component in small vessel vasculitis. In these disorders, inflammation and necrosis affects primarily glomerular capillaries and renal biopsy specimens will demonstrate a focal necrotizing glomerulonephritis (1). Necrosis of the glomerular capillary wall results in exudation into Bowman's space and stimulates crescent formation. Within the same biopsy specimen, lesions of differing age and severity are characteristic as is some interstitial inflammation. This interstitial infiltration consists of eosinophils, plasma cells and lymphocytes. The lesions which are seen on light microscopy are non-specific and occur in a number of different syndromes (1).

The three clinical disorders in children in which a focal necrotizing glomerulonephritis plays an important role are Systemic Lupus Erythematosus, Henoch-Schonlein Purpura and Wegener's Granulomatosis. Although the renal lesion on light microscopy may be quite similar in each of these entitites, findings on immunofluorescent and electron microscopy may differentiate between them (Figure 2). However, some caution must be exercised since the characteristic features may not be present on renal biopsy specimens in many cases. Thus, we do not recommend renal biopsy for the purpose of documenting a specific vasculitic syndrome. Rather, evaluation of renal tissue should be used to determine the extent and severity of renal involvement.

Clinical disorders with a focal necrotizing glomerulonephritis often have cutaneous involvement. Characteristically, these skin lesions have arterioles and venules with breakdown of nuclei which produces karyorrhectic fragments. Thus, the leukocytoclastic angiitis of the skin represents the same pathologic process as the focal necrotizing glomerulonephritis in the kidney (1).

In this chapter, we will discuss three vasculitic syndromes, Systemic Lupus Erythematosus (SLE), Henoch-Schonlein Purpura (HSP) and Wegener's Granulomatosis, with special emphasis on diagnostic criteria. For the clinician who may see children with one of these disorders, the diagnosis at initial presentation may be obscure. This occurs, not because of a lack of recognition of the disorder,

FIGURE 1

VASCULITIC SYNDROMES

INFLAMMATION AND NECROSIS OF BLOOD VESSELS

Systemic Lupus Erythematosus

Schonlein-Henoch Syndrome

Wegener's Granulomatosis

Hypersensitivity Angiitis

Giant Cell Arteritis

Takayasu Arteritis

Infantile Polyarteritis

Polyarteritis

Mucocutaneous Lymph Node Syndrome

Rheumatoid Arthritis

Rheumatic Fever

Mixed Connective Tissue Disease

Dermatomysitis

but because the cardinal clinical manifestations do not present simultaneously or in a consistent pattern and may occur over several months. Thus, when such patients are referred to a consultant, the constellation of clinical findings necessary to establish a diagnosis may be evident.

SYSTEMIC LUPUS ERYTHEMATOSUS

Systemic Lupus Erythematosus is a well described clinical disorder which affects predominantly young women (2). The initial manifestations are quite varied and include: fever, fatigue, skin rash, photosensitivity and arthritis. The classical butterfly rash occurs on the malar eminence and includes areas of atrophic skin with telangiectasia which will help differentiate this lesion from a malar flush. The American Rheumatism Association has established diagnostic criteria which are helpful in differentiating SLE from other rheumatic diseases such as rheumatoid arthritis, juvenile rheumatoid arthritis, Reiter's syndrome and ankylosing spondylitis (3). Since these criteria were generated from adult patients in rheumatology clinics, strict adherence to the ARA criteria in young patients presenting with renal disease may be misleading. Several studies have shown that renal disease may be the initial manifestation of SLE. Also, renal disease may precede the onset of clinical SLE in other cases. Evidence of renal disease as an initial manifestation of SLE was present in 3.1% of 520 cases reported by Dubois (4), 5% of the 138 cases reviewed by Harvey and coworkers (5), 2.9% of 275 cases reported by Haserick (6), and 6% of 200 cases surveyed by Larson (7). Reports by Libit and associates (8) and Kallen et al. (9) have focused attention on the subsequent development of SLE in young patients who presented with nephrotic syndrome secondary to a membranous nephropathy.

SLE is the only vasculitic syndrome for which specific laboratory confirmation of the diagnosis is possible. In 1948 Hargraves and coworkers (10) described the LE cell test. Subsequently this serum factor was identified as an immunoglobulin directed against DNA histone and desoxyribonucleoprotein. Although a positive LE cell test was initially considered specific for SLE, a number of other conditions - including cirrhosis, scleroderma, polyarteritis, and polymyositis - have been reported to have a positive LE cell preparation.

The presence in serum of a nonspecific antinuclear factor (ANF) is quite sensitive but not specific for any one antinuclear antibody. Accordingly, the ANF is used as a screening test. A peripheral pattern of immunofluorescence, however, appears to be more specific for SLE and correlates reasonably well with the degree of clinical activity (11). Koller and associates (12) observed an interesting incongruity in 20 patients who had a positive LE cell preparation, but an ANF could not be demonstrated in their sera by standard immunofluorescent techniques. These patients all had multisystem disease, and in several patients the ANF was seen after special treatment of their sera.

Antibodies directed against double stranded DNA are considered specific for the diagnosis of SLE. The most commonly used method for the assessment of anti-DNA antibodies is based on the ammonium

FIGURE 2

FOCAL NECROTIZING GLOMERULONEPHRITIS

	IMMUNOFLUORESCENCE	ELECTRON MICROSCOPY
SLE	CAPILLARY LOOP AND MESANGIAL IgG, M, A & Cl, C3	SUBEPITHELIAL, MESANGIAL, SUBENDOTHELIAL DEPOSITS
HSP	MESANGIAL IgG, IgA	MESANGIAL, OCCASIONAL SUBENDOTHELIAL DEPOSITS
WEGENER'S GRANULOMATOSIS	MESANGIAL AND CAPILLARY LOOP IgG, M, C3	OCCASIONAL DEPOSITS

sulfate techniques described by Farr (13). In this method a mixture of serum and radioactive DNA is rendered half-saturated in ammonium sulfate, and radioactivity is detected in the precipitate only if DNA is bound to antibody. Using this technique, high titers of anti-DNA antibodies have been found to be highly specific for SLE (14), to correlate well with clinically active renal disease (4,15,16), and to provide a sensitive diagnostic aid in the evaluation of suspected cases of SLE. Adler et al. (17) showed that sera from patients with active and untreated SLE exhibited DNA binding capacity (DNA-bc) greater than 20% in 19 of 21 samples, while DNA-bc values of less than 20% and usually less than 10% were obtained with sera from 100 normal controls, 21 patients with rheumatoid arthritis, and 19 patients with cases of rheumatoid variants. In addition to providing an important adjunct in the diagnosis of SLE, serial determination of DNA-bc in patients with lupus nephritis have also provided a good index of response to therapy, and the pattern of DNA-bc has been of prognostic significance (17,18). In some instances, changes in DNA-bc have preceded clinical exacerbation of disease activity by three to six months.

In addition to these antibody tests, the serum complement profile in patients with active SLE usually shows evidence of classical pathway activation. Clinically, this is manifest as a low CH_{50}, low C_3 and low C_4 complement protein levels. To a certain extent, these values may be helpful as an index of disease activity (18).

The incidence of renal involvement in SLE varies with the criteria used to define "renal involvement". Using standard clinical criteria such as decreased renal function or the presence of proteinuria or cells and casts in urinary sediment, the reported incidence varies from 40% to 75% of cases (4,19-21). On the average, approximately 50% of patients with SLE have or will develop renal involvement. Using histopathologic criteria, however, the incidence of renal disease appears to be much greater and may approach 90% when immunofluorescent and electron microscopic techniques are employed (22-24). Houghton (25) evaluted 19 patients in whom clinical signs of renal disease were absent, histopathologic alterations were noted in 16 patients. Of these 16 cases, 9 showed moderately severe proliferative changes by light microscopy and subendothelial deposits on ultrastructural examination. Mahajan and associates (26) have reported that of 27 patients without clinical evidence of renal involvement at the time of initial evaluation, 3 had minimal glomerular involvement, 12 had focal proliferative changes, and 12 had a diffuse proliferative glomerulonephritis. Hecht reported an analysis of 31 cases of renal disease in which a proliferative lesion was revealed by light microscopy and subendothelial deposits were discovered by electron microscopy, 5 did not have proteinuria when first examined and 3 of these had a normal urinary sediment (18). These observations suggest that not only is the incidence of renal involvement in SLE underestimated when standard clinical criteria are used but that clinical features alone are not sufficient to predict the type or severity of renal histopathologic alterations.

HENOCH SCHONLEIN PURPURA

Henoch Schonlein Syndrome is well known to most pediatricians. Despite recognition of the clinical manifestation of HSP as early as 1782, its etiology and pathogenesis remain unclear (27). Schonlein first described children with joint pain and purpura while Henoch recognized the other typical features of the syndrome: abdominal colic, bloody diarrhea and nephritis. This syndrome - abdominal pain, bloody diarrhea, arthritis/arthralgia, purpura and renal disease - has also been termed anaphylactoid purpura.

The diagnosis of HSP must rest solely on the clinical manifestations since laboratory confirmation is non-specific and mostly useful to exclude other possibilities. Skin lesions are described in almost all patients and demonstrate a leukocytoclastic angiitis on biopsy. The purpura in this syndrome which are associated with a normal platelet count, usually occur predominantly on the lower extremities and buttocks but may not be present at initial presentation (28). Serologic tests for SLE are negative and serum complement levels are normal or elevated. Since IgA is characteristically deposited in the skin and glomeruli of patients with HSP, the finding of elevated serum levels of IgA in 10 of 20 patients reported by Trygstad and Stiehm (29) was of interest. Unfortunately, elevated serum IgA levels have been observed in a variety of other conditions as well (27).

Renal involvement in children with HSP is usually present but of highly variable severity (30). It has been estimated that 50-100% of children will demonstrate microscopic hematuria sometime in the course of their disease. Twenty percent of patients may present as an acute nephritis while 10% will manifest nephrotic syndrome and a small proportion will follow a rapidly progressive clinical course. Similarly, the spectrum of histopathologic involvement varies from mild focal lesions to a severe necrotizing and crescentic lesion (30,31). Meadow has demonstrated a fairly good correlation between the severity of clinical presentation and morphologic appearance (31). In his group of 88 patients, children with only microscopic hematuria had no more than focal lesions while patients with diffuse crescent formation invariably had nephrotic syndrome. Thus, in HSP there is a good correlation between the clinical manifestation of renal disease and the underlying histopathologic changes.

WEGENER'S GRANULOMATOSIS

In 1936 Wegener described a multisystem disease characterized by widespread necrotizing and granulomatosis vasculitis (32). This is a relatively uncommon disorder that has been reported infrequently in children (33-34). The diagnosis of this syndrome rests on the clinical documentation of 1) necrotizing granuloma of the upper and lower respiratory tract, 2) generalized focal necrotizing vasculitis of arteries and veins, and 3) a glomerulonephritis with focal necrosis (35). The diagnosis is secured by demonstrating the presence of necrotizing granuloma which consists of perivascular infiltrates accompanied by giant cells with a histiocytic reaction. These lesions may appear in the nasopharyngeal mucosa, pulmonary tissue or kidney. Since granuloma are necessary to document this condition, percutaneous renal biopsy specimens may be too limited in terms of tissue sample and biopsy specimens of other tissues may have a higher yield of establishing a definitive diagnosis (36).

The upper respiratory tract symptoms associated with this disease include persistent rhinorrhea, recurrent epistaxis, nasal obstruction, chronic sinusitis, tracheobronchial or nasopharyngeal ulcers, nasal deformities, serous otitis, recurrent laryngitis, and shortness of breath (34). Lower respiratory findings include chronic cough, hemoptysis, migratory pulmonary infiltrates and pulmonary cavitation. The persistence of these symptoms, particularly in an adolescent patient, and associated evidence of renal disease such as microscopic hematuria or minimal proteinuria should suggest the possibility of this diagnosis. Although early reports indicated that this disease was nearly uniformly fatal, more recent evidence suggests that early treatment with cyclophosphamide may have a dramatic effect in both children (33,34) and adults (37). Consequently, a high index of suspicion and concomitant early diagnosis are of importance to maximize the prognosis for these patients.

REFERENCES

1. Spargo, B., Seymour, A.E. and Ordonez, N.G.: Renal biopsy pathology with diagnostic and therapeutic implications: Chapter 12, VASCULITIS, John Wiley and Sons, New York, 1980.
2. Siegel, N.J. and Hayslett, J.P.: Renal involvement in systemic lupus erythematosus. In: The Kidney in Systemic Disease, Second Edition, Suki, W.N. and Eknoyan, G. (eds), John Wiley and Sons, New York, p. 55, 1981.
3. Cohen, A.S., Reynolds, W.E., Franklin, E.C., et al: Preliminary criteria for the classification of systemic lupus erythematosus. Bull Rheum. Dis., 21:643, 1971.
4. Dubois, E.L.: Lupus Erythematosus, Second Edition, McGraw-Hill, New York, 1974.
5. Harvey, A.M., Shulman, L.E., Tumulty, A., et al: Systemic lupus erythematosus: Review of the literature and clinical analysis of 138 cases. Medicine, 33:291, 1954.
6. Haserick, J.R.: Unpublished data.
7. Larson, D.L.: Systemic Lupus Erythematosus. Little Brown & Co., Boston, 1961.
8. Libit, S.A., Burke, B., Michael, A.F., et al: Extramembranous glomerulonephritis in childhood: Relationship to systemic lupus erythematosus. J. Pediatr., 88:394, 1976.
9. Kallen, R.J., Soo-Kwang, L., Arsonson, A.J., et al: Idiopathic membranous glomerulopathy preceding the emergence of systemic lupus erythematosus in two children. J. Pediatr., 90:72, 1977.
10. Hargraves, M.M., Richmond, H. and Morton, R.: Presentation of two bone marrow elements: The "tart" cell and "L.E." cell. Proc. Staff Mayo Clin., 23:25, 1948.
11. Gonzales, E.N. and Rothfield, N.F.: Immunoglobulin class and pattern of nuclear fluorescence in systemic lupus erythematosus. N. Engl. J. Med., 274:133, 1966.

12. Koller, S.R., Johnston, C.L., Moncure, C.W., et al: Lupus erythematosus cell preparation: Antinuclear factor incongruity. Am. J. Clin. Pathol., 66:495, 1976.
13. Farr, R.S.: A quantitative immunochemical measure of the primary interaction between I BSA and antibody. J. Infect. Dis., 103:239, 1958.
14. Hughes, G.R.: Significance of anti-DNA antibodies in systemic lupus erythematosus. Lancet, 2:861, 1971.
15. Casals, S.P., Friou, G.P. and Myers, L.L.: Significance of antibody to DNA systemic lupus erythematosus. Arthritis Rheum., 7:379, 1964.
16. Tan, E.M., Schur, P.H., Carr, R.I., et al: Deoxyribonucleic acid (DNA) and antibodies to DNA in serum patients with systemic lupus erythematosus. J. Clin. Invest., 45:1732, 1966.
17. Adler, M.K., Baumgarten, A., Hecht, B., et al: Prognostic significance of DNA-binding capacity patients with lupus nephritis. Ann. Rheum. Dis., 35:444, 1975.
18. Hecht, B., Siegel, N.J., Adler, M., et al: Prognostic indices in lupus nephritis. Medicine, 55:163, 1976.
19. Dubois, E.L. and Tuffanelli, D.L.: Clinical manifestations of systemic lupus erythematosus: Computer analysis of 520 cases. JAMA, 190:104, 1964.
20. Rothfield, N.F., McClusky, R.T. and Baldwin, D.S.: Renal disease in systemic lupus erythematosus. N. Engl. J. Med., 269:537, 1963.
21. Meislin, A.G. and Rothfield, N.: Systemic lupus erythematosus in childhood. Pediatrics, 42:37, 1968.
22. Koffler, D., Agnello, V., Carr, I., et al: Variable patterns of immunoglobulin and complement deposition in the kidneys of patients with systemic lupus erythematosus. Am. J. Pathol., 56:305, 1969.
23. Dujovne, I., Pollak, V.E., Pirani, C.L., et al: The distribution and character of glomerular deposits in systemic lupus erythematosus. Kidney Inter., 2:33, 1972.
24. Dillard, M.G., Tillman, R.L. and Sampson, C.C.: Lupus nephritis: Correlations between clinical course and presence of electron-dense deposits. Lab. Invest., 32:261, 1975.
25. Houghton, D., Bennett, W., Bardana, E., et al: Silent renal involvement in systemic lupus erythematosus. Kidney Inter., 8:499, 1975.
26. Mahajan, S.K., Ordonez, N.G., Feitelson, P.J., et al: Diffuse lupus glomerulonephritis without clinical renal involvement, abstracted, Am. Soc. Nephrology, 9th Annual Meeting, Nov. 1976, p. 17.
27. Crumb, C.: Renal involvement in Schonlein-Henoch Syndrome: In: The Kidney in Systemic Disease, Suki, W.N. and Eknoyan, G. (eds), John Wiley and Sons, New York, p. 99, 1981.
28. Gairdner, D.: The Schonlein-Henoch syndrome (anaphylactoid purpura). Q. J. Med., 17:95, 1948.
29. Trygstad, C.W., Stiehm, E.R.: Elevated serum IgA globulin in anaphylactoid purpura. Pediatrics, 47:1023, 1971.
30. Meadow, S.R., Glasgow, E.R., White, R.H.R., et al: Schonlein-Henoch nephritis. Q. J. Med., 163:241, 1972.

31. Meadow, S.R., Glasgow, E.F., White, R.H.R., et al: Schonlein-Henoch nephritis. In: Glomerulonephritis, Kincaid-Smith, P., Matthew, T.H., Becker, E.L. (eds), John Wiley & Sons, New York, vol. 2, p. 1089, 1973.
32. Wegener, F.: Uber generalisierte, septische Gefasserkrankunjen Vesh. Dtsch Ges. Pathology, 29:202, 1936.
33. Baliga, R., et al: Wegener's granulomatosis in childhood. Pediatrics 61:286, 1978.
34. Moorthy, A.V., Chesney, R.W., Segar, W.E. and Groshong, T.: Wegener granulomatosis in childhood: Prolonged survival following cytotoxic therapy. J. Pediatr., 91:616, 1977.
35. Fahey, J., Leonard, E., Churg, J. and Godman, G.C.: Wegener's granulomatosis. Am. J. Med., 17:168, 1954.
36. Appel, G.B., Gee, B., Kashgarian, M. and Hayslett, J.P.: Wegener's granulomatosis: Clinical-pathological correlations and long-term course. Am. J. Kidney Dis., 1:27, 1981.
37. Fauci, A.S., Haynes, B.F., Katz, P. and Wolff, S.M.: Wegener's granulomatosis: Prospective clinical and therapeutic experience with 85 patients for 21 years. Ann. Internal Med., 98:76, 1983.

THE KIDNEY IN SICKLE CELL DISEASE

Jose Strauss, M.D., Carolyn Abitbol, M.D., Gaston Zilleruelo, M.D. and Michael Freundlich, M.D.

Sickle cell disease (SCD) and trait (SCT) are acknowledged as existing in North America and Africa but often overlooked is the fact that they also are found in Central America and northern South America, primarily in those areas into which blacks were brought from Africa. Hemoglobin A is the normal hemoglobin which has a glutamic acid in position 6, while hemoglobin S is the characteristic hemoglobin of sickle cell disease and has a valine in position 6 (1). In an SCD or SCT patient in crisis, hemoglobin gels and leads to the formation of the classically sickled shape red blood cell (RBC); when hemoglobin S remains in its gel status, the RBC's become irreversibly (or permanently) sickled (2).

We shall review here some of the histological, functional, clinical, etiopathogenic, and therapeutic/prophylactic characteristics of the nephropathy associated with SCD and SCT. The classical anatomic and histological changes in SCD have consisted of glomerular hypertrophy (Fig. 1) (3), medullary congestion, cortical infarctions (Fig. 2) (3), papillary necrosis (Fig. 3) (3), renal vein and artery thrombosis, and tubulo-interstitial nephropathy. The glomerular hypertrophy was accurately described by Bernstein (4). Medullary congestion was documented by Bukalew (5); it has stasis in the Vasa Rectae which can be severe enough to lead to papillary necrosis with profuse hematuria. The latter more often originates in the left than in the right kidney, and may be more frequent in SCT than in SCD; various series report conflicting statistics (6, 7). Patients with SCD tend to have interstitial deposits of iron which may play a pathogenetic role in functional or morphological changes.

Histological changes in SCD or SCT patients in Miami have consisted exclusively of membranoproliferative glomerulonephritis (MPGN) type I, with its characteristic double contour best seen on silver stain and electron microscopy (8). This is almost the only type of patient in whom we diagnose MPGN; i.e., 9 of 10 patients in which the diagnosis of MPGN is made, will have SCD or SCT. Other centers have also found focal-segmental sclerosis (FSS) (9), membranous glomerulonephritis (MGN), etc., associated with HbS.

This study was funded in part under an agreement with the Department of Health and Rehabilitative Services, State of Florida Children's Medical Services.

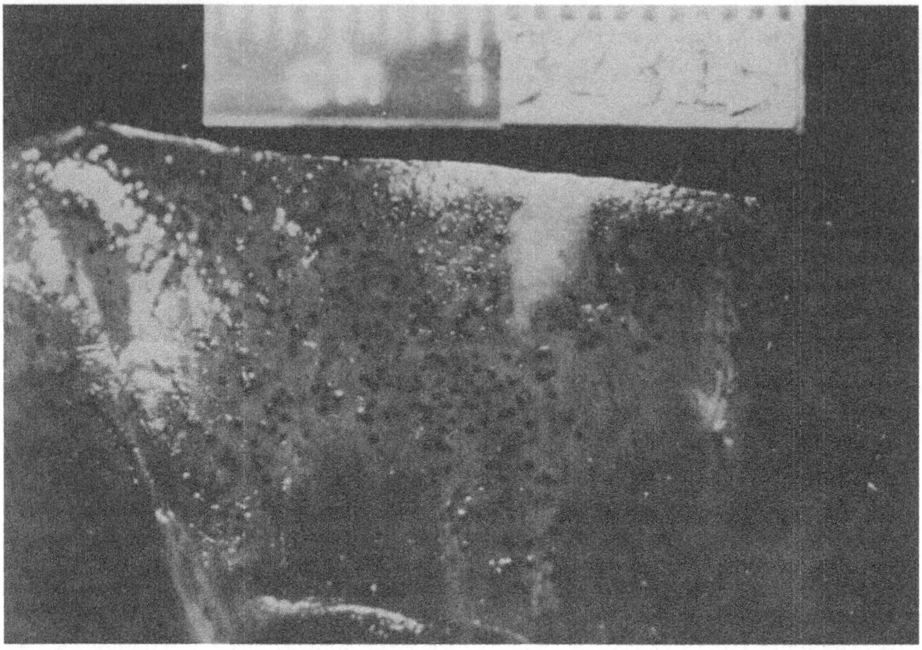

Figure 1. Glomerular hypertrophy. From Heptinstall, R.H.: Pathology of the Kidney, Second Edition. Boston: Little, Brown and Company, 1983, p. 1674, with permission.

We also have found in SCD patients glomeruli with immunofluorescence positive for IgG; when the eluate of the kidney of one of those patients was put in contact with normal kidney, proximal tubule epithelium was stained, with preferential staining of the brush border, suggesting that the brush border is the source of what other people and we have called renal tubular epithelial antigen (RTE antigen). The findings may be summarized as follows: 1) RTE antigen was localized on the renal glomerulus in association with immunoglobulins and complement components; 2) diluted antibody fixed to renal tubules but not to glomeruli; 3) fixation of diluted antibody to renal tubules was abolished by absorption with RTE antigen prior to exposure of the normal kidney; (4) blocking studies supported the presence of RTE antibody in the glomeruli; (5) circulating antigen-antibody complexes (RTE - anti RTE, IgG - anti IgG) were identified in the serum cryoprecipitate. We concluded that these findings suggest an autologous immune-complex pathogenesis with hypoxic/ischemic tubular damage release of the RTE antigen, and autosensitization (10).

The sequence of events which we proposed has been put into a schematic form by Thompson et al. (11) which states that there are hypoxia, high osmolality and acid pH in the renal medulla under normal conditions. When a sickle cell crisis develops, these conditions worsen and lead to sickling in the renal medulla with stasis, severe hypoxia and ischemia, renal tubular damage, release of RTE antigen into the circulation with antibody formation, circulating immune-complexes, deposition in the glomeruli with complement fixation which leads to a glomerulonephritis, and in most of these patients, to a nephrotic syndrome.

Very likely there are other situations involving HbS in which there is not an immunological mechanism. That may be the case of the hyperperfusion/hyperfiltration hypothesis which has been proposed as a cause of progression of renal disease in general and has been presented recently as a possible mechanism in SCD patients (12).

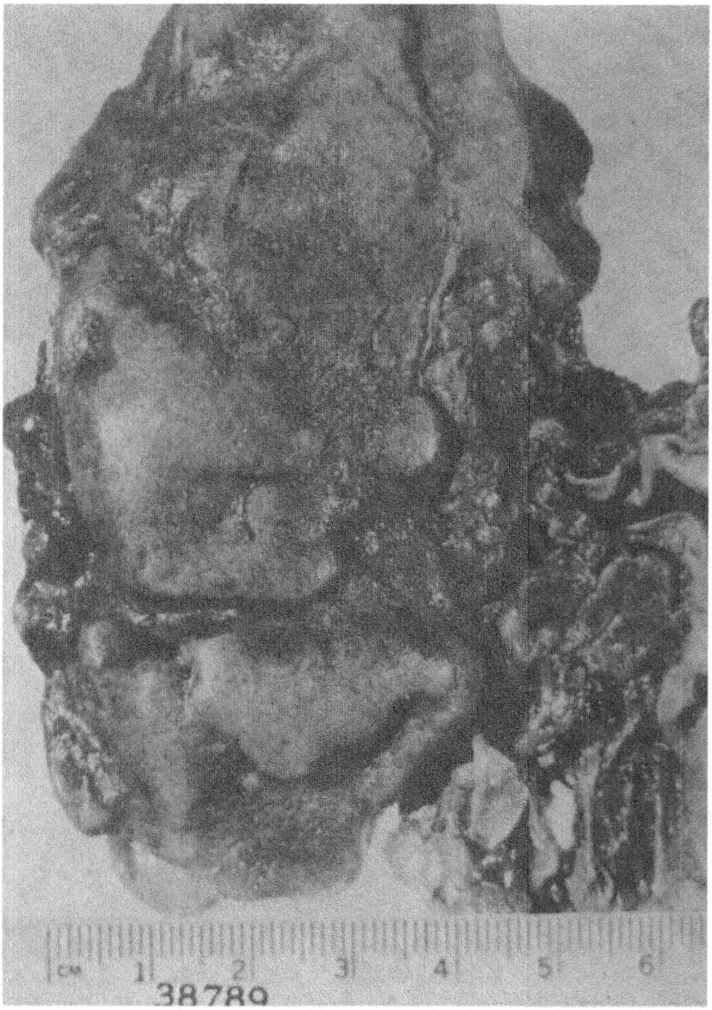

Figure 2. Cortical infarctions. From Heptinstall, R.H.: Pathology of the Kidney, Second Edition. Boston: Little, Brown and Company, 1983, p.1676, with permission.

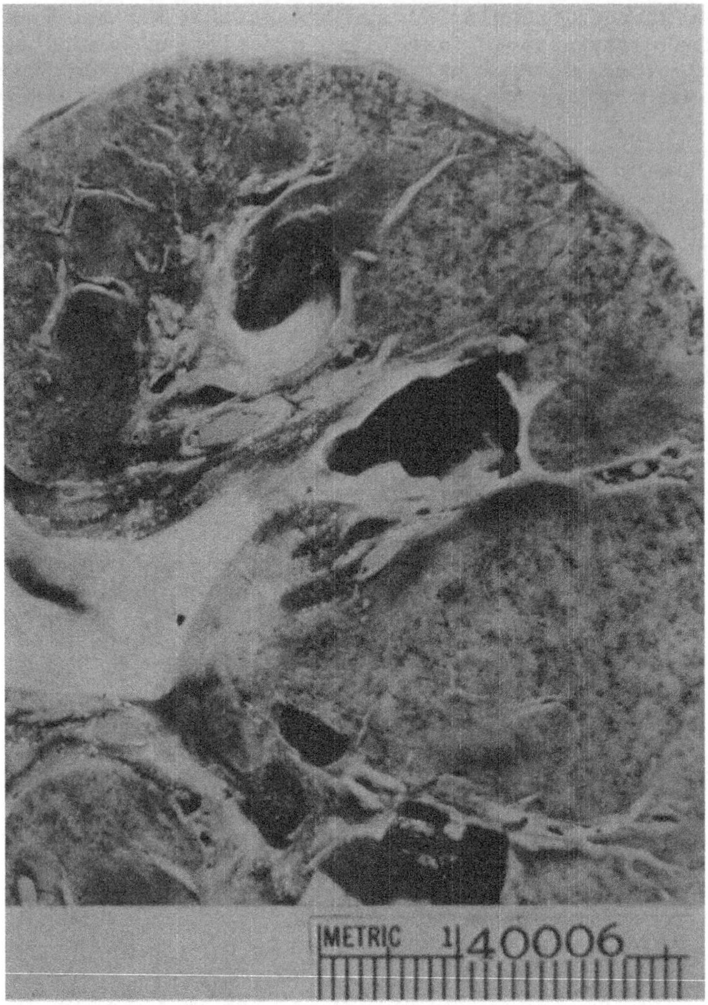

Figure 3. Papillary necrosis. From Heptinstall, R.H.: Pathology of the Kidney, Second Edition. Boston: Little, Brown and Company, 1983, p. 1675, with permission.

Functional Changes

Here, we shall assess functional changes without entering in details which we (7) and de Jong (13) already have extensively reviewed. Characteristically, there is an increase in renal blood flow, an increase in glomerular filtration rate (GFR), and a decrease in urinary concentrating ability. Probably, urinary dilution is normal but the status of tubular permeability and ADH response by the tubules is still controversial. Some people believe that there is a good response to vasopressin, but others cannot elicit that response; this needs to be clarified because a form of therapy has been recommended for SCD patients on the basis of this response being present (14). Hydrogen ion production has been extensively studied in our Medical Center by Dr. C. Vaamonde and his group. It seems that in SCD there is a decreased production of hydrogen ions under most conditions and with most stimuli; conversely, in SCT, that response is normal (15). Tubular excretion of uric acid clearly seems to be increased; this increase is probably related to increased intravascular and total body water (16).

The renal handling of sodium and potassium has been traditionally regarded as normal but now questions have been raised. Some investigators have shown rather convincingly that there is a decreased potassium excretion, with a fractional excretion of potassium (FEK^+) which is lower in SCD patients than in controls at comparable GFR levels (17). The increase in urine sodium excretion and decrease in serum sodium during a crisis have been postulated to be consistent with inappropriate secretion of ADH (SIADH) (18). Tubular reabsorption of phosphorus seems to be increased, although there are still some questions (7).

At the clinical level, arterial blood pressure (BP) seems to have been only recently studied in adults; the findings reflect lower systolic and diastolic BP's in these patients (Fig. 4) (19). It has been suggested that the BP changes are prostaglandin related, and that there may be vasodilatation which lowers BP in the presence of an increased intravascular volume (13, 19, 20).

At a more basic etiopathogenic level, the Adherence Ratio of the sickle cells to the vascular endothelium correlates well with a Clinical Severity Score (21), suggesting that the vessels actively contribute to the crisis. Photographs have shown even the entrapment of sickled RBC's by cells of the vascular endothelium (22).

Treatment

Handling of sodium is at the center of some therapeutic maneuvers which have been suggested. Some believe that SCD patients have problems maintaining normonatremia because of excessive sodium losses in the urine (23). Others think that sodium excretion needs to be enhanced in order to induce hyponatremia which in turn would expand the sickled RBC's and shift the hemoglobin oxygen dissociation curve (HODC) to the left (14). Presumably, the curve's shift is desirable in order to increase O_2 affinity by hemoglobin, which then ensures a greater O_2 transport to the tissues. Even though it was reported that fewer crises and better hemoglobin oxygenation ensue, others have failed to duplicate those results and some have even reported serious side effects (24), probably because of decreased O_2 release to the tissues (7).

The attempts at increasing hemoglobin affinity for O_2 may be based on the finding that patients with hemoglobinopathies of higher O_2 affinity have higher serum erythropoietin and blood hematocrit levels than patients with a lower O_2 affinity hemoglobin like hemoglobin S. However, blood level of hemoglobin may be too rough an assessment since SCD patients who are anemic also have a high reticulocyte count and a high rate of hemolysis. It may be that the right shifted hemoglobin S could be improved or corrected by a further shift to the right and by protecting RBC's flow and membrane, preventing gelation, and minimizing the vascular component of a crisis (25).

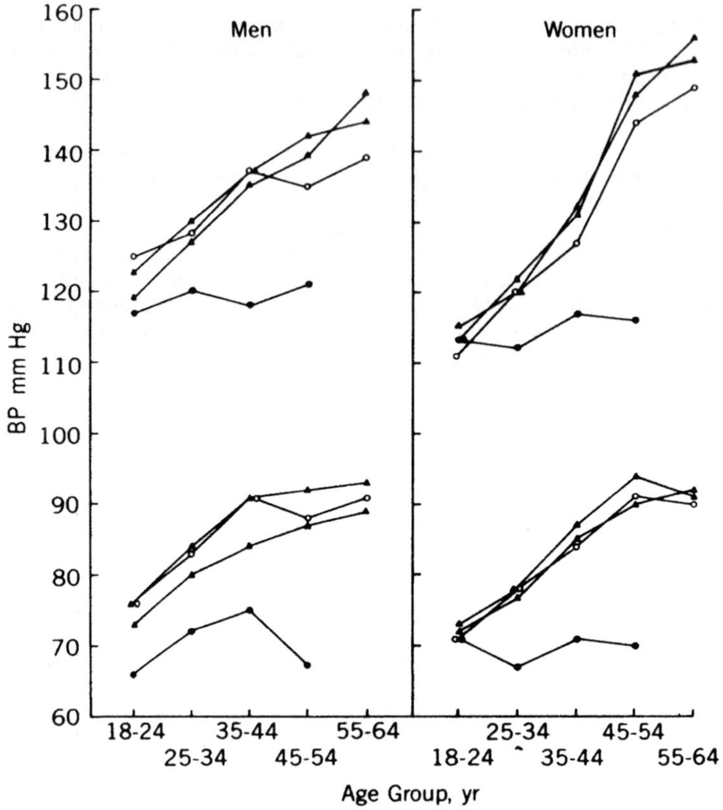

Figure 4. Mean systolic and diastolic arterial blood pressures (BP) in SCD patients (closed circles), persons in large metropolitan areas (open circles) and other controls (triangles). From Johnson, C.S. and Giorgio, A.J.: Arterial blood pressures in adults with sickle cell disease. Arch. Int. Med. 141:892, with permission.

If increased plasma erythropoietin levels are taken as a reflection of poor tissue oxygenation, high O_2 affinity hemoglobin seems to perform less well than normal blood (26), since the former prevented the fall in erythropoietin induced by normal fresh blood in an anemic patient (27), and increased erythropoietin blood levels in rats (28). Also, the erythropoietin increase in hypobaric (high altitude) hypoxia is greatest in alkalosis (highest hemoglobin O_2 binding with left shift) and least in acidosis (lowest hemoglobin O_2 binding with right shift of the HODC). In addition, induction of a left shift in the O_2 dissociation curve of hemoglobin by chemical means (cyanide, urea, etc.) have failed to improve the patient's condition, decrease the frequency of crises, or prevent the development of crises (7). Thus, treatment of SCD patients by modification of the hemoglobin physico-chemical properties has not yet been successful.

The various therapies which have been proposed can be classified as molecular, cellular, and microvascular (25). At the molecular level, the key words are "gelation inhibition". These are changes in hemoglobin which are required for the sickling episode to occur. Approaches have been directed toward inhibition of contacts of the S hemoglobin, and to decreasing the hemoglobin concentration. As stated above, one way of attaining the latter has been to enlarge the RBC's by inducing hyponatremia; thus, the hemoglobin concentration per unit of volume decreases, the HODC moves to the left, and the P50 (the PaO_2 at which hemoglobin is 50% saturated) is lowered (14). At the cellular level, basically the efforts are directed at modifying the RBC's membrane in order to diminish or avoid sickling. At the microvascular level, the goal is to modify the relationship between the vascular endothelium and the sickled cell (21, 22).

Prophylaxis

Since SCD and SCT patients have difficulty in concentrating their urine, this fact should be emphasized and they should be encouraged to drink extra amounts of fluids, particularly in hot weather and when engaged in strenuous exercise. Some disagree with this approach on the basis of psychological concerns; we believe that making the patient aware of his limitations and use of this simple preventive measure, are highly desirable. Once an individual's handling of electrolytes during and between crises is known, appropriate recommendations should be made, encouraging intake of those ions lost in excess and discouraging excessive intake of those poorly excreted.

Other general measures must include avoidance of nephrotoxic agents, administration of extra amounts of fluids when radio-opaque solutions must be administered for diagnostic purposes, and avoidance of acidosis, hypoxia, hypo- or hypertension, hyperosmolarity, and extreme anemia or polycytemia. Administration of vaccines or prophylactic antibiotics is recommended by various groups but others avoid vaccines for fear of antibody development which could affect a future organ transplantation. GU anomalies which interfere with renal function should be corrected following general indications.

Finally, a humanistic approach should be followed when dealing with these patients. They need to be well informed regarding their limitations but should be encouraged to lead as normal lives as possible while applying the recommended prophylactic measures. The natural barriers which prevent these patients from reaching the health system, must be overcome through education of the general population and health providers.

REFERENCES

1. Pauling, L. Itano, H. A., Singer, S. J. et al.: Sickle cell anemia, a molecular disease. Science 110:543-548, 1949.

2. Jain, S. K. and Shohet, S. B.: A novel phospholipid in irreversibly sickled cells: evidence for in vivo peroxidative membrane damage in sickle cell disease. Blood 63:362-367, 1984.

3. Heptinstall, R. H.: Pathology of the Kidney, Second Edition. Boston: Little, Brown and Company, 1983, pp. 1671-1680.

4. Bernstein, J. and Whitten, C. F.: A histologic appraisal of the kidney in sickle cell anemia. Arch. Pathol. (Chicago) 70:407-418, 1960.

5. Buckalew, V. M., Jr. and Someren, A.: Renal manifestations of sickle cell disease. Arch. Intern. Med. 133:660-669, 1974.

6. Eknoyan, G., Qunibi, W. Y., Grissom, R. T. et al.: Renal papillary necrosis: An update. Medicine 61:55-73, 1982.

7. Strauss, J., Zilleruelo, G. and Abitbol, C.: The kidney and hemogloblin S. Nephron 43:241-245, 1986.

8. Pardo, V., Strauss, J., Kramer, H. et al.: Nephropathy associated with sickle cell anemia: An autologous immune complex nephritis. II. Clinicopathologic studies in seven patients. Am. J. Med. 59:650-659, 1975.

9. Tejani, A., Phadke, K., Adamson, O. et al.: Renal lesions in sickle cell nephropathy in children. Nephron, In Press.

10. Strauss, J., Pardo, V., Koss, M. N. et al.: Nephropathy associated with sickle cell anemia. An autologous immune complex nephritis. I. Studies on the nature of the glomerular-bound antibody and antigen identification in a patient with sickle cell disease and immune deposit glomerulonephritis. Am. J. Med. 58:382-387, 1975.

11. Thompson, A. M., Lessin, L. and Antonovych, T. T.: The sickle cell nephropathies. In W. Fried (ed.): Comparative Clinical Aspects of Sickle Cell Disease. New York: Elsevier North Holland, Inc., 1982, pp. 131-146.

12. Brenner, B. M.: Mechanisms of progression of renal disease. Ninth International Congress of Nephrology, Los Angeles, Cal., June 1984, Program and Abstracts, p. 6A.

13. de Jong, P. E., Landman, H. and Statius van Eps, L. W.: Blood pressure in sickle cell disease (letter). Arch. Int. Med. 142:1239-1240, 1982.

14. Rosa, R. M., Bierer, B. E., Thomas, R. et al.: A study of induced hyponatremia in the prevention and treatment of sickle-cell crisis. N. Engl. J. Med. 303:1138-1143, 1980.

15. Vaamonde, C. A., Oster, J. R. and Strauss, J.: The Kidney in Sickle Cell Disease. In Suki, W.N. and Eknoyan, G. (eds.): The Kidney in Systemic Disease. New York:John Wiley & Sons, 1981, pp: 159-195.

16. Diamond, H. S., Meisel, A., Sharon, E. et al.: Hyperuricosuria and increased tubular secretion of urate in sickle cell anemia. Am. J. Med. 59:796-802, 1975.

17. DeFronzo, R. A., Taufield, P. A., Black, H. et al.: Impaired renal tubular potassium secretion in sickle cell disease. Ann. Inter. Med. 90:310-316, 1979.

18. DeFronzo, R. A., Siegel, N. J. and Pearson, H. A.: More on the pathogenesis and management of hyponatremia in the crisis of sickle cell disease (letter). J. Pediatr. 89:1038-1040, 1976.

19. Johnson, C. S. and Giorgio, A. J.: Arterial blood pressure in adults with sickle cell disease. Arch. Int. Med. 141:891-893, 1981.

20. de Jong, P.E., de Jong-van den Berg, L.T.W. and Statius van Eps, L.W.: The tubular reabsorption of phosphate in sickle cell nephropathy. Clin. Sci. Mol. Med. 55:429-434, 1978.

21. Hebbel, R. P., Booogaerts, M.A.B., Eaton, J.W. et al.: Erythrocyte adherence to endothelium in sickle cell anemia. A possible determinant of disease severity. N. Engl. J. Med. 302:992-995, 1980.

22. Hebbel, R. P., Yamada, O., Meldow, C.F. et al.: Abnormal adherence of sickle erythrocytes to cultured vascular endothelium: possible mechanism for microvascular occlusion in sickle cell disease. J. Clin. Invest. 65:154-160, 1980.

23. Radel, E. G., Kochen, J. A. and Finberg, L.: Hyponatremia in sickle cell disease. A renal salt-losing state. J. Pediatr. 88:800-805, 1976.

24. Leary, M. and Abramson, N.: Induced hyponatremia for sickle-cell crisis (letter). N. Engl. J. Med. 304:844-845, 1981.

25. Dean, J. and Schechter, A. N.: Sickle-cell anemia: molecular and cellular bases of therapeutic approaches. N. Engl. J. Med. 299:752-763, 804-811, and 863-870, 1978.

26. Jelkmann, J.: Renal Erythropoietin: Properties and Production. Rev. Physiol. Biochem. Pharmacol. 104:139-215, 1986.

27. Napier, J.A.F.: Effect of age and 2, 3-DPG content of transfused blood on serum erythropoietin. Vox Sang 39:318-321, 1980.

28. Miller, M.E., Garcia, J.F., Shive, G.G. et al.: Humoral regulation of erythropoiesis. In Killman, S.A., Cronkite, E.P. and Muller-Berat, C.N. (eds.).: Haempoietic stem cells. Munksgaard, Copenhagen, 1983 pp. 217-228.

29. Dunn, C.D.R. and Lange, R.D.: Erythropoietin: assay and characterization. In Roath, S. (ed.).: Topical Reviews in Haematology. Bristol:Wright, 1980, pp. 1-32.

RENAL CHANGES IN CHILDREN WITH CONGENITAL HEART DISEASE

Alan B. Gruskin, M.D.

Fundamental anatomical and functional differences in the kidney exist in some children with congenital heart disease (1). Acquired changes in renal function related to angiography, cardiac surgery and bacterial endocarditis also occur. Both sets of alterations constitute the subject of this report. The impact of congestive heart failure on renal function will not be considered.

RENAL CHANGES RELATED TO CONGENITAL HEART DISEASE

ANATOMICAL LESIONS:

Exclusive of renal and cardiac defects seen in children with chromosomal and recognized congenital syndromes, the incidence of non-microscopic renal anomalies in patients with acyanotic or cyanotic congenital heart disease is reported as being similar to or slightly higher than the incidence in children without congenital heart disease (1). Conversely, the incidence of congenital heart disease in those with "primary" congenital renal defects is significant. In one report, the incidence of congenital heart disease associated with Potter syndrome, unilateral renal agenesis, horseshoe kidney and adult polycystic kidney was 71%, 17%, 44% and 18% respectively (2,3). The cardiac lesions most often found were VSD, followed by cushion defects, tetralogy and PDA.

A number of microscopic renal changes occur in children with cyanotic congenital heart disease (1). The most prominent lesions are large glomeruli with dilated capillaries. The etiology of these lesions is thought to be related to prolonged hypoxemia and perhaps polycythemia. Other, less often observed, lesions include mesangial hypercellularity, enlarged juxtaglomerular apparatus, mesangial deposits of IgG, and thickened glomerular basement membranes. A few patients have been reported to have focal segmental glomerulosclerosis, diffuse sclerotic lesions and renal hemosiderosis (4). It is not known whether the sclerotic lesions are a result of glomerular hyperperfusion or whether the numbers of glomeruli are normal or reduced in children with congenital heart disease. Relatively few, if any, microscopic alterations in renal structure occur in patients with acyanotic congenital heart disease.

URINALYSIS:

The routine urinalysis in most children with congenital heart disease is usually benign (1). Some children with cyanotic congenital heart disease develop mild to moderate degrees of proteinuria. Some believe that the incidence of nephrotic syndrome is increased in children with cyanotic congenital heart disease. Although no data are available on the incidence of bacteriuria in children with congenital heart disease, no reason exists to assume it is increased. In a few children with cyanotic congenital heart disease, phlebotomy has reduced urinary protein excretion (5).

RENAL FUNCTION IN CONGENITAL HEART DISEASE:

Renal clearances in children with congenital heart disease are variable (Table 1). Most reports indicate that GFR is normal in children with acyanotic congenital heart disease and normal to depressed in those with cyanotic congenital heart disease. Levels of effective renal plasma flow (C_{PAH}) parallel those of GFR. In both groups, the mean filtration fraction is elevated and suggests that renal vascular resistance is increased in children with congenital heart disease. The abnormalities are more pronounced in those with cyanotic congenital heart disease.

Table 1: Renal Clearances - In Children With Congenital Heart Disease

Lesion	GFR*	C_{PAH}*	RBF*	FF*	TM_{PAH}**
Acyanotic	114-138	431-538	736-849	0.25-0.29	71
Cyanotic	68-145	271-711	643-1997	0.21-0.37	83
Coarctation	103-154	434-519	869-945	0.24-0.30	—
Normal	100-104	500-700	1200	0.20	65-78

*ml/min/1.73m^2 - range

**mg/min/1.73m^2

Studies of renal blood flow and its distribution by means of xenon^{133} washout studies indicate that, compared to normal, the outer cortical blood flow rate is reduced in children with acyanotic congenital heart disease, further reduced in those with cyanotic congenital heart disease, and markedly reduced in children with heart failure and with an elevated LVED (6,7). Fractional flow to the outer cortex is similarly reduced. In contrast, outer cortical renal blood flow is reduced in children with coarctation of the aorta while fractional flow remains unchanged.

The specific etiology of these changes is unclear. Influencing factors may include the impact of malnutrition, reduced salt intake, hypoxemia, and stress. These factors may alter renal blood flow, its distribution, and/or normal developmental processes. It may also be that the usually expected decrease in renal vascular resistance occurring after birth does not occur in patients with congenital heart disease. In fully recovered post-operative patients with congenital heart disease, some have experienced a return to normal renal clearances; others continue to display deviations from normal (1).

Some of the biochemical changes observed in children with congenital heart disease may be explained by alterations in renal functions: proximal renal tubular acidosis, somewhat lower levels of serum bicarbonate and a reduced capacity to excrete hydrogen ion after ammonium chloride loading (1). Hyperuricemia, uricosuria, and uric acid lithiasis have also been described in children with congenital heart disease (8,9).

COARCTATION HYPERTENSION:

A number of factors, hormonal, renal and mechanical, may influence the hypertensive process in coarctation (10). Support for a central role of the kidney in this process is provided by renal transplantation studies. If the kidney is transplanted to a site above an experimentally produced coarctation, hypertension does not develop. Data relative to the mechanisms leading to coarctation hypertension are consistent with that obtained from both the classical one- and two-kidney models of hypertension. Initially, hyperreninemia develops. Next, post stenosis induced changes in renal function lead to salt and water retention. Finally, renin secretion is reduced; however, it fails to fall to absolutely suppressed levels and results in "relative" hyperreninemia.

This concept of relative hyperreninemia in children with coarctation is supported by studies which have demonstrated increases in extracellular volumes, decreases in blood pressure in response to angiotensin blocking agents, and a renal renin secretory rate similar to that of children with acyanotic congenital heart disease. When measured by the $xenon^{133}$ washout technique, outer cortical renal blood flow is reduced in children with coarctation (11). Such changes may lead to an increase in renal renin secretion.

ACQUIRED CHANGES IN RENAL FUNCTION

CONTRAST MEDIA:

Multiple studies demonstrate that contrast media can be nephrotoxic (1,12, 13). The clinical manifestations of contrast nephrotoxicity include: hematuria; proteinuria; transient and permanent reductions in renal function: acute renal insufficiency; vascular involvement leading to medullary, corticomedullary and renal venous thrombosis. The pathogenesis of contrast induced nephrotoxicity has been attributed to the dose, concentration, site of injection, injection time, and structure (sodium versus non-sodium) of contrast. Injection of contrast media directly into renal arteries in animals leads initially to vasoconstriction and is followed by vasodilation. Proximal tubular vacuolization has been attributed to the osmotic effect of contrast. Tubular blockade can occur secondary to contrast mediated precipitation of intraluminal protein. Changes in renal renin release localized to individual nephrons and increases in its systemic release have been noted. Catecholamine release may also be increased. Dehydration should be anticipated as a result of the osmotic effect of contrast.

Groups of patients at risk for developing contrast mediated nephrotoxicity can be identified in adult populations (14). At risk are patients with preexisting renal insufficiency; diabetics, especially those with diminished renal function; patients in congestive heart failure; and those who undergo contrast studies while dehydrated. In children with congenital heart disease undergoing cardiac angiography, additional factors may influence their response to contrast administration. These include congenitally related changes in renal function, the impact of hypoxemia and hyperviscosity, a developmentally reduced level of GFR in infants below 1-1½ years of age, and renal blood flow. Available data lead to the conclusion that the vasculature of the newborn kidney, in contrast to the adult kidney, responds with a more intense vasoconstriction when stressed. In neonatal piglets, infusions of contrast lead to increases in filtration fraction subsequent to reductions in renal plasma flow (13). GFR remains unchanged. Post-mortem examinations of the kidney in some piglets revealed proximal tubular vacuolization.

In children, creatinine clearances apparently do not change in the 15-30 minutes following angiocardiography (1). Post angiographic studies of renal blood flow rates and its distribution by xenon^{133} washout techniques almost uniformly reveal reductions in total renal blood predominantly outer cortical in location (6,7). Fractional distribution does not change significantly. Following angiocardiography renal renin release fails to fall to levels one might anticipate given the degree of acute extracellular volume expansion that occurs with the addition of hyperosmotic contrast to the extracellular compartment. Thus, it appears that relative hyperreninemia exists after angiocardiography and may, in part, explain the observed decreases in outer cortical blood flow.

Following angiocardiography, young infants appear to be at greater risk for developing overt nephrotoxicity than older children (13). They also tend to receive more contrast per unit of bodyweight because of the need to accurately define complex cardiac anomalies. Neonates undergoing angiocardiography and receiving more than 3 ml/kg may be at risk for developing corticomedullary necrosis. In 30 infants less than 3 months of age, 8 developed microhematuria after angiography. Conversely, in 80 children over 3 months none developed microhematuria when given less than 3 ml/kg of contrast.

BACTERIAL ENDOCARDITIS:

Bacterial endocarditis affects the kidney in a number of ways (1,15,16,17); the clinical course is usually that of a post-infectious nephritis. Clinical syndromes range from that of microhematuria and proteinuria, to acute and/or chronic renal failure. The hypertension and edema may occur, and a few children with SBE have presented with acute rapidly progressive renal failure (18). Infectious agents causing SBE nephritis include: streptococcus viridans, and hemolytica, staphylococcus and candida. Noteworthy is the fact that renal insufficiency secondary to SBE nephritis contributed significantly to mortality in the preantibiotic era. Appropriate antibacterial therapy or the removal of infected endocardial vegetations result in renal recovery. The most common renal histopathology is a focal segmental proliferative lesion. Other changes include extra- and endocapillary proliferation, subepithelial humps, and IgG, IgM, IgA, and C_3 deposits. A less commonly observed SBE related problem is embolization to the kidney of infected vegetations leading to infarction and microabcesses.

RENAL CHANGES ASSOCIATED WITH CARDIAC SURGERY:

In studies involving 456 and 418 children undergoing cardiopulmonary bypass, acute renal insufficiency occurred in 5.3 and 3.6% children respectively (19,20). Mortality rates ranged from 18 to 100% in those requiring dialysis. Predisposing risk factors for developing acute renal insufficiency include age, the complexity of the cardiac lesion, hypoxia, malnutrition, polycythemia, length of bypass, and post-operative low output states. Death was usually the result of post-operative low output states, or infectious complications rather than renal failure.

The most frequent form of bypass post-surgery renal insufficiency is acute tubular necrosis secondary to hypotension and/or hypoxemia. Hemoglobinuric renal failure also occurs secondary to hemolysis following prolonged bypass, usually more than 120 minutes. Adequate pre-operative hydration may prevent its onset when the judicious use of intra-operative mannitol is used. Rarely, the development of post-operative endocarditis leads to renal failure. Of interest are recent observations that hyperuricemia is present pre-operatively in many cyanotic polycythemic, hypoxemic children (8,9,21,22). The pre-operative use of allopurinol to lower serum uric acid in such children may favorably influence their post bypass course.

Specific guidelines for initiating dialysis vary. Indications for initiating dialysis include volume overload, hyperkalemia, hyperphosphatemia and hyperuricemia. Available data suggest that survival following early dialysis is significantly better than prolonged medical management subsequently followed by dialysis. The acute renal failure seen in children after open heart surgery is usually accompanied by a hypercatabolic state and consideration ought to be given to some form of hyperalimentation. Evidence has been presented that the careful provision of energy and amino acids in patients with acute renal failure may reduce the length and magnitude of acute renal failure.

Both hemodialysis and peritoneal dialysis have been successfully used. Also, continuous arteriovenous ultrafiltration can be used to control volume overload. Most pediatric nephrologists prefer peritoneal dialysis because of the risk of hemorrhagic complications associated with hemodialysis. It should be remembered that sustained ultrafiltration is difficult to accomplish in infants less than 3-4 months of age. The most often used form of peritoneal dialysis is repeated acute peritoneal dialysis. Others prefer a form of continuous dialysis with cycle lengths adjusted according to ultrafiltration requirements and to the need to remove solute. The use of smaller than usual volumes of dialysate may be helpful in controlling the impact of peritoneal volume on respiratory function. The use of peritoneal dialysis can be associated with problems in ultrafiltration related to poor peritoneal perfusion, the rapid absorption of glucose and age. Also, peritoneal fluid frequently enters the child's pleural cavity causing respiratory embarrassment. Pleural collections can usually be drained through a chest tube and peritoneal dialysis continued. However, peritoneal dialysis may need to be discontinued and hemodialysis tried. In those requiring acute hemodialysis, a subclavian access is often helpful. Meticulous attention directed toward controlling hemostasis during hemodialysis is mandatory.

REFERENCES:

1. Gruskin, A.B.: The kidney in congenital heart disease. Advances in Pediatrics. Yearbook Publishers, Chicago, 1978, p. 133.

2. Leier, C.V., Baker, P.B., Kilman, J.W., Wooley, C.F.: Cardiovascular abnormalities associated with adult polycystic kidney disease. Ann Intern Med 100(5):683, 1984.

3. Greenwood, R.D., Rosenthal, A., Nadas, A.S.: Cardiovascular malformations associated with congenital anomalies of the urinary system. Observations in a series of 453 infants and children with urinary system malformations. Clin Pediatr (Phila), 15(12):1101, 1976.

4. Roberts, W.C.: Renal hemosiderosis (blue kidney) in patients with valvular heart disease. Hm J Pathol 48(3):409, 1966.

5. deJong, P.E., Weening, J.J., Donker, A.J.M., van der Hem, G.K.: The effect of phlebotomy on renal function and proteinuria in a patient with congenital cyanotic heart disease [letter]. Nephron 33(3):225, 1983.

6. Gruskin, A.B., Auerbach, V.H., Black, I.F.S.: Intrarenal blood flow in children with normal kidneys and congenital heart disease: Changes due to angiocardiography. Pediatr Res 8:561, 1974.

7. Gruskin, A.B., Auerbach, V.H., Black, I.F.S.: Clinical assessment of renal blood flow in children using ^{133}Xenon changes due to congenital heart disease, angiocardiography and heart failure. In: Winkel, K., Blaufox, M.D., and Funck-Brentano, J-L., (eds.). Radionuclides in Nephrology. Proceedings of the IIIrd International Symposium, Berlin, April 1974, Georg Thieme Verlag, Stuttgart, 1975, p. 51.

8. Hencz, P., Deverall, P.B., Crew, A.D., Steel, A.E., Mearns, A.J.: Hyperuricemia of infants and children: a complication of open heart surgery. J Pediatr 94:774, 1979.

9. Hsu, A.C., Kooh, S.W., Izukawa, T., Fox, I.H.: Uric-acid lithiasis in an infant with cyanotic congenital heart disease [letter]. J Pediatr 91(6):1021, 1977.

10. Bagby, S.P.: Dissection of pathogenetic factors in coarctation hypertension. In: Loggie, J.M.H., Horan, M.J., Gruskin, A.B., et al (eds.). NHLBI Workshop on Juvenile Hypertension. Proceedings of Symposium, Bethesda, Maryland, May 26 and 27, 1983, p. 253.

11. Gruskin, A.B., Auerbach, V.H., Black, I.F.S., Sapire, D.W.: Intrarenal blood flow distribution (IRBFD) and renal renin secretory rates (RRSR) in children with coarctation. Pediatr Res 12:383, 1978.

12. Mudge, G.H.: Nephrotoxicity of urographic radiocontrast drugs. Kidney Int 18:540, 1980.

13. Gruskin, A.B., Oetliker, O., Wolfish, N.M., Gootman, N., Edelmann, C.M. Jr.: Effects of Angiography on Renal Function and Histology in Infants and Children. J. Pediatrics 76:41, 1970.

14. D'Elia, J.A., Gleason, R.E., Alday, M., et al: Nephrotoxicity from angiographic contrast material. A Prospective Study. Am J Med 72: 1982.

15. Johnson, C.M., Rhodes, K.H.: Pediatric endocarditis. Mayo Cln Proc 57:86, 1982.

16. Johnson, E.H., Rosenthal, A., Nadas, A.S.: A forty year review of bacterial endocarditis in infancy and childhood. Circulation 51:581, 1975.

17. Mendelsohn, G., Hutchins, G.M.: Infective endocarditis during the first decade of life. An autopsy review of 33 cases. Am J Dis Child 133(6):619, 1979.

18. Schleman, M., Casta, A., Balsara, R.K.: Bacterial endocarditis and renal failure in a 10 year old boy. Ped Cardiol 2:259, 1982.

19. Rigden, S.P.A., Barratt, T.M., Dillon, M.J., de Leval, M., Stark, J.: Acute renal failure complicating cardiopulmonary bypass surgery. Arch Dis Child 57:425, 1982.

20. Book, K., Ohqvist, G., Bjork, V.O., Lundberg, S., Settergren, G.: Peritoneal dialysis in infants and children after open heart surgery. Scan J Thor Cardiovasc Surg 16:229, 1982.

21. Yip, W.C.L., Tay, J.S.H.: Hyperuricaemia as a cause of acute renal failure complicating cardiopulmonary bypass surgery [letter]. Arch Dis Child 58(2):159, 1983,

22. Yip, W.C.L., Tay, J.S.H., Ho, T.F.: Serum uric acid level in congenital heart disease (abstract). Proceedings of the Fourth Asian Congress of Paediatrics, Seoul, 1982:159.

RENAL INJURY FROM CHEMOTHERAPEUTIC AGENTS

J.R. Ingelfinger, M.D.

Drugs and toxins may produce a variety of renal injuries including isolated tubular abnormalities, acute renal failure and chronic renal failure. Syndromes associated with toxic nephropathies are shown in Table I.

Table I: SYNDROMES ASSOCIATED WITH TOXIC NEPHROPATHIES

Acute Renal Failure
Chronic Renal Failure
Proteinuria/nephrotic syndrome
Abnormalities of diluting/concentrating mechanisms
Abnormalities of acid base balance
Abnormalities of individual tubular functional components
Obstruction
Laboratory test abnormalities induced by drugs

This paper will present examples of these various clinical syndromes. Nephrotoxicity is a common complication of drug therapy, and continual awareness of its possible occurrence is important in patient management.

SUSCEPTIBILITY OF THE KIDNEY TO INJURY

Multiple aspects of renal physiology lead to the susceptibility of the kidney to toxic substances (1,2). Twenty-five percent of cardiac output passes through the kidneys every minute. Furthermore, the glomerular capillary endothelium has a large surface area which may be exposed to drugs, many of which are organic acids or bases with high protein affinity rapidly leading to high concentrations of drug. Furthermore, drug-mediated renal cell injury may occur either through mitochondrial respiratory chain uncoupling, or changes in enzyme activity. Because of the medullary countercurrent mechanism, abnormal accumulation of various agents and their metabolites may also occur. Furthermore, since renal acidification and concentration occur in distal segments of the nephron, certain agents or metabolites which undergo solubility change in an acid medium may precipitate within the lumen of the renal tubule, contributing to acute renal failure. Osmotic diuretics may deplete a patient of electrolytes and minerals, and secondarily cause renal problems. For instance, drug-induced chronic hypokalemia leads to secondary tubular changes. Some drugs may have an endocrine action which may mimic certain endogenous hormones, competing for receptor sites and interfering with intracellular mechanisms.

Multiple renal enzymes may be involved in drug metabolism and are listed in Table II.

Table II: RENAL ENZYMES INVOLVED IN DRUG METABOLISM

- Oxidative (cytochrome P-450 dependent; aromatic and aliphatic hydroxylation, N-, S-, dealkylation, expoxidation)
- Reductive (reduction of aldehydes and ketones to alcohols; glutathione-dependent reactions)
- Hydrolytic (esters and amides; epoxide hydrase)
- Synthetic
- Conjugative (glucuronides, sulfate esters, glutathione conjugates)

Thus there are many aspects of cellular metabolism which may be affected by drugs to which the kidney is exposed. Cytochrome P-450 dependent oxidation is localized to the smooth endoplasmic reticulum or microsomal fraction of renal cells. Cytochrome P-450 must be in a reduced state to bind oxygen, so the involvement of a reductase is also obligatory. Reduced cytochrome P-450 may also serve as an electron donor in some reductions without binding oxygen. It has been known for some time that mixed function oxidase activities are present in renal tissue. The highest concentrations of the P-450 system are in the kidney cortex, and certain drugs may induce their activity. Two groups of enzymes are involved in the oxidation of alcohols to aldehydes or ketones, and of aldehydes to carboxylic acids. These are common reactions and two groups of enzymes are involved - purine nucleotide linked oxidases and aldehyde oxidase. Hydrolytic esters and amides and epoxide hydrase are also present. Conjugation reactions also occur in the kidney. Glucuronide formation in the kidney is an important pathway of drug metabolism. A variety of drugs induce renal glucuronyl transferase activity. Thus it is clear that in addition to its susceptibility to exposure to toxic agents, the kidney participates in drug metabolism in vivo, making it further subject to direct toxicity.

CLINICAL PROBLEMS RELATED TO TREATMENT WITH CHEMOTHERAPEUTIC AGENTS

Antibiotics:

Acute renal failure (oliguric or polyuric) has been well reported with a variety of antibiotics, especially aminoglycosides. All aminoglycosides have potential for nephrotoxicity. There are three main groups of aminoglycosides which differ in their amino sugar: the kanamycin group, the neomycin group, and the gentamicin group. (See References 3-7 for review). Gentamicin will serve as an example for this discussion.

Gentamicin (and other aminoglycosides) are bacteriocidal due to their binding irreversibly to specific proteins in the smaller 30S segment of bacterial ribosomes. On a cellular level it would appear that aminoglycosides interfere with mitochondrial function (8,9). Gentamicin, which is the most frequently and completely studied aminoglycoside, appears to enhance monovalent cation uptake with relatively greater effect on sodium permeability than potassium. Gentamicin uncouples mitochondrial respiration.

The water-soluble aminoglycosides are strongly cationic and bound by change interaction to the brush border and are transported across the lipid membrane by pinocytosis. Aminoglycosides are concentrated within cellular lysosomes. Hydrolysis of phospholipids by lysosomes appears to be impaired, and as complex polar lipids accumulate, whorls of multilamellar osmiophilic material (called myeloid bodies) appear (10-12).

GFR AND AMINOGLYCOSIDES

Glomerular filtration rate has been shown to fall with aminoglycoside therapy even without obvious renal tubular damage (13-14). Micropuncture experiments in Munich-Wistar rats have demonstrated a drop in K_f, the ultrafiltration coefficient, though no change in capillary wall permeability was seen by transmission electron microscopy. Renal plasma flow also becomes reduced with decrease in filtration fraction and increased pre-glomerular arteriolar resistance. Volume expansion partially corrects these findings, and captopril has been shown to prevent them, which implies that angiotensin II may mediate toxicity.

In acute renal failure, the tubular injury may also cause some obstruction and backleak which decreases renal blood flow. Additionally, there may be vascular effects which will further decrease renal blood flow (13,14). The combination will then decrease the driving force for glomerular filtration. Gentamicin has been shown to cause a dose dependent intrarenal vasoconstriction after chronic administration. So both vascular and tubular effects are seen.

The incidence of gentamicin nephrotoxicity varies between 0.5 and 30% of patients (1-3, 7, 15-16). Nine percent of courses of gentamicin treatment were associated with increase in blood urea nitrogen in the study by the Boston Collaborative Drug Survey (16). However, young animals and children seem relatively resistant to aminoglycoside nephrotoxicity (17-19).

The spectrum of renal toxicity is shown in Table III. Clinical changes in renal function usually occur after 1 week of therapy. A number of markers in the urine may be seen. Typically, patients excrete brush border and lysosomal enzymes including N-acetyl-glucose aminidase (NAG), Betagalactosidase, alanine aminopeptidase and alkaline phosphatase (20-23).

Table III: AMINOGLYCOSIDE NEPHROTOXICITY MAY INCLUDE

Enzymuria:	brush border membrane lysosomal
Tubular proteinuria and aminoaciduria	
Transport abnormalities:	glycosuria
	Mg^{2+} wasting
	K^{+} wasting
Vasopressin resistant concentrating defect	
Decreased glomerular filtration rate	

Such enzymuria is less often seen with other agents which cause acute renal failure such as cephalosporins, ampicillin, cloxacillin, sulfonamides and tetracycline. β_2-microglobulin is also seen after a week or so of aminoglycoside therapy. Proteinuria, sometimes reaching the nephrotic range, may also occur. Prior to renal insufficiency, a vasopressin-resistant urinary concentrating defect and increase in fractional excretion of sodium may be seen (24-26). Then a progressive decrease in renal function occurs. Yet most patients recover fully and dialysis is rarely needed.

HISTOLOGY

When histology is available in cases of aminoglycoside toxicity, patchy necrosis of the proximal tubule may be found. As mentioned, ultrastructural studies in both animals and man show cytosegrasomes containing myelin-like material (1,27). It is thought that these are a marker of ingestion and not diagnostic. Because aminoglycosides do not undergo metabolic degradation, they are excreted primarily unchanged. Thus their damage is direct.

FACTORS MODIFYING TOXICITY (1,3-5)

It is possible to moderate gentamicin toxicity by altering the dosage schedule by following drug levels and using the lowest possible dose. Metabolic acidosis worsens toxicity, and thus alkalinization may protect against gentamicin toxicity.

Aminoglycosides administered with cephalosporins may cause increased renal toxicity (28-30), especially if also combined with cis-platinum use or associated temporarily with blood loss. When aminoglycosides are combined with cancer chemotherapy or with methoxyflurane anesthesia, amphotericin, or clindamycin, renal toxicity may be enhanced. Furosemide and other diuretics may worsen gentamicin toxicity in the presence of volume depletion. See Table IV.

NEPHROTOXICITY FROM OTHER AGENTS (See Table IV)

Tetracyclines: (31-35)

Tetracyclines are an infrequent cause of acute renal failure. High tetracycline concentrations, especially if the tetracycline is given intravenously, may lead to renal insufficiency and renal damage. All tetracyclines appear to be anti-anabolic (except possibly doxicycline) and may therefore increase urea production. The antianabolic effect occurs because of an induced effect in amino acid utilization of protein synthesis and urea production thereby increases.

Tetracycline-induced Fanconi syndrome was reported in the 1960's but is reported only with outdated, degraded tetracycline (33). The occurrence of this syndrome in children is extremely rare.

Table IV: ANTIMICROBIAL-INDUCED NEPHROTOXICITY: POTENTIATING FACTORS	
CLINICAL:	Underlying disease
	Pre-extant renal disease
	Sepsis
	Dehydration/hypovolemia/hemorrhage
	Acidosis
	Advanced age
PHARMACOLOGIC:	
Concomitant Drugs -	
	Antineoplastic (cis-platinum)
	Diuretics (furosemide)
	Concomitant antibiotics (cephalothin, clindamycin, amphotericin B with aminoglycosides)
	Anesthetic agents (methoxyflurane, enflurane)
Dosage Regimens -	
	Amount
	Frequency

Amphotericin B: (36-47)

Nephrotoxicity resulting in renal dysfunction from amphotericin, a polyene antimicrobial produced by streptomyces nodosus is related to the length of therapy. After 2-3 grams of amphotericin (cumulative dose) renal abnormalities appear in most patients. However, renal insufficiency (41) and permanent renal failure (45) are rare, though isolated renal tubular defects are more common. Proximal or distal renal tubular acidification defects may occur (39,40). Renal potassium wasting (46), leading to hypokalemia may also occur and is usually accompanied by renal concentration abnormalities (36).

Amphotericin is bound to cell membranes, and leads to increased permeability to ions and small charged molecules. Vasoconstriction may also play an important role in the pathophysiology of amphotericin nephrotoxicity. Alkalinization (37) and watching the cumulative dose are most important in preventing toxicity.

Cephalosporin Nephrotoxicity: (48-55)

A variety of cephalosporins have been reported to cause nephrotoxicity including cephaloradine (51,54,55) (the most common), cephalothin (51) and cephalexin (53). These agents are actively carried into proximal tubule cells by the PAH transport system and trapped intracellularly. Inhibitors of organic acid secretion seem to inhibit both transport and toxicity (53-54). When cephalosporin nephrotoxicity is seen, other nephrotoxic agents or diuretics may have been used concomitantly. Nephrotoxicity is at least partially mediated by inhibitory effects of cephalosporins on mitochondrial respiration. Dosages, therefore, must be adjusted with renal insufficiency.

ANESTHESIA AND RENAL DYSFUNCTION (56-65)

Surgical anesthesia leads to transient changes in renal function related to decrease in renal blood flow and increases in renal vascular resistance (57). Furthermore, the trauma of surgery and possibly dehydration may also lead to such changes. Very frequently, the concomitant changes in cardiovascular function related to the surgery itself may combine to cause problems. Methoxyflurane (60, 61, 64), has been associated with a renal concentrating defect and with severe toxicity with oliguric acute renal failure. This is quite rare in the pediatric population. It would appear that fluoride mobilization may lead to the nephrotoxicity on its own (59). Increased oxalate excretion has accompanied the nephrotoxicity. Maximum serum fluoride concentration seems to correlate well with the clinical changes such as polyuria. Additional suggestions that fluoride may mediate the nephrotoxicity come from the fact that fluoride treated hyperthyroid patients have been reported to suffer similar nephrotoxicity (65). Neither halothane (56,57) nor enflurane (58) have been associated with renal failure except on rare occasions. Most of the time, fluorinated anesthetics are associated with mild renal concentrating defects resistant to vasopressin. Oliguric renal failure associated with deposition of calcium oxalate occurs much less frequently.

RADIOCONTRAST AGENTS (66-74)

The radiocontrast materials iothalamate and diatrizoate are most commonly used and associated with renal dysfunction. The patient groups seemingly at risk are those with pre-existing decreased renal function, history of multiple exposure to radiocontrast agents or previous dehydration (67,68). Though the presence of medical ultrasound makes it less likely that children have routine intravenous pyelography, an increasing number of patients are undergoing other procedures (e.g. CAT scans) where the radio-contrast agents are administered. Thus, it is worthwhile to discuss contrast agents as a chemotherapeutic agent. The incidence of acute renal dysfunction related to radio-contrast material in normal patients appears to be very low. However, in at-risk patients, it may be as high as 10-12% (66-67). The occurrence of renal failure may present itself within 24 hours with pathologic changes usually seen in the proximal tubule. Some studies suggest that previous proteinuria is a risk factor for contrast induced nephropathy as is hyperuricemia (66). Volume contraction may predispose to nephropathy, and care to avoid dehydration may be helpful in lessening nephrotoxicity.

Nephrotoxicity appears to be mediated by direct effect of the contrast agent or by increases in urinary uric acid and oxalate caused by the contrast agent.

There is a biphasic hemodynamic response and it has been shown that there is a marked early rise in renal blood flow followed by a period of decreased renal flow (74). The vasoconstriction appears to be mediated by the renin angiotensin system and may be somewhat attenuated by volume expansion (74). Additionally, changes in the microcirculation due to red blood cell morphologic changes may also play a role (74).

CANCER THERAPY CAUSING ACUTE RENAL FAILURE

Anti-cancer agents causing acute renal failure include cis-platinum, nitrosoureas such as streptozotoin and Methyl CCNU, methotrexate, mitomicin C, mithramycin and 5-azacytidine. Radiation therapy may also be associated with acute renal failure. Additionally, the nitrosoureas and radiation therapy may cause chronic renal failure in time (see references 75 and 76 for general review).

<u>Cis-Platinum</u>: (77-84)

Cis-platinum interacts with nucleophilic sites in DNA similar to other bifunctional alkylating agents (80,84). The spectrum of renal dysfunction caused by cis-platinum ranges from minor damage to acute tubular necrosis. It would appear from animal studies that administration of cis-platinum leads to uncoupling of mitochondrial oxidative phosphorylation which disrupts energy production in the renal cells (78). Furthermore, defects in medullary solute accumulation may be seen. It is felt that primary mitochondrial toxicity underlies both of these findings (78). Use of prehydration and diuretics as well as probenacid may be helpful in preventing toxicity (81). Radioprotective compounds (79) or chelator diethyldithiocarbamate or sodium thiosulfate (80) may be protective.

Nitrosoureas: (85)

Nitrosoureas are cell cycle non-specific agents which are effective in treating many neoplasms. Both streptozotocin and Methyl CCNU have been reported to be associated with nephrotoxicity.

Streptozotócin (85) acts through inhibiting DNA synthesis secondarily blocking RNA and protein synthesis. Proteinuria often follows administration with renal tubular damage thereafter characterized by Fanconi syndrome or individual tubular defects. Regardless of the dosage, proteinuria must be monitored, and intravenous hydration or the use of diuretic programs may be helpful.

Methyl CCNU (86-87) is a lipid soluble nitrosourea, which has been associated with acute renal failure, but also insidiously with chronic renal failure. High dose therapy may lead to glomerulosclerosis and irreversible renal failure. The majority of reported cases of end stage renal disease due to sulfonoureas receive drug doses greater than 1.5 gm/M^2, thus it appears important to discontinue this therapy when a total of 1,000 mg/M^2 to 1,250 mg/M^2 has been achieved (86-89).

Methotrexate:

Methotrexate, a structural analogue of folic acid, competitively binds to dihydrofolate reductase, which is the enzyme that converts folic acid to reduce folate cofactors (90). These reduced cofactors are essential for metabolic transfer of 1-carbon units for biosynthesis of thymidylic acid (specific DNA nucleotide) and inosinic acid (purine precursor for DNA and RNA synthesis). Methotrexate, as a result, is cell-cycle dependent, acting mainly during DNA synthesis. The dihydrofolate reductase inhibition may be circumvented by providing metabolites such as citrovorum factor and thymidine acting distal in the folate pathway, which "rescues" the cell from methotrexate effect.

In conventional dosages, methotrexate does not often cause renal failure. However, high dose methotrexate followed by "rescue therapy" with citrovorum is associated with renal failure unless a vigorous program of hydration and alkalinization is followed (90-92). Severe toxicity can usually be anticipated in patients who have 100% or more rise in their serum creatinine within 48 hours after methotrexate administration. Usually the renal failure is non-oliguric so that hydration and alkalinization can be maintained. However, rescue factors should be increased if there is any question about severe toxicity onset.

ACUTE INTERSTITIAL NEPHRITIS (AIN) (93-98)

AIN has been reported with a variety of antimicrobial agents, and is generally immunologically mediated. Hypersensitivity-related AIN has been reported with methicillin, oxacillin, nafcillin, penicillin G, ampicillin, and carbenicillin and also with rifampin. The reader is referred to reviews for additional information. (93-98)

RADIATION NEPHRITIS

The reader is referred to other references for discussion of radiation nephritis. (1,99)

SPECIAL CONSIDERATIONS IN THE CHILD (100)

A number of other problems should be anticipated in the child receiving potentially toxic drugs. One is that of the youngster with malignancy who has a high likelihood of developing acute uric acid nephropathy. In this instance, starting allopurinol, ensuring hydration, and maintaining water diuresis can be very beneficial. When there is a very large tumor burden as with Burkitt's lymphoma, it is important to arrange for anticipated need for acute hemodialysis. Additional problems include hypertension and volume overload due to iatrogenic volume expansion.

End-stage renal disease occasionally may occur in a child with malignancy either because of chemotherapeutic toxicity or because of surgical removal of the kidneys. In these situations, planning in advance is mandatory, though the outcome is often complicated.

REFERENCES

1. Coggins, C.H. and Fang, L.S.T. Acute renal failure associated with antibiotics, anesthetic agents, and radiographic contrast agents. In: Brenner, B.M. & Lazarus, M. Acute Renal Failure, 1983, p. 283.
2. Anders, M.W. Metabolism of drugs by the kidney. Kidney Int. 18:636, 1980.
3. Rozek, S.L. The aminoglycoside antibiotics. The antimicrobial newsletter. 1:51, 1984.
4. Blumer, J.L. and Reed, M.D. Clinical pharmacology of aminoglycoside antibiotics in pediatrics. Ped. Clin. N. Amer. 30:195, 1983.
5. Schentag, J.J. Aminoglycoside pharmacokinetics as a guide to therapy and toxicology. In: Whelton, A. and Neu, H.D. The aminoglycosides: microbiology clinical use and toxicology, NY, Marcel Dekker, 1983, pp. 143-167.
6. Morin, J.P. Viotte, G. Vandervalle, A. et al. Gentamicin-induced nephrotoxicity: a cell biology approach. Kidney Int. 18:583, 1980.
7. Hewitt, W.L. Reflections on the clinical pharmacology of gentamicin. Acta. Path. Micro. Scand. B81, Suppl. 241:151, 1977.
8. Simmons, C.F. Bogusky, R.T. and Homes, H.D. Inhibitory effects of gentamicin on renal mitochondrial oxidative phosphorylation. J. Pharm. Exp. Ther. 214:709, 1980.
9. Weinberg, J.M. and Humes, H.D. Mechanisms of gentamicin-induced dysfunction of renal cortical mitochondria. Arch. Biochem. Biophys. 205:222, 232, 1980.
10. Whelton, A. Renal tubular transport and intrarenal aminoglycoside distribution. In: Whelton, A. and Neu, H.C. The aminoglycosides: microbiology, clinical use and toxicology, NY, Marcel Dekker, Inc, 1982, pp. 191-222.
11. Kaloyanides, G.J. and Pastoriza-Munoz, E. Aminoglycoside nephrotoxicity, Kidney Int. 18:571, 1980.
12. Kornguth, M.D. Bayer, W.H. and Kunin, C.M. Binding of gentamicin to subcellular fractions of rabbit kidney: Inhibition by spermine and other polyamines. J. Antimicrob. Chemother. 6:121, 1980.
13. Baylis, C. The mechanism of the decline in glomerular filtration rate in gentamicin-induced acute renal failure in the rat. Antimicrob. Chemother. 6:381, 1980.
14. Baylis, C. Rennke, H.G. Brenner, B.M. Mechanism of the defect in glomerular ultrafiltration associated with gentamicin administration. Kidney Int. 12:344, 1977.
15. Dellinger, P. Murphy, T. Pinn, V. et al. Protective effect of cephalothin against gentamicin-induced nephrotoxicity in rats. Antimicrob Agents Chemother. 9:172, 1976.
16. Fanning, W.J. Gump, D. and Jick, H. Gentamicin-and cephalothin-associated rises in blood urea nitrogen. Antimicrob. Agents. Chemotherap. 10:80, 1976.
17. Cowan, R.H. Jukkola, A.F. and Arant, B.S. Jr. Pathophysiological evidence of gentamicin (G) nephrotoxicity in the neonatal puppy. Kidney Int. 14:628, 1978.
18. Karniski, L. Chonko, A. Stewart, R. et al. The effects of gentamicin (G) on renal function in the sexually mature vs. sexually immature rabbits. Kidney Int. 14:726, 1978.
19. Zakavddin, S. and Adelman, R. Urinary enzyme activity in neonates receiving gentamicin therapy. Clin. Res. 26:142A, 1978.

20. Keys, T.F. Kurtz, S.B. Jones, J.D.and Mullen, S.M. Renal toxicity during therapy with gentamicin or tobramycin. May Clin. Proc. 56:556, 1981.
21. Mondorf, A.W. Zegelman, M. Kose, J. et al. Comparative studies of the action of aminoglycosides and cephalosporins on the proximal tubule of the human kidney. J. Antimicrob. Chemother. 4 (Suppl): 53, 1978.
22. Welwood, J.M. Simpson, P.M. Tighe, F.R. et al. Evidence of gentamicin nephrotoxicity in patients with renal allografts. Brit. Med. J. 3:278, 1975.
23. Schentag, J.J. and Plaut, M.E. Patterns of urinary beta-2 microglobulin excretion by patients treated with aminoglycosides. Kidney Int. 17:654, 1980.
24. Hsu, C.H. Maletz, R.M. Rozas, V.V. et al. Renal tubular sodium and water excretion in antibiotic-induced nephrotoxicity. Renal function in antibiotic nephrotoxicity. Nephron. 20:227, 1978.
25. Anderson, F.J. Linas, S.L: Bearns, A.S. et al. Non-oliguric renal failure. N. Engl. J. Med. 296:1-34, 1977.
26. Gary, N.E. Buzzeo, L. Salaki, J. et al. Gentamicin-associated acute renal failure. Arch. Intern. Med. 136:1101, 1976.
27. Luft, F.C. and Evan, A.P. Comparative effects of tobramycin and gentamicin on glomerular ultrastructures. J. Infect. Dis. 142:910, 1980.
28. Barza, M. The nephrotoxicity of cephalosporins: an overview. J. Infect. Dis. 137 (suppl):560, 1978.
29. Luft, F.C. Patel, V. Yom, M.N. et al. Nephrotoxicity of cephalosporin-gentamicin combination in rats. Antimicrob. Agents. Chemother. 9:831, 1976.
30. Moellering, R.C. Jr., And Swartz, M.N. The newer cephalosporins. N. Engl. J. Med. 294:24, 1976.
31. Casteel, D.O. and Sparks, H.A. Nephrogenic diabetes insipidus due to demethylchlortetracycline hydrochloride. J.A.M.A. 193:237,1965.
32. Fulop, M. and Dropkin, A. Potassium depletion syndrome secondary to nephropathy apparently caused by "outdated tetracycline." N. Engl. J. Med. 272:986, 1965.
33. Gross, J.M. Fanconi Syndrome (adult type) developing secondary to ingestion of outdated tetracycline. Ann. Intern. Med. 58:523, 1963.
34. Shils, M.E. Renal disease and the metabolic effects of tetracycline. Ann. Intern. Med. 58:389, 1963.
35. Falloon, W.W. Downs, J.J. Duggan, K. et al. Nitrogen and electrolyte metabolism and hepatic function and histology in patients receiving tetracycline. Am. J. Med. Sci. 233:563, 1957.
36. Barbour, G.L. Straub, K.D. O'Neal, B.L. et al. Vasopressin-resistant nephrogenic diabetes insipidus - a result of amphotericin B therapy. Arch. Intern. Med. 139:86, 1979.
37. Olivero, J.J. Lozano-Mendex, J. Ghafory, E.M. et al. Mitigation of amphotericin B nephrotoxicity by mannitol. Brit. Med. J. 1:550, 1975.
38. Gouge, T.H. and Andriole, V.T. An experimental model of amphotericin B nephrotoxicity with renal tubular acidosis. J. Lab. Clin. Med. 78:713, 1971.
39. Douglas, J.B. and Healy, J.K. Nephrotoxic effects of amphotericin B, including renal tubular acidosis. Am. J. Med. 46:154, 1969.
40. McCurdy, D.K. Frederic, M. and Elkinton, J.R. Renal tubular acidosis due to amphotericin B. N. Engl. J. Med. 278:124, 1968.

41. Butler, W.T. Bennett, J.E. Alling, D.W. et al. Nephrotoxicity of amphotericin B. Early and late effects in 81 patients. Ann. Intern. Med. 61:175, 1964.
42. Butler, W.T. Hill, G.J. Szwed, C.F. et al. Amphotericin B renal toxicity in the dog. J. Pharmacol. Exp. Ther. 143:47, 1964.
43. Holeman, C.W. Jr. and Einstein, H. The toxic effects of amphotericin in man. Calif. Med. 99:90, 1963.
44. Iovine, G. Berman, L.B. Halikis, D.N. et al. Nephrotoxicity of amphotericin B: A clinical-pathological study. Arch. Intern. Med. 112:853, 1963.
45. Takacs, F.J. Tomkiewicz, A.M. and Merrill, J.P. Amphotericin B nephrotoxicity with irreversible renal failure. Ann. Intern. Med. 59:716, 1963.
46. Ekroyan, G. and Roberts, A.D. Nephrotoxicity of amphotericin B: Observations on the mechanism of hypokalemia. Antimicrob. Agents Chemother. 2:497, 1962.
47. Rhoades, E.R. Ginn, H.E. Muchmore, H.G. et al. Effect of amphotericin B upon renal function in man. Antimicrob. Agents Ann. 1960:539, 1961.
48. Lentnek, A.L. Rosenworcel, E. and Kidd, L. Case report: acute tubular necrosis following high-dose cefamandole therapy for hemophilus parainfluenzae endocarditis. Am. J. Med. Sci. 281:164, 1981.
49. Tune, B.M. Wu, K.Y. Fravert, D. et al. Effect of cephaloridine on respiration by renal cortical mitochondria. J. Pharm. Exp. Ther. 210:98, 1979.
50. Swain, R.R. and Briggs, S.L. Positive interference with the Jaffe reaction by cephalosporin antibiotics. Clin. Chem. 23:1340, 1977.
51. Foord, R.D. Cephaloridine, cephalothin and the kidney. J. Antimicrob. Chemother. 1 (Suppl): 119, 1975.
52. Tune, B.M. Relationship between the transport and toxicity of cephalosporins in the kidney. J. Infect. Dis. 132:189, 1975.
53. Verma, S. and Kieff, E. Cephalexin-related nephrotoxicity. J.A.M.A. 234:618, 1975.
54. Tune, B.M. Effect of organic acid transport inhibitors on renal cortical uptake and proximal tubular toxicity of cephaloridine. J. Pharm. Exp. Ther. 181:250, 1972.
55. Rosenthal, T. and Boichis, H. Nephrotoxicity of cephaloridine. Br. Med. J. 4:115, 1971.
56. Cotton, J.R. Jr., Schwartz, M.M. Lindley, J.D. et al. Acute renal failure following halothane anesthesia. Arch. Pathol. Lab. Med. 12:628, 1976.
57. Deutsch, S. Effects of anesthetics on the kidney. Surg. Clin. North Am. 55:775, 1975.
58. Hartnett, M.N. Lane, W. and Bennett, W.M. Non-oliguric renal failure and enflurane. Ann. Intern. Med. 81:560, 1974.
59. Fry, B.W. Taves, D.R. and Merin, R.G. Fluorometabolites of methoxyflurane. Anesthesiology. 38:38, 1973.
60. Halpren, B.A. Kempson, R.C. and Coplon, N.S. Interstitial fibrosis and chronic renal failure following methoxyflurane anesthesia. J.A.M.A. 223:1239, 1973.
61. Frascino, J.A. Varamee, P. and Rosen, P.P. Renal oxalosis and azotemia after methoxyflurane in man. N. Engl. J. Med. 283:676: 1970.
62. Beutsch, S. Bastron, R.D. Pierce, E.C. et al. The effects of anesthesia with thiopentone, nitrous oxide, narcotics and neuromuscular blocking drugs on renal function in normal man. Brit. J.

Anaesth. 41:807, 1969.
63. Deutsch, S. Pierce, E.L. and Vandam, L: Cyclopropane effects on renal function in normal man. Anaesthesiology. 28:547, 1967.
64. Crandell, W.B. Pappas, S.G. and MacDonald, A. Nephrotoxicity associated with methoxyflurane anesthesia. Anesthesiology. 27:591, 1966.
65. Goldenberg, L. Tratamiento de la enfermedad de Basedow y del hipertiroidismo por fluor. Rev. Soc. Med. Int. Soc. Tsiolog. 6:217, 1980.
66. Harkonen, S. and Kjellstrand, C. Contrast nephropathy. Am. J. Nephrol. 7:69, 1981.
67. Mudge, G.H. Nephrotoxicity of urographic radiocontrast drugs. Kidney Int. 18:540, 1980.
68. Byrd, L. and Sherman, R.L. Radiocontrast-induced acute renal failure a clinical and pathophysiological review. Medicine. 58:270, 1979.
69. Gelman, L.M. Rowe, J.W. and Coggins, C.H. Effects of an angiographic contrast agent on renal function. Cardiovasc. Med. 4:313-1978.
70. Heneghan, M. Contrast-induced acute renal failure. Editorial Am. J. Roentgenol. 131:1113, 1978.
71. Hanaway, J. and Black, J. Renal failure following contrast injection for computerized tomography. J.A.M.A. 238:2956, 1977.
72. Ansari, Z. and Baldwin, D.S. Acute renal failure due to radiocontrast agents. Nephron. 17:28, 1976.
73. Garber, G.L. and Read, R.C. Protective effect of hypervolemia in cardioangiography. J.A.M.A. 180:376, 1962.
74. Caldicott, W.J.H. Hollenberg, N.K. and Abrams, H.L. Characteristics of response of renal vascular bed to contrast media. Evidence for vasoconstriction induced by renin-angiotensin system. Invest. Radiol. 5:539, 1970.
75. Abelson, H.T. and Garnick, M.B. Renal failure induced by cancer chemotherapy. In: Rieselbach, R.E. and Garnick, M.B. (eds), Cancer and the Kidney, Philadelphia, Lea & Febiger, 1982, pp. 769-813.
76. Garnick, M.B. and Mayer, R.J. Management of acute renal failure associated with neoplastic disease. In: Yarbro, J.W. and Bornstein, R.S. (eds): Oncologic Emergencies, NY, Grune and Stratton, 1981,pp.247-271.
77. Lyman, N.W. Hemalatha, C. Viscuso, R.L. et al: Cisplatin-induced hypocalcemia and hypomagnesemia. Arch. Intern. Med. 140:1513, 1980.
78. Weinberg, J.M. Simmons, C.F. and Humes, H.D. Renal mitochondrial injury is an early pathogenetic event in cis-platinum (CP) nephrotoxicity. Clin. Res. 28:464A, 1980.
79. Yuhas, J.M. and Culo, F. Selective inhibition of the nephrotoxicity of cis-dichlorodiamine platinum (II) by WR-2721 without altering its anti-tumor properties. Cancer Treat. Rep. 64:57, 1980.
80. Filipski, J. Kohn, K.W. Prather, R. et al. Thiourea reverses crosslinks and restores biological activity in DNA treated with dichlorodiamminoplatinum (II) Science 294:181, 1979.
81. Frick, G.A. Ballentine, R. Driever, C.W. et al. Renal excretion kinetics of high dose cis-dicnlorodiammine-platinum (II) administered with hydration and mannitol diuresis. Cancer Treat. Rep. 63:13, 1979.
82. Ross, D.A. and Gale, G.R. Reduction of the renal toxicity of cis-dichlorodiammine-platinum (II) by probenecid. Cancer Treat. Rep. 63:781, 1979.
83. Shilsky, R.L. and Anderson, T. Hypomagnesemia and renal magnesium wasting in patients receiving cisplatin. Ann. Intern. Med. 90:929, 1979.

84. Madias, N.E. and Harrington, J.T. Platinum nephrotoxicity. Am. J. Med. 65:397, 1978.
85. Weiss, R.B. Streptozotocin: a review of its pharmacology, efficacy and toxicity. Cancer Treat. Rep. 66:427, 1982.
86. Harmon, W.E. Cohen, H.J. Schneeberger, E.E. et al. Chronic renal failure in children treated with methyl-CCNU. N. Engl. J. Med. 300:1200, 1979.
87. Nichols, W.C. and Moertel, C.G. Nephrotoxicity of methyl-CCNU. N. Engl. J. Med. 301:1181, 1979.
88. Kundaria, B. Armentrout, S. Margileth, D. et al. Nephrotoxicity of semustine. Proc. Am. Soc. Clin. Oncol. 22:352, 1981.
89. Schacht, R.C. and Baldwin, D.S. Chronic interstitial nephritis and renal failure due to nitrosourea (NU) therapy. Kidney Int. 14: 661, 1978.
90. Pitman, S.W. and Frei, E. III. Weekly methotrexate-calcium leukovorin rescue: Effect of alkalinization on nephrotoxicity, pharmacokinetics and use in CNS-non-Hodgkins lymphoma. Cancer Treat. Rep. 61:695, 1977.
91. Weinstein, G.D. Methrotrexate. Ann. Intern. Med. 86:199, 1977.
92. Link, D.A. Fosburg, M.T. Ingelfinger, J.R. et al. Renal toxicity of high dose methotrexate. Pediatr. Res. 10:455, 1976.
93. Cotran, R.S. Tubulointerstitial diseases. In: Brenner, B.M. and Rector, F.C. The Kidney, 2nd Edit., Philadelphia, WB Saunders, 1981. pp. 1633-1667.
94. Kleinknecht, D. Kanfer, A. Morel-Maroger, L. et al. Immunologically mediated drug induced acute renal failure. Contrib. Nephrol. 10:42.
95. Ditlove, J, Weidmann, P, Bernstein, M, et al: Methicillin nephritis, Medicine. 56:483, 1977.
96. Gabow, P.A. Lacher, J.W. and Neff, T.A. Tubulointerstitial glomerular nephritis associated witn rifampin. Report of a case. J.A.M.A. 235:2517, 1976.
97. Mattson, K. Riska, H. Forsström, J. et al. Acute renal failure following rifampin administration. Scand. J. Resp. Dis. 55:291, 1974.
98. Kleinknecht, D. Homberg, J.D. and Decroix, G. Acute renal failure after rifampin. Lancet. 1:1238, 1972.
99. Arneil, G.L. Emmanuel, I.G. Flatman, G.E. et al. Nephritis in two children after irradiation and chemotherapy for nephroblastoma. Lancet. 1:960, 1974.
100. Avner, E.D. and Ingelfinger, J.R. Special considerations in the Pediatric Patient. In: Rieselbach, R.E. and Garnick, M.B. Cancer and the Kidney, Philadelphia, Lea and Febiger, 1982, pp. 275-302.

DISCUSSION: SYSTEMIC DISEASES

PANELISTS: Alan Gruskin, M.D., Julie Ingelfinger, M.D., Gwendolyn Scott, M.D., Norman Siegel, M.D. and Carlos Vaamonde, M.D.

MODERATOR: Jose Strauss, M.D.

MODERATOR: Does anyone want to challenge any of the statements which were made? Any questions?

QUESTION: Do you biopsy all your patients with lupus (SLE)? When you treat them, how do you determine how long to treat with high dose corticosteroids or whatever regimen you use? Do you follow the clinical response? Do you follow any particular parameters?

RESPONSE: I have to admit that we have been fairly liberal in biopsing patients who have SLE. I guess we can blame it on the disease since there is a silent SLE lesion which has always worried us, particularly in the younger children. I would say that most of our patients have been biopsied almost on routine bases. I am not sure that I can extend that to all patients who have SLE. I think that, as we say for so many situations, you have to individualize based on the patient's clinical presentation. I would say that any patient who has clinical evidence of renal involvement should have a renal biopsy done. It is not easy to predict which one of the lesions will be present. There are certain clinico-pathologic correlates but there are enough exceptions to any of those correlates to make a biopsy relevant in SLE. Certainly, the patient who has no clinical evidence of renal involvement but who has serological evidence of a very active disease which persists over a short period of time, a month or so, would be a candidate for biopsy and perhaps for altering treatment accordingly. I cannot prove to you that the early treatment of the clinically silent proliferative lesion is more effective than the treatment started when the lesion becomes clinically apparent. But we do biopsy children fairly regularly who have good documentation of SLE.

QUESTION: Specifically, what in the biopsy makes you change from treating the non-renal manifestations to getting the big guns out and treating the kidney? What specific features in the biopsy do you follow as significant? What are you looking for?

RESPONSE: I think that evidence of a diffuse proliferative involvement with or without glomerular necrosis would be very important. A second finding would be crescent formation. Certainly, the patient who on electron microscopy has subendothelial deposits which are seen in more than one capillary loop is at high risk for progressive renal disease. In those situations where we find a diffuse proliferative lesion particularly associated with subendothelial deposits on EM, we go to fairly aggressive therapy with corticosteroids and immunosuppressive agents, and continue that therapy even when the clinical manifestations of the disease, other than renal disease, are under control. We follow the DNA binding capacity and the serum complement levels; although they are not always predictive of the relapse of the disease, they are a helpful indicator if they have been abnormal initially and begin to return to normal levels, that the patient is responding to therapy. Usually, it is also evident that the patient is feeling better. However, the proteinuria can persist for a very long time. Since many of these patients will not have a reduced renal function on the initial presentation, the serologic tests can offer you a good handle. We do not alter the immunosuppressive regimen so as to normalize the SLE serologically, but we do like to see a pattern of return toward normal values and then a stabilization of that within about two months of starting therapy.

COMMENT-QUESTION: I would like to ask the audience, since we have a large number of practicing pediatric nephrologists, how many of you recommend biopsy in every patient you see who has SLE? I think that most do, from the number of raised hands. This may be the only thing that we all agree upon.

COMMENT-QUESTION: We have a split decision in our Unit, two of us do and only one does not; that is why I did not raise my hand. I have a Chairman who believes that it is not necessary and he is beginning to persuade me.

QUESTION-COMMENT: First, I want to know if in some patients who have a negative ANA titer you have searched for deficiencies of complement components as it is known that congenital deficiency of C_2 and C_4 may present with a picture similar to SLE. Second, I was surprised because of the statement of the questionable value of plasmapheresis. Personally, I am very impressed with the results obtained in our Unit on patients who did not respond to cytotoxic agents. The third comment and a question is that in one of our patients who was already on peritoneal dialysis with a serum creatinine of 8 mg/dl, after a couple of months of plasmapheresis the serum creatinine started to come down and currently the patient is off dialysis. I would like to know your thoughts on that.

COMMENT-RESPONSE: I would agree that it is unusual to see a patient who has SLE and is ANA negative. I think that we definitely see patients who have a lupus-like syndrome who are ANA positive but DNA negative or do not elevate their anti-DNA antibody substantially above normal. In the ANA negative patient in whom you feel that the clinical complex is SLE, I think you are right in that you want to look for another immunodeficiency, a complement deficient syndrome. The second thing you want to do is to ask the laboratory to do the ANA with an anti-IgM rather than with an anti-IgG. There are a handful of patients who have been reported as having an IgM anti-nuclear antibody but not an anti-IgG anti-nuclear antibody. We have had that happen to us twice and we have seen one patient with the congenital complement deficiency syndrome with a lupus-like clinical disease. We will begin to see these patients who do not have the extractable nuclear antigen. With regard to plasmapheresis, like so many therapies in SLE, it is a very emotionally charged area. I think that in the published studies that are available, both in the abstracts of the American Society of Nephrology last year and this year and in the poster presentations, it has not been an overwhelmingly impressive therapy. We have all seen a patient who responds, and I am not saying that I would necessarily deny that to a patient, but I am just not convinced that that is going to be the solution for these patients. My great frustration is the inability of the nephrologists in this country to come to some reasonable collaborative effort to study what is a rare disease. Each one of us has one or two patients with whom we struggle very hard, and sometimes we see them improve with a variety of therapies, but we need a nationwide collaborative study to answer that question. The last question you asked was about the patient with SLE, who while on dialysis, begins to get better; that is as you know, relatively unique. There is an interstitial nephritis that can have an almost purely interstitial component to a SLE nephritis which can recover like a prolonged ATN. Maybe that is what that patient had; I do not know whether or not a biopsy was done. That type of a patient was discussed five or ten years ago at a New England Journal CPC; I do not know why they got the correct diagnosis since it is such an unusual renal involvement in SLE.

MODERATOR: What about the study being carried out in Chicago? At our last exchange a couple of years ago they thought that plasmapheresis was working well. Do you know how it is coming along?

RESPONSE: I do not know the people there personally. I know that there was one paper presented by the group at the American Society of Nephrology in 1984; their conclusion was that if you have diffuse proliferative lesions on biopsy, you are at high risk for progressive renal disease. They did not present any data on plasmapheresis. They may still be collecting it because it is a very slow process to collect information on treated and control patients.

QUESTION: The biopsy finding on the patient I mentioned was diffuse proliferation. That patient was hypertensive and the hypertension was controlled with several antihypertensive agents before his creatinine started to decrease.

COMMENT: In relation to the use of plasmapheresis in Chicago, they stated recently that this issue is still unsettled. With respect to your patient, we all have seen such a patient. A year or two ago at the EDTA meeting, some investigators reported following patients with Acute Renal Failure who were on dialysis for at least three months; some patients who were transplanted were included. After a number of months on dialysis or after transplantation, those patients regained the renal function they had lost. When the causes of the renal disease were looked at, the vasculitides were at the top of the list. So, if you have a patient who has one of these disorders, particularly if he has hypertension and then the hypertension is controlled, do not be surprised if he regains his renal function. I would call that a successful therapy. These physicians even changed their rules for transplanting patients; now they wait at least one year before transplanting somebody who has one of those diseases since he may regain function of his kidneys.

COMMENT-QUESTION: I would like to ask one of the panelists to comment on the concept of one form of SLE nephropathy converting to another. Certainly there have been reports of that. Earlier in this session it was asked, "Who biopsies patients?" For those of us following patients with SLE who might get the disease at a very young age, the question is: "When do we re-biopsy them and what leads us to be suspicious that the histological changes have converted?" Of course, when things all seem better, you do not really want to pick up a biopsy needle to show that the disease has gone away, unless you are going to stop something like cytotoxic drugs, perhaps. I would like to hear your comments on that.

RESPONSE: I think that the conversion of the lesions occurs in two different settings. One is within the natural history of the disease. There is good documentation that with a mild proliferative lesion, either without therapy or with minimal amounts of therapy, the extra-renal manifestations of the disease can be controlled. Then there may be a marked and persistent change in the serological tests, like the anti-DNA which may have been minimally active suddenly becomes very active, or the C_3 and C_4 levels which had been near normal, become very low and it looks again like the patient's initial presentation. Under those conditions, I would be suspicious that an histological conversion has occurred. This would especially be true if there were any changes in renal presentation or clinical manifestations. The other instance in which we have seen conversion of lesions is under therapy where a patient begins with a diffuse proliferative and necrotizing lesion with subendothelial deposits, there is a quieting down of the renal disease, there is a normalization or near normalization of the serological tests, and the patient remains with proteinuria. The patient comes in with four grams of protein in the urine, is treated but the proteinuria persists at one or two grams/day, the serum complement is normal, and 18 months to two years into his course of therapy, one asks: "Should I continue with the immunosuppressive agent at this point? Could I get along just with low dose corticosteroids?" We have tended to biopsy such a patient; frequently, we have found a conversion of the original diffuse proliferative and necrotizing SLE to a membranous pattern. We cannot prove that this was drug induced since it was an uncontrolled study. Because those patients began with a fairly severe lesion, they all were treated initially, so whether or not the conversion was because of the natural course of the disease cannot be known. That is the second circumstance in which one can use a biopsy to help the patient. We feel that a conversion from a diffuse proliferative lesion toward a membranous lesion and the disappearance of sub-endothelial deposits, are very good prognostic signs for the patient. At that point, we do take them off of their immunosuppressive agent (if they are on one) because, obviously, the long term immunosuppressive risk factor, especially the risk factor related to tumors even with azathioprine usage, is important for these very young patients who are going to have a life-long SLE disease, and probably a waxing and waning pattern. Those are the two situations where interconversion of lesions has been well documented.

MODERATOR: A few years ago the group from Mexico presented a couple of patients at the Workshop of this Seminar. In those patients, the nephrotic syndrome associated with or due to membranoproliferative changes did not have a good correlation between the clinical course and the histological changes. In other words, as one patient improved clinically, his renal biopsy findings worsened; the other patient was just the reverse, with clinical worsening and renal biopsy improvements. How often do you see, or have you seen it at all, or has anybody here seen patients with SLE who have followed such a course? Or, do the biopsy changes always correlate well with clinical changes?

RESPONSE-QUESTION: There is one paper that describes progressive renal insufficiency without much in the way of clinical manifestations in a group of children. I have the impression that the clinical course may not necessarily fit with the histopathology. We have seen a few children who looked like they had terrible pathology but clinically were reasonably benign. In response to a previous question, we have seen one adolescent who sounds just like the patient described: he came in like he had Rapidly Progressive Glomerulonephritis, had a biopsy with crescents and diffuse proliferation, was hypertensive, was put on a lot of drugs, was dialyzed for a month or two, came off dialysis, but subsequently developed persistent renal failure. He may have been a compliance problem with therapy as well. Did your patient subsequently redevelop renal failure?

RESPONSE: No.

COMMENT: One other comment. A government agency asked the Executive Committee of the Council on Clinical Nephrology, Dialysis and Transplantation of the National Kidney Foundation to report on the current status of plasmapheresis in the treatment of various renal diseases, including transplantation rejection. The questions were circulated to about 25 nephrologists around the country and elsewhere. There were two situations for which the respondents agreed that there were clear indications for plasmapheresis: Goodpasture's Disease and some of the myeloma-renal failure syndromes. As for any of the other diseases, the consensus was that there are no hard data in any prospective controlled fashion that would suggest that plasmapheresis positively influences outcome. The final statement was that there are a number of issues which require appropriate study.

QUESTION: I do not want to belabor a point but there is the observation, at least in adult patients, published in the Annals of Internal Medicine that while patients are receiving hemodialysis, many of the other symptoms of SLE tend to resolve, and the immunological activity of the disease reflected in the serology, tends to quiet down. That raises the question of whether or not there may be some improvement in renal function which is associated with changes in the immunology while the patient is undergoing hemodialysis. Have you seen that in children who reach End-Stage Renal Disease and go on dialysis? What about changes in the other symptoms of SLE?

RESPONSE: There has been the concept that if the patient has bad renal involvement and goes into End Stage Renal Disease, he will burn out his SLE and become asymptomatic. While that observation is real clinically, if one keeps some of those patients on dialysis long enough, they will have recrudescence of their SLE. We have had two patients who have been for relatively long terms on hemodialysis therapy, both have had clear relapses of their SLE, with polyserositis, arthritis, and an elevated anti-DNA titer. I think what happens is that an acute exacerbation, during which they've lost their renal function, burns out. It just follows the natural history of the disease which is to wax and wane in terms of its clinical course. But there are good examples, besides our two anecdotal ones, of SLE patients who have recrudescence of their disease while on dialysis therapy. So, I do not think that dialysis itself is doing anything against recurrence of the disease.

COMMENT: We also have seen a couple of patients who have done the same thing. After several months of dialysis the renal function has returned and we have been able to discontinue dialysis. My question pertains to your last comment regarding SLE's characteristic of waxing and waning. Would that then preclude transplantation in your view?

RESPONSE: No, I do not think so but I certainly can stand to be corrected. It is interesting that in our last review, we did not find a patient who had a recurrence of SLE nephritis in a transplanted kidney. I would point out that for the kidney transplant patient the most commonly used drugs before cyclosporine were a combination of prednisone and azathioprine, also a treatment regimen that has been used long term for the treatment of SLE. Some data in the NZB mouse suggest that if one begins immunosuppressive therapy before clinically apparent SLE in that animal model, one will not see renal involvement. Thus, it may be that we do not see recurrence of SLE nephritis in the transplanted kidney because we are treating the patient with drugs which have some effect on their native disease.

MODERATOR: Are we ready to leave SLE for a little bit? The answer seems to be "yes".

COMMENT: I want to discuss two or three other topics. I was struck by the fact that the renal lesion in AIDS in young children and infants was quite different from the renal lesion that has been described in adults. One of the intriguing possibilities is that the adult patients described were largely an addict population. They had the focal sclerosing lesion alluded to in the first Panel Discussion. A number of us have heard these data presented at various places, including the ASN and the International Meeting in Los Angeles in 1984. I am beginning to wonder now whether or not their observation is a heroin nephropathy, if there is such a thing.

MODERATOR: I was at the ASN when a couple of papers on AIDS in adults were presented, one of them from Miami. There is no question that some places seem to have more focal and segmental sclerosis than others. I do not know why; maybe they are following the patients longer. Those places seem to have that histological picture with greater frequency also in association with other disorders, not only AIDS. Here, pathologist Dr. Victoriano Pardo and the adult nephrologists have found that histology, but in fewer patients. The hypothesis that we have come to agree upon is that besides the influence of heroin on that population, the duration of AIDS may have something to do with the finding. The adults obviously have had more time than the children have to develop some reaction to immune complexes or other deposits.

COMMENT: You also may be looking at something immunologically different in the children than in the adults. We find, in general, that children have a poor antibody formation to many different types of antigens. For instance, even if they develop severe cytomegalovirus infection, it is rare that we can pick up cytomegalovirus antibody. Although they have high immune complexes, we do not know against what those complexes are directed. We do find, at least in the younger children, that they have difficulty making antibody to some of the common antigens, particularly polysaccharide antigens. It may have something to do with the immune system of the infants and their response.

COMMENT-QUESTIONS: I wanted to ask about the clinical findings of hematuria and proteinuria in the little children with AIDS. Under what concomitant circumstances were they there? Since all of us are going to be seeing patients like these, it is critical for us to know: did they have any evidence of clotting abnormalities at the time? Were they treated with or affected by anything that would cause temporary proteinuria? What can you tell us about the on-going situation?

MODERATOR: We got involved with these questions because we had exchanges with some of the people in New York who were involved in the early reports of AIDS. I asked them if they were seeing renal disorders, and if not, why did they think that there were no renal changes with such a quantity of circulating immune complexes? I could not get a clear explanation. When I came back to Miami, I marched into Dr. Gwendolyn Scott's office and said: "Gwen, we need to start looking at the urine of those AIDS patients because there must be something going on in the kidneys!". She said: "What else is new? Sure, they have proteinuria, and sure, we are finding urinary abnormalities." She had the data carefully maintained and had filed all the information. Then it was a matter of getting organized and finding somebody as reliable as Dr. Brenda Sanchez-Montane to systematically study the patients. There may be something else that is causing those problems; these are very complex patients who are very sick and have several problems going on at the same time. Somebody else within Pediatric Nephrology or Infectious Diseases who knows those patients more intimately should comment on this. One of the points made earlier pertained to the temperature of these patients; we looked into that and all but one turned out to be afebrile at the time of the study. Some call this non-specific proteinuria. We also need to look into the other illnesses present since they are dismally ill. Most of these patients have been studied subsequently in an out-patient setting, where the GFR's were done.

COMMENT-RESPONSE: It is of interest that in general their basic kidney function seemed to be fairly normal. We found exacerbation of proteinuria during times of acute illness or when they were admitted to the hospital with fever and infection. With the clearing of the infection and fever, in those patients with intermittent proteinuria, the latter would also clear. In those with persistent proteinuria, it remained even after the infection cleared; but these were the minority of patients we saw.

COMMENT: Although I do not know much about it, there is an entity called "febrile proteinuria" which supposedly occurs mainly in older children, usually with high fever, usually with bacterial infections, and it usually goes away in two to three weeks. I am not aware of any data in children below one year of age.

MODERATOR: The other point that needs discussion is the degree of proteinuria. The people in Jamaica have called attention to the fact that in patients with sickle cell disease they find quite often 1+ proteinuria but not so often larger amounts. We have seen gross proteinuria in some of these AIDS patients at times when they really were not so sick. It is not in most of them, but it can be something striking.

COMMENT: People talk about febrile proteinuria being able to have up to 1 gm/day, which is a rather significant amount.

COMMENT-QUESTION: I want to question the documentation that the Hepato-Renal Syndrome is so rare in children. I personally have seen several cases which I thought perhaps had that syndrome. I would like to briefly describe the situation. I didn't even think that it was important to write them up. Two patients were children with cystic fibrosis who had cirrhosis, bleeding esophageal varices, end-stage hepatic disease, and obviously, they also had severe pulmonary disease. They went into a condition which we felt was not just Acute Tubular Necrosis because of urinary findings, etc. The third was a girl who ultimately died of acetaminophen poisoning with hepatic toxicity. Her urinary findings and urinary indices were compatible with what we thought was Hepato-Renal Syndrome. Her kidneys were used for a transplant and functioned as any other transplanted kidneys. These were older adolescents and one may choose not to consider them as children. I would like your comments on that.

RESPONSE: As you know, I am not a pediatrician, so I looked carefully in the world's literature as far as the search would go. If you look at any major text of pediatrics or nephrology, you will not find any reports. If you feel strongly, you can prove to an Editorial Board that you do have pediatric patients with Hepato-Renal Syndrome and you should be able to have that material published. This is precisely the kind of information we all need. That was the reason I said that probably there are unreported anecdotal cases. Of course, there are cases of acetaminophen poisoning that are called Pseudo-Hepato-Renal Syndrome; I agree with that. What we do not seem to see, is this form of renal failure which occurs in well-established cirrhosis of the liver, in end of the line VA patients or municipal hospital patients, which every large city has. These patients, without any precipitating event, evolve into this form of lingering Acute Renal Failure for a few weeks until they die, as Dr. Solomon Papper used to say, "not <u>of</u> renal failure but <u>in</u> renal failure". They usually die of something like massive bleeding, hepatic coma, sepsis, etc. These patients do evolve into Acute Tubular Necrosis, do have nephrotoxicity, do have dehydration despite expanded blood volumes, and so on. It is a very hard issue to prove in the adult, but it is even harder to prove its presence in children. I have asked other pediatric nephrologists; they have assured me that it is very hard to come by one of these cases. If you feel that you have, by all means you should go ahead and publish them.

COMMENT: I would echo what was said earlier, since I was going to say the same thing. I have seen three or four cases, two in cystic fibrosis, and at least one in a child who had Hepatic Fibrosis with renal insufficiency. The liver disease in the last one was worse than in the others; he had a couple of episodes which seemed to be superimposed on his renal failure--an Hepato-Renal Syndrome kind of picture, although we never stressed him or tested it. That does not fit the diagnosis; I realize that.

COMMENT: But you should join efforts with the previous commentator and publish those cases. In one month at this Medical Center, we may see somewhere from four to ten cases of Hepato-Renal Syndrome in adults. Not all are going to be; that is going to be discussed in the differential diagnosis. This is a fairly common event in the hospitals that deal with chronic patients or with poor people coming to Community Hospitals. I'm sure that this happens also in hospitals that deal with more well-to-do people, because alcoholism doesn't have a price tag, as we see in this country. There is a great difference in prevalence and frequency, and there are no publications on children. So, please write them down.

COMMENT: I was sitting here, nudging my colleague who is saying that in our chronic cystic fibrosis population, our group has seen a number of patients who really would fit the diagnosis. Of course, a lot of them could be qualified as young adults but it is a unique population, probably not seen by internists. Therefore, it is something that we all ought to look into.

MODERATOR: We need to diversify the subject matter but we have another comment.

COMMENT-QUESTION: I have one more question about the Hepato-Renal Syndrome. Could you describe for me the relationship between the BUN and serum creatinine in the adult population? Do they parallel each other?

RESPONSE: Regarding a person with the Hepato-Renal Syndrome, you may be facing one of several situations: if there is no blood in the GI tract, there is no bleeding process, of course, and the BUN would tend to be much lower (proportionately) than the serum creatinine or, better said, the increase in the BUN would be proportionately smaller due to the inability of the liver to synthesize albumin. Somebody is saying "No", but there are data from human liver biopsies done by Surgery Department members here in Miami showing that the liver of people with cirrhosis cannot synthesize albumin normally. This is counteracted by the presence of blood in the GI tract or elsewhere, or by a hypercatabolic state. It is a difficult question to answer. Most of our patients are admitted with a BUN of 3-5 mg/dl if they are not bleeding. The serum creatinine also will be relatively low, a bit like a cancer patient, in whom the serum chemistries mask the true level of GFR because their muscle mass is grossly decreased due to the fact that these are chronic wasting diseases. So, their pool of creatinines is low. If I see a serum creatinine of 1.2 mg/dl in a severe cirrhotic, I am worried; his GFR may be only 30-40 ml/min/1.73m^2. I do not know whether or not I answered your question; I assume that in children it should not be much different, even when considering the low serum values that they have.

COMMENT: I would like to make a couple of random comments addressed primarily to the audience and not to the elite panel. The first I'd like to say is I'd like very much to vote for legalizing bias. As Dr. Strauss indicated, he presented some material which was biased; he went so far as to indicate that one group in Chicago has some interesting data to report but nobody has seen the data yet. I think that is fascinating! Really, what I need to comment on is the Report on Congenital Heart Disease. Again, some random thoughts. I was a little horrified at what we are doing to children with congenital heart disease as I looked at the data presented. As I listened to the other people, I had some time to calm down and realize that maybe there is a little bias in the presentation too. As the presenter knows, and I just want to point out to the audience, you have to be careful about lumping patients with Cyanotic Congenital Heart Disease and Acyanotic Congenital Heart Disease since they are miles apart. Individuals with lesions who are acyanotic or cyanotic are as different as different can be, depending on the severity of the lesion. We all know this. But there are other things which you need to keep in mind: that is, who is the surgeon? What happened in the operating room? When was this done? Were these procedures done 20 years ago, five years ago, or when? There is a tremendous difference among surgeons who are doing this kind of work and they refer to themselves as differentiating between the men and the boys. All the boys can do coronary bypass surgery; it takes the men to do Congenital Heart Disease surgery. Known from a lot of experience accumulated through the years, what happens to the patient, 90% of it happens in the operating room. Not only how long is the procedure, but how good is the repair? I think that it is very difficult to do any retrospective studies in this group of patients; they have to be done prospectively.

There were two comments made which I would like to share and emphasize: one has to do with the importance of biologic maturation and what happens early in life to the development of some of these homeostatic processes. It is in this context that the general approach to Congenital Heart Disease at the present time is early surgical repair. By early surgical repair, I mean in the first months of life. The men are doing this extremely well; I'd be leary of the boys attempting to do this. The second very interesting point which was made and which I'd like to emphasize, is the similarity between the vasculature in the lung and the kidney. Those interested in Congenital Heart Disease have had a lot of experience and have made a lot of observations on what happens in the lungs and what happens to pulmonary pressure when the individual is exposed to various noxious stimuli. For example, if individuals are exposed to hypoxia, what happens to the pulmonary artery tree? There is tremendous individual variability in terms of how much pulmonary hypertension results from similar levels of hypoxia. I cannot help but wonder if similar things do not happen in the kidney, and not only whether the kidney vasculature responds to noxious stimuli but whether there is tremendous individual variation in terms of the nature of the response. It is the kind of information that I would hope gets reviewed and explored. Thank you.

MODERATOR: Thank you! For those of you who do not know the last commentator, he is a statesman and a very good friend of mine who played a key role in my coming to Miami. He always brings out the questions of ethics, behavior, statistical relevance, bias, and so on. In my own defense, it was interesting to me to find that the data I was looking for had been stored prospectively as raw data. With that data we can ask the statisticians to set in motion the processing which will yield meaningful results. Even more, they can request the additional points which are missing because those patients are still being followed.

COMMENT-RESPONSE: I agree with everything you have said. First of all, I put the data together on one slide, mixing acyanotic with cyanotics in terms of the numbers, trying to show basal patterns which happen to exist. Clearly, they are not comparable groups. I wonder, for example, in the acyanotic group, whether the shunts, the obstructions and the coarctations are really three different situations and whether or not only the complex cyanotics are different. Second, in terms of the data on surgery, the two studies quoted looking at the incidence of Acute Renal Failure came from very fine centers; a lot of their patients are young, and a lot of them have complex lesions. This is what you would expect as you work your way back. That is not to imply that all of those who developed Acute Renal Failure needed dialysis. We are talking about rises in serum creatinine which may reverse. The point I was trying to make simply was that those who came to dialysis had a very difficult time; but, in reality, that is a small fraction. Thirdly, in terms of the pulmonary-kidney vasculature, this is something that I have always found fascinating. There are a number of parallels with the placenta. It is not just a lung but a lung-kidney. When you remove that "artificial" organ, the two organs in the body that undergo this vasodilatation with some of the anatomical changes which have been described, are the lung and the kidney. Their responses to stress in the newborn period seem to be much more extensive than that of the older individual; as aging occurs, they become less responsive to stress. If you think in terms of one of my favorite forms of science, teleology, it makes great sense. This is an area that is worthy of additional exploration. The surgeons are clearly doing better. The other thing that is fascinating is this uric acid business, the fact that maybe it plays some kind of role in what happens post-operatively. It makes sense; if you have lots of uric acid floating around, perhaps the post-op cardiac patient is sort of like the chemotherapeutically treated leukemic: they are set to make a lots of uric acid; if they get stressed, they make it. Some people think that uric acid is a vasoactive drug; other people think it is a useless substance.

COMMENT: I am glad that the previous comments were made, in that I wanted to comment about some of the interesting and provocative data on piglets which one of the speakers has. I was grateful that he was talking about it, and thought that the renal failure induced by contrast material was something I should have put in my slides. I was glad that he put that in his. Part of what was described earlier today in those youngsters who were getting high doses of contrast media is something which is quite likely age-related. I would like to mention some comparable studies that were done in Boston looking at immature rabbits. The investigator had a kidney preparation where he could look at A-V differences of iodothalamate and also do PAH clearances. With that set-up and an on-line computer, he was able to look at GFR minute to minute. What he found, using the usual radio-contrast material that we are used to (Renografin®), was that these rabbits, especially the very immature ones, had an immediate massive drop in GFR which took some time to recover, and that later, renal plasma flow seemed to decrease, as you found that it did. Interestingly, there are some experimental and not yet released radio contrast agents which are not so hypertonic, which will be released within the next year or two, and which cause not so much diminution in GFR, just some.

MODERATOR: I know that one of the panelists has reviewed the subject of nephrotoxicity on many occasions, and has included contrast material among his interests. Could you discuss briefly gentamicin nephrotoxicity in the newborn?

RESPONSE: I have been studying for the last five years a model of contrast media nephrotoxicity in the diabetic rat. We concluded, after a long study, that there is a tremendous specie difference in the Acute Renal Failure response. In particular, for contrast media, the rat is not a good model. We still do not know why there is contrast media nephrotoxicity. What somebody can show after radiocontrast injection in mice is that within 30 minutes the GFR drops. But the question as to whether or not they are going to get Acute Renal Failure, nobody can answer. A number of these patients do not . You have to do more long range studies; but, of course, there are lots of limitations to doing that in humans. And again, there are a lots of specie differences; it is very difficult to interpret the literature. We are more aware of contrast media nephrotoxicity but what it is, I do not have the least idea because there are, among others, rheological, hemodynamic, and toxic factors.

COMMENT: Theoretically, it seems to me that there should be much more gentamicin toxicity in the newborn period; and yet, it is not reported. As far as I know, some of the animal studies which have been reported would also suggest that the very young are resistant to it. That has always surprised me.

MODERATOR: But some would say that it depends on how you define nephrotoxicity and what changes you follow: enzymes (which ones?), serum creatinine, etc.

COMMENT: That is true. It has been a while since I was a House Officer but there was gentamicin back in those days, and we always gave a slightly lower dose so we may have "biased" the results in a way that was clinically fortunate.

COMMENT: Chronic lithium therapy for the manic depressive disorders may cause, in the long run, some form of chronic interstitial nephritis. Recently, the question of End Stage Renal Disease was brought up in a study, but the study itself has been questioned because it was not a longitudinal one. Now that the data are coming back from longitudinal assessments, it is clear that 1) psychiatric patients, without receiving lithium therapy, do have renal function and histology abnormalities; 2) up to a follow-up of two years, there are no manifestations. For up to eight years we have followed patients receiving continuous lithium treatment at low doses to avoid nephrotoxicity; they have no changes in GFR. I know of no study in children in this regard; such studies may need to be done.

COMMENT: Clearly, manic depressive diseases in childhood are not very well understood. Indeed, depression in childhood is only being discussed now. The longitudinal studies which could come out of this age group might be very important since there are going to be some patients on treatment for a very long time.

MODERATOR: Our colleagues, mates, and the sunshine are all waiting for us. Our time is up. Thank you.

III

NUTRITIONAL ASPECTS OF HYPERTENSION AND ATHEROSCLEROSIS

THE ROLE OF SODIUM IN CHILDHOOD HYPERTENSION

Alan B. Gruskin, M.D., Gary Lerner, M.D. and Larry E. Fleischmann, M.D.

Even though controversial, much data supports a relationship between sodium and blood pressure regulation. Despite such support, the precise role of the sodium ion in the hypertensive process remains elusive and many are not able to demonstrate positive correlations (1). Also, relatively few studies of this relationship in pediatric populations exist. To be considered here are mechanisms by which sodium and blood pressure may be related, the impact of altering sodium balance on blood pressure in normotensive and hypertensive adults and children, genetic influences on sodium homeostasis, and the treatment, control and prevention of hypertension by means of reducing one's sodium load. Not considered here are studies demonstrating a role in the hypertensive process for calcium, (2), magnesium, (3), and chloride (4). This article focuses on the view that sodium plays an important role in primary hypertension.

Population Studies. Studies in multiple societies suggest that sodium influences blood pressure. In many unacculturated groups ingesting a diet containing approximately 60 mM of salt daily throughout life, blood pressure values in the elderly are similar to those of young adults (5,6). Upon migration to areas where the salt intake is much higher, a large fraction of such groups develop hypertension. Unacculturated groups exposed to a high sodium intake do develop hypertension in the absence of obesity (7). Noteworthy is the observation that blood pressure increases during the childhood years in all societies.

Mechanism of Hypertension. The mechanism(s) by which blood pressure increases when salt is ingested is multifactorial and not simply that of volume expansion. Differences exist in salt sensitive compared to salt-resistant individuals. For example, peripheral resistance in salt-sensitive Dahl rats increases after the animals are fed a high salt diet. Conversely, peripheral resistance appropriately falls in salt resistant rats fed a similar diet (8).

The increase in blood pressure associated with salt loading may result from increases either in cardiac output and/or peripheral resistance. In patients with end stage renal disease both mechanisms may be operative with 80% of patients developing hypertension as a consequence of increases in peripheral resistance and 20% experiencing an increased cardiac output (9).

The ability of the kidney to excrete sodium is another factor influencing blood pressure responses when sodium is ingested. In isolated perfused whole kidney studies, less sodium is excreted at a given level of blood pressure in salt-sensitive versus salt-resistant rats.

This occurs in groups of rats fed both low and high salt diets (10). Explanations for these differences in salt sensitive rats include difference in a circulating humoral factor, perhaps a natriuritic hormone, in prostaglandin activity in the kidney, and in papillary blood flow (11).

The level of activity of the sympathetic nervous system influences salt mediated increases in blood pressure. Surgical sympathectomy of nerves innervating the hindquarters in salt sensitive Dahl rats lowers by 50% the blood pressure response to salt loading (12). Chemical sympathectomy in infantile Dahl salt-sensitive rats prevents the onset of salt mediated hypertension. The full expression of salt induced hypertension appears to require catecholamine containing neurons in the brain (13). Infusions of angiotensin II into the lateral ventricle of the brain in Dahl sensitive rats increases blood pressure twice as much as that occurring in salt resistant rats. Artificially induced lesions in the AV3V area of the third ventricle inhibit salt induced rises in susceptible animals.

<u>Studies in Experimental Animals</u>. A number of studies in animals demonstrate a clear relationship between sodium and the onset and/or the persistence of hypertension. Investigators have developed groups of inbred rats whose mature blood pressure is not only salt dependent but genetically determined. The most extensively studied model is the Dahl rat. The salt sensitive Dahl rat becomes irreversibly hypertensive only when its diet contains a certain amount of sodium; otherwise it remains normotensive (14). Additionally, rats fed a high salt diet for six weeks, compared to two weeks after weaning display significantly higher blood pressure levels at 12 months. Those started on a high salt diet at weaning, in contrast to those fed a similar salt diet beginning either three or six months after weaning, develop higher blood pressures even though all become hypertensive and die as a consequence of their disease (15). In short, not only is sodium induced hypertension genetically determined, in this model the time of exposure as well as its duration is critical.

The central role of the kidney in generating hypertension in the Dahl rat is demonstrable by organ transplantation studies. Transplanting a kidney from a salt-sensitive to a salt-resistant rat leads to hypertension; transplanting a kidney from a salt-resistant to a salt-sensitive rat lowers blood pressure. These studies indicate that even though the sympathetic nervous system can play a major role in blood pressure regulation as noted above, there are other models and mechanisms that operate in the absence of sympathetic innervation. Similar effects are demonstrable in the Milan rat model of hypertension (11).

<u>The role of sodium in regulating blood pressure in adults</u>. When considering recommendations relative to salt intake, an important issue to understand is the degree to which alterations in the dietary intake of sodium and perhaps potassium influence blood pressure in normotensive as well as hypertensive individuals. Of equal importance is the degree to which such responses are influenced by race, genetics and age.

Sodium restriction to a mean level of 69.5 mEq/day in normotensive adults is associated with a dual response. In a group of 31 normotensive adults most lowered both systolic, x = -6.3 mmHg, and diastolic, x = -5.5 mmHg. Some (7/31) failed to lower their blood pressure and even experienced increases. Such changes can occur in the absence of demonstrable alterations in either potassium excretion or body weight (16).

Normotensive blacks may be at greater risk for increasing their blood pressure than whites when dietary sodium intake is increased. When blood pressures in normotensive blacks and whites are evaluated after being allowed to stabilize on sodium intakes ranging from 10 to 1500 mEq/day, blood pressure increases to a lesser degree (13 mmHg) at a higher sodium intake (1200 mEq/day) in whites than in blacks (21 mmHg at a sodium intake of 800 mEq/day) (17). Of interest is the finding that virtually all adults challenged with enough sodium for a number of days experience a rise in blood pressure (18). The blood pressure increase related to sodium intake can be attenuated in some by replacing simultaneously experienced potassium losses. The mechanism by which blood pressure increases in these individuals involves increases in cardiac output, and plasma levels of norepinephrine. As expected, aldosterone and renin activity fall.

Not only does the level of sodium intake influence blood pressure in normotensive adults, it alters the effect of norepinephrine on blood pressure. In adults ingesting a 10 or 800 mEq sodium diet daily, a positive linear correlation is observed between the amount of norepinephrine infused and the increment in mean arterial blood. The threshold response to norepinephrine infusion is less and plasma levels higher in those ingesting the low sodium diet and vice versa (19). In another group of 52 normotensive young adults ages 20 to 25 years, 22 were shown to be salt sensitive. Compared to 30 salt resistant subjects, salt sensitive individuals display the following characteristics: pressor responses to norepinephrine are double, salivary sodium concentrations are less, and the incidence of a positive family history is 2.5 fold higher. The salt sensitivity in this group was attributed to an enhanced sympathetically mediated increase in the proximal tubular reabsorption of sodium (20).

Two types of response to salt restriction occur in hypertensive adults. When adults with essential hypertension are given a daily sodium diet containing either 9 or 249 mEq/day, salt sensitive and salt resistant groups can be identified (21). Some patients fail to lower their blood pressure when their sodium intake is lowered; others experience a paradoxical increase in blood pressure presumably because of the stimulation of either the sympathetic nervous system and/or the renin angiotensin system (22).

It is difficult to demonstrate sustained lowering of blood pressure in hypertensive adults when salt intake is modestly lowered. Different responses to sodium loading are observed in hypertensive adults. When given a progressively increasing sodium intake of up to 1500 mEq/day, greater amounts of sodium are retained and blood pressure increases to a greater degree in some. In others no increase in blood pressure occurs (23). Blacks exhibit a greater increase in blood pressure than whites. Potassium may be as important as sodium in mediating the observed changes in blood pressure. When the sodium related kaliuresis is corrected by administering potassium, blood pressure does not increase as significantly (24).

Insofar as sodium homeostasis influences blood pressure regulation, changes in either the size and/or composition of various body compartments ought to exist in hypertensive subjects. Such differences have been reported and have been correlated by some with age and the presence or absence of hypertension. In hypertensive adults, exchangeable and total body sodium correlates positively with blood pressure and increasing age; also total body and exchangeable potassium correlate inversely with blood pressure and age (25).

Recent studies suggest that the blood pressure longevity effect on weight loss is due to changes in sodium balance. When sodium is given to dieting obese individuals, blood pressure does not fall as weight is lost. Others feel that the mean exchangeable total body sodium is normal in hypertensive adults.

The question arises as to whether one's salt appetite is inherited or acquired and whether differences exist in hypertensive populations. Most data suggest that salt appetite is acquired. For example, primitive and/or non-westernized societies normally ingesting low salt diets uniformly dislike added salt when first offered yet eventually accept the added salt as part of their routine diet. Also, individuals known to be heavy users of salt after a few weeks are easily able to adapt to a diet containing a few hundred milligrams of salt; others feel that they not only exhibit an increased desire for salt but when exposed to salt ingest greater amounts than normotensive individuals (26). It is not clear whether genetically at risk offspring of hypertensive parents have an altered oral threshold for salt.

Therapeutic studies. Support for sodium influencing blood pressure is provided by therapeutic studies showing that reducing the body burden of sodium either by reducing its intake or increasing its output reduces blood pressure in some hypertensive individuals. Dietary reductions in sodium intake influence blood pressure acutely and chronically. Reducing the dietary intake of sodium in adults from 200 to 100 mmol/day has a small effect on blood pressure whereas further reduction in sodium intake more significantly lowers blood pressure. Based on population studies it is probable that the relationship between sodium and blood pressure is semilogarithmic rather than linear. Thus the impact of lowering sodium intake becomes increasingly more apparent when salt intake is reduced from 90 to 10-25 mEq/day (27). A major problem with dietary reductions in sodium intake as a therapy for lowering blood pressure is the unwillingness of most individuals to chronically ingest such diets. Also, not all individuals respond.

Increasing sodium excretion through the use of diuretics effectively lowers blood pressure in many hypertensive individuals (28). The blood pressure lowering effect of some diuretics can be either blunted or eliminated by providing extra sodium when the diuretic is administered. Others have shown that part of the effect of diuretics may be through mechanisms other than their impact on renal sodium excretion even though diuretic therapy may effectively lower blood pressure. Chronic diuretic therapy in hypertensive children should not necessarily be viewed as the first agent to use in treating mild primary hypertension in children. Their long term effect on electrolyte homeostasis, uric acid metabolism, carbohydrate and lipid metabolism may place individuals at increased risk (28, 29). In large populations, the impact of these risk factors is less compared to that of an increased blood pressure (30).

The reduction in blood pressure seen in obese subjects during the first few weeks of dieting may be the result of salt restriction rather than weight loss per se. In dieting adults maintained on 10 gm of salt daily, blood pressure falls only after weight falls to 20% below their ideal (26).

The role of sodium in childhood blood pressure. Data on the role of sodium influencing blood pressure levels in children are unclear. Studies evaluating the impact in drinking water of high concentrations of sodium on blood pressure in children yield conflicting results (31). Also, available information provides conflicting data on the issue as to whether reductions in sodium intake chronically lowers blood pressure in hypertensive children (32). Intakes of sodium in children far in excess of those found in most hypertensive children can be shown to elevate blood pressure (33). Changing sodium intake in 20 children ages 6-9 with a blood pressure above the 95% but less than 130/90 mmHg, lowered sodium excretion from 130 to 87 mEq/day, but failed to significantly lower blood pressure (34). In a group of eight children ages 8-19 years with primary hypertension studied for 15 consecutive days while ingesting diets containing amounts of sodium initially normal, next low (<10 mEq m^2 day), and finally high (>150 mEq m^2 day) mean systolic and diastolic blood pressure fell from 134/87 to 125/82 mmHg and increased minimally with the higher salt intake (35).

Racial differences in cation excretion can be demonstrated in the offspring of hypertensive parents. Rates of sodium excretion in black children were increased and potassium excretion reduced in a single center study comparing the offspring of black and white hypertensive families (36). The blacks also had lower levels of plasma renin activity. Approximately 25% of black hypertensive adolescents when compared to black controls excreted excessive amounts of sodium thereby exhibiting an "exaggerated" natriuresis (28, 37).

When either normal or hypertensive children are placed on diets containing low, normal or high amounts of sodium, a curvilinear relationship between either plasma renin activity and urinary or plasma aldosterone levels can be demonstrated (28, 37). Adolescent children with primary hypertension exhibit three types of hypertension: hypertension associated with low or suppressed, normal or elevated plasma renin activity (28, 37) or aldosterone (38). In one study, low renin hypertension in hypertensive black adolescents was associated with a reduced sodium excretion (39). Evidence exists suggesting that individuals with low renin hypertension are salt sensitive. When the renin angiotensin system is acutely stimulated by giving furosemide orally, a significant fraction of hypertensive adolescents ingesting low sodium diets compared to those ingesting normal sodium diets respond by lowering rather than further increasing their plasma renin activity (37). The explanation for the dissociation between sodium balance and renin is unknown.

Finally, salt loading influences the blood pressure response to mental stress in adolescents. When teenagers with a positive family history of hypertension were compared to an age matched group without a family history of hypertension, a statistically significant increase in blood pressure in response to solving mathematical problems occurred in the offspring of hypertensive parents. Post-stress plasma catecholamine levels were also higher. After ingesting 10 gram sodium tablets for 14 days, the offspring of hypertensive parents developed a higher baseline blood pressure and a greater elevation after being mentally stressed. The blood pressure as well as the response to stress in the control group did not change (40, 41).

A logical question based on the role of sodium in generating and sustaining hypertension in the experimental animal is whether the magnitude of sodium intake during the neonatal period influences blood pressure in humans. Since very high intakes of salt potentially lead to increases in blood pressure in many normal adults, another issue is that of deciding what is a "normal" salt intake in the human neonate. Neonates receiving breast milk ingest an average of 7-8 mEq of sodium per day (1 mEq/100 kcal) and often excrete less than 2 mEq of sodium per day. By six months of age infants ingesting breast milk alone imbibe 1 mEq/kg/day of sodium. Until the past few years most commercially available infant formulas contained sodium in concentrations approximately two to three times that of breast milk. Most American suppliers have altered their manufacturing process so that formulas whose sodium content is similar to breast milk are available. Cow's milk contains 22.5 mEq/L of sodium.

Prior to the reduction of sodium in commercially processed baby food beginning in the early seventies, infants ingested approximately 6-8 mEq/kg/day of sodium (35). Despite even further lowering of the sodium content in processed foods, 40-50% of infants still have a sodium intake exceeding 4 mEq/kg/day (42). Homemade baby food may contain up to ten times the amount of sodium in processed food.

Debate as to whether salt appetite in children is acquired or learned continues. Differences in salt threshold in children cannot be correlated with levels of "normal" blood pressure. Available data suggest that most of a child's salt intake is determined by that of the adult members of the family. Infants ingest equal quantities of food whether salted or not. By early childhood, most children prefer food that contains significant quantities of salt, most likely because of social influences. Black compared to white children prefer higher concentrations of salt.

A most important issue is whether the quantity of sodium ingested during the neonatal period influences the normal maturationally associated increase in blood pressure. In one carefully done study in which a group of infants ingested a sodium diet equal to that of breast milk for 12 weeks followed by the addition of solid foods containing 2-14 mEq/L for 12 more weeks, mean blood pressure was 2.1 mmHg less than that of a group whose mean sodium intake was approximately three times higher (43). Additionally, the rate of rise of blood pressure was significantly less in the group ingesting less sodium. The degree to which the observed changes will persist as these children mature and what if any effect such differences will ultimately have on adult blood pressure levels and salt preference need long term study. Others have not found that sodium intake during the first years of life influences blood pressure levels. Clearly the ingestion of lower amounts of sodium associated with artificial neonatal feeding practices during the rapid growing phases ought not to constitute a significant risk if the amount of sodium ingested is similar to that obtained from breast milk feeding alone.

In summary, available data derived from epidemiologic, genetic, experimental and clinical studies support the conclusion that sodium plays an important role in influencing the onset and sustaining components of hypertension. Studies of societies suggest that salt intake in "acculturated" groups is high. Genetically driven studies demonstrate a relationship between sodium intake and blood pressure. Unfortunately the precise manner by which sodium influences the hypertensive process remains elusive as does our ability to unequivocally identify those individuals with or at risk for developing primary hypertension who might benefit were their sodium intake to be significantly altered. Still to be decided is whether a societal thrust ought to be a reduction in sodium intake and whether such a reduction ultimately favorably impacts on cardiovascular disease.

REFERENCES

1. Nicholls, M.G.: Reduction of dietary sodium in western society, benefit or risk? Hypertension, 6:795, 1985.
2. Perlman, S.A., Prebis, J.W., Gruskin, A.B., et al: Calcium homeostasis in adolescents with essential hypertension. Seminars in Nephrology 3:149, 1983.
3. Resnick, L.M., Laragh, J.H., Sealey, J.E., Alderman, M.H.: Divalent cations in essential hypertension: Relations between serum ionized calcium, magnesium and plasma renin activity. N Eng J of Med, 309:888, 1983.
4. Kotchen, T.A., Luke, R.G., Ott, C.E., Galla, J.H., Whitescarver, S.: Effect of chloride on renin and blood pressure responses to sodium chloride. Ann Int Med 398:817, 1983.
5. Olivier, W.J., Cohen, E.L., Neel, J.V.: Blood pressure, sodium intake, and sodium related hormones in the Yanomamo Indians, a "no-salt" culture. Circulation 52:146, 1975.
6. Prior, I.A.M., Evans, J.G., Harvey, H.P.B., Davidson, F., Lindsey, M.: Sodium intake and blood pressure in two Polynesian populations. N Engl J Med 279:515, 1968.
7. Page, L.B., Damon, A., Moellering, R.C., Jr.: Antecedents of cardiovascular disease in six Solomon Island societies. Circulation 49:1132, 1974.
8. Canguli, M., Tobian, L., Iwai, J.: Cardiac output and peripheral resistance in strains of rats sensitive and resistant to NaCl hypertension. Hypertension 1:3. 1979.
9. Onesti, G., Kim, K.E., Greco, J.A., Del Guericio, E.T., Fernandes, M., Swartz, C.: Blood pressure regulation in end-stage renal disease and anephric man. Circ Res 36:I-145, 1975.
10. Tobian, L., Lange, J., Azar, S., Iwai, J., Koop, D., Coffee, K., Johnson, M.A.: Reduction of natriuretic capacity and renin release in isolated, blood-perfused kidneys of Dahl hypertension prone rats. Circ Res 43:I-92, 1978.

11. Tobian, L.: Salt and Hypertension: The role of the kidney in hypertension. In Genest, J., Kuchel, O., Hamet, P., Cantin, M., (eds.): Hypertension, Second Edition. McGraw-Hill, New York, 1983, pp 73-83.
12. Takeshita, A., Mark, A.L.: Neurogenic contribution to hindquarters vasoconstriction during high sodium intake in Dahl strain of genetically hypertensive rats. Circ Res 43:I-86, 1978.
13. Goto, A., Ikeda, T., Tobian, L., Iwai, J., Johnson, M.A.: Brain lesions in the paraventricular nuclei and catecholaminergic neurons minimize NaCl hypertension in Dahl salt-sensitive rats. Clin Sci 61:53s, 1981.
14. Dahl, L.K., Heine, M., Tassinari, L.: Role of genetic factors in susceptibility to experimental hypertension due to chronic excess salt ingestion. Nature 194:480, 1962.
15. Dahl, L.K., Knudsen, K.D., Heine, M.A., et al: Effects of chronic excess salt ingestion: Modification of experimental hypertension in the rat by variations in the diet. Circ Res 22:11, 1968.
16. Miller, J.Z., Daugherty, S.A., Weinberger, M.H., Grim, C.E., Christian, J.C., Lang, C.L.: Blood pressure response to dietary sodium restriction in normotensive adults. Hypertension 5:790, 1983.
17. Weinberger, M.H., Luft, F.C., Bloch, R., Henry, D.P., Pratt, J.H., et al: The blood pressure-raising effects of high dietary sodium intake: Racial differences and the role of potassium. J of Am College of Nutr 1:139, 1982.
18. Murray, R.H., Luft, F.C., Bloch, R., Weyman, A.E.: Blood pressure responses to extremes of sodium intake in normal man. Proc Soc Exp Biol Med 159:432, 1978.
19. Rankin, L.I., Luft, F.C., Henry, D.P., Gibbs, P.S., Weinberger, M.H.: Sodium intake alters the effects of norepinephrine on blood pressure. Hypertension 3:650, 1981.
20. Skrabal, F., Herholz, H., Neumayr, M., Hamberger, L., Ledochowski, M., Sporer, H.: Salt sensitivity in humans is linked to enhanced sympathetic responsiveness and to enhanced proximal tubular reabsorption. Hypertension 6:152, 1984.
21. Kawasaki, T., Delea, C.S., Bartter, F.C., Smith, H.: The effect of high sodium and low sodium intakes on blood pressure and other related variables in human subjects with idiopathic hypertension. 64:193, 1978.
22. Longworth, D.K., Drayer, J.I.M., Weber, M.A., Laragh, J.H.: Divergent blood pressure responses during short-term sodium restriction in hypertension. Clin Pharmacol Ther 27:544, 1980.
23. Luft, F.C., Rankin, L.I., Bloch, R., Weyman, A.E., Willis, L.R., Murray, R.H., Grim, C.E., Weinberger, M.H.: Cardiovascular and humoral responses to extremes of sodium intake in normal black and white men. Circulation 80:617, 1979.
24. Luft, F.C., Weinberger, M.H.: Sodium intake and essential hypertension. Hypertension 4(Suppl 3):III-14-III-19, 1982.
25. Lever, A.F., Beretta-Piccoli, C., Brown, J.J., Davies, D.L., Fraser, R., Robertson, J.I.S.: Sodium and potassium in essential hypertension. Br Med J 283:1, 1981.
26. Dahl, L.K.: Salt intake and hypertension. In Genest, J., Kuchel, O., Hamet, P., Cantin, M.,(eds.): Hypertension, Second Edition. McGraw-Hill, New York, 1977, pp. 548-559.

27. Brown, J.J., Lever, A.F., Robertson, J.I.S., Beretta-Piccoli. C., Davies, D.L., Fraser, R., McAreavey, D., Semple, P.F.: Blood pressure and sodium: A personal view. In Genest, J., Kuchel, O., Hamet, P., Cantin M., (eds.): Hypertension, Second Edition McGraw-Hill, New York, 1983 pp 632-645.
28. Gruskin, A.B.: The adolescent with hypertension. In Blumenthal, S. (ed.): Hypertension: Prevention, Diet and Treatment in Infancy and Childhood. Proceedings from a symposium, Bethesda, Maryland, May 25, 1983. Biomedical Information Corporation. pp. 35-39, 1983.
29. Gruskin, A.B.: Antihypertensive drug usage in children with primary hypertension. 88th Ross Conference on Pediatric Research, May 13-15, 1984. (In press).
30. Narins, R.G.: Mild hypertension: A therapeutic dilemma. Kidney International, 26:881, 1984.
31. Hofman, A.: Editorial Review: Blood pressure in childhood: An epidemiological approach to the etiology of hypertension. Hypertension 2:323, 1984.
32. Costa, F.V., Ambrosioni, E., Montebugnoli, L., Paccaloni, L., Vasconi, L., Magnani, B.: Effects of a low-salt diet and of acute salt loading on blood pressure and intralymphocytic sodium concentration in young subjects with borderline hypertension. Clin Sci 61:21s, 1981.
33. McQuarrie, I., Thompson, W.H., Anderson, J.A.: Effects of excessive ingestion of sodium and potassium salts on carbohydrate metabolism and blood pressure in diabetic children. J Nutr 1936;11:77-101.
34. Gillum, R.F., Elmer, P.J., Prineas, R.J., Surbey, D.: Changing sodium intake in children. The Minneapolis Children's Blood Pressure Study. Hypertension 3:698, 1981.
35. Rauh, W., Levine, L.S., New, M.I.: The role of dietary salt in juvenile hypertension. In Giovanneli, G., et al. (eds.): Hypertension in Children and Adolescents. Raven Press, New York, 1981, pp. 34-44.
36. Hohn, A.R., Riopel, D.A., Keil, JE., Loadholt, C.B., Margolius, H.S., et al: Childhood familial and racial differences in physiologic and biochemical factors related to hypertension. Hypertension 5:56, 1983.
37. Gruskin, A.B., Baluarte, H.J., Kaiser, B.A., Polinsky, M.S., Morgenstern, B.Z., Perlman, S.A.: Hypertension in the adolescent; Physiologic studies and treatment issues. Proc. Sixth Int. Symp. Paed. Neph., Hannover, FRG. Brodehl, J. and Ehrich, J. (eds.) pp. 372-377, 1984.
38. New, M.I., Baum, C.J., Levine, L.S.: Nomograms relating aldosterone excretion of urinary sodium and potassium in the pediatric population: their application to the study of childhood hypertension. Am J of Cardiol, 37:658, 1976.
39. Kilcoyne, M.M., Thomson, G.E., Branche, G., Williams, M., Garnier, C., Chiles, B., Soland, T.: Characteristics of hypertension in the black population. Circulation 50:1006, 1974.
40. Falkner, B., et al: The role of sodium in essential hypertension in genetically hypertensive adolescents. In Onesti, G., et al. (eds.): Hypertension in the Young and the Old. New York, Grune & Stratton, 1981, p 29.

41. Falkner, B.: Cardiovascular reactivity and psychogenic stress in juveniles. In NHLBI Workshop on Juvenile Hypertension, Loggie, J.M.H., Horan, M.J., Gruskin, A.B., et al. Proceedings from a Symposium, Bethesda, Maryland, May 26-27, 1983, pp 161-171.
42. Pediatric Hypertension Subgroup to the Hypertension Task Force, National Heart, Lung, and Blood Institute. (1979): DHEW publication no. (NIH) 79-1628.
43. Hofman, A., Hazebroek, A., Valkenburg, H.A.: A randomized trial of sodium intake and blood pressure in newborn infants. JAMA 250:370, 1983.
44. Supported in part by NIH Grants #HL 23511 and 19869.

HORMONAL FACTORS IN JUVENILE HYPERTENSION

J.R. Ingelfinger, M.D.

Both cardiac output and peripheral vascular resistance are involved in the determination of blood pressure level. Peripheral vascular resistance depends on a number of factors including local factors (ionic, humoral and autoregulatory); the adrenergic nervous system; and circulating humoral agents, both vasoconstrictor (renin, angiotensin, aldosterone and catecholamines) and vasodilator (prostaglandins and kinins). In this seminar, some of the hormonal aspects of blood pressure control as they relate predominantly to primary hypertension, will be considered. A variety of hormones are involved, but this presentation will focus on the renin-angiotensin-aldosterone system. (For reviews, the reader is referred to references (1-4).)

RENIN ANGIOTENSIN FUNCTIONS

Renin is produced in the juxtaglomerular cells in the macula densa of the kidney (1-4). In the kidney, secretion is affected by renal nerves, adrenergic receptors and by renal tubular sodium (1-4). In the human and most other mammalian species, renin appears to be relatively high in the perinatal period in the plasma, and falls with age (5). The significance of the elevated plasma renin activity in early life is as yet unknown.

The renin angiotensin system (RAS) plays a pivotal role in blood pressure control. In the normal individual, different physiologic states such as sodium depletion, upright posture and hemorrhage all stimulate renin secretion. Factors which inhibit or stimulate renin release are shown in Table I. It is well known that in pathologic situations such as renovascular hypertension (6), renin is stimulated, and in some forms of essential hypertension, renin is elevated (7).

For some time it has been known that renin is present in a variety of extrarenal tissues in many mammals (8). In addition to evidence that the

TABLE I: FACTORS WHICH INFLUENCE RENIN RELEASE

Decrease	Increase
Beta adrenergic blockade	Beta adrenergic stimulators
Alpha adrenergic stimulators	Diuretics
Mineralcorticoids	Vasodilators
Angiotensin II	EDTA (Ca^{2+} efflux)
Vasopressin	Glucogon
Salt load	Prostaglandins
Volume expansion	Catecholamines
	Salt loss
	Volume loss

kidney is most important in renin secretion, renin has been found in the adrenal (9), in vascular tissue (both endothelium and smooth muscle cells) (10), in the brain (11), the uterus (12), testis (13), salivary gland (14), and in a variety of extrarenal tumors (15).

In order to begin to understand why the RAS is present in multiple sites, and why it appears to be so active early in life, it may be important to examine not only renin biochemistry and physiology, but also to examine renin molecular biology.

Renin is an acid protease with a heavy chain of 31,000 daltons and light chain of about 5,000 connected by a single disulfide bond. Renin acts on its substrate, angiotensinogen, which is produced in the liver, to produce a decapeptide, angiotensin I. Angiotensin converting enzyme removes 2 amino acids to produce angiotensin II, which is a very potent vasoconstrictor substance. Various angiotensinases break down AII into largely inactive fragments, although angiotensin III, which is a 7 amino-acid compound, does have some activity.

RENIN PROCESSING

Studies on renin synthesis and secretion have shown a great deal about the intracellular processing of renin. Since the mouse salivary gland contains large amounts of renin, much concerning renin cell biology has been discovered by studying this organ. It would appear that renin is synthesized from its messenger RNA as a preproenzyme and is rapidly translocated into the lumen of the endoplasmic reticulum (16,17). Subsequently, renin is processed to a proform and then in the Golgi apparatus to the final mature, active enzyme which is packaged and stored in secretory granules. For the processing and maturation of prorenin to renin, 2 proteolytic cleavages are necessary, the first at an arginine-serine (arg-ser) bond, which converts prorenin to a single chain polypeptide, and the 2nd at a site which removes the dipeptide (arg-arg) resulting in 2 chains. Studies in the mouse salivary gland using the pulse chase technique (17), where labeled S-35 methionine can be incorporated into protein and renin identified by specific antirenin antibody, suggest that renin is translated very quickly from the preproform which is inactive to prorenin which is inactive (16). Prorenin is relatively quickly changed to one chain renin; only slowly is the one chain form turned into the two chain form. It would also appear that 1 and 2 chain forms are secreted in the mouse. In addition to the slow processing in granules (a "regulated" pathway), there seems to be a constitutive pathway where one chain renin may be rapidly secreted from the Golgi under circumstances which remain to be defined.

It may be asked whether the kinetics of cellular renin processing change under various stimuli and whether the amount of renin specific messenger RNA (mRNA) changes under certain circumstances. For example, Dzau and colleagues have shown that a low salt diet will stimulate both renal and cardiac renin mRNA production (18).

Is it possible that levels of renin-specific mRNA vary during ontogeny in different mammalian species? It may be that post-translational processing also changes during growth and development.

In a non-human model, the mouse (13,19), differences in renin processing occur during growth and development. In male mice carrying 2 renin genes (some strains have just one) renal renin appears to remain at constant levels (per mg of protein) during development. However, extrarenal renin (salivary gland, testes, adrenal) appears to be relatively high in the immediate newborn period, to drop down thereafter, and to rise again only after puberty. Furthermore, there are apparent differences pre- and post-puberty in the proportion of one and two-chain renin secreted by mouse salivary glands (19-20). This may suggest that prior to puberty, the constitutive pathway quickly responds when renin is needed whereas afterward, the more mature system is utilized. Whether similar extrarenal events occur in other mammals during growth and development awaits investigation.

Once active renin has acted upon its substrate producing angiotensins, angiotensin II (AII) has effects in a variety of ways (1-4). It causes vascular smooth muscle to contract and also has effects on the renal tubules, glomerular mesangial cells, adrenal cortex and central nervous system (1-4). A variety of studies using pharmacologic interruption of the renin angiotensin system has made it possible to learn something of responses. For example, infusions of angiotensin II will decrease renal blood flow and increase blood pressure (21). Saralasin, an angiotensin II partial agonist, but primarily antagonist, blunts this response (22). Using inhibitors of angiotensin converting enzyme such as captopril, the effects of AII are also blunted (23). Recent studies by Norman Hollenberg and Gordon Williams and their colleagues, would suggest that certain individuals with essential hypertension appear to have a blunted response to AII infusion (24). Some of these individuals would appear to be the same population who are salt sensitive essential hypertensives. These individuals with salt sensitive essential hypertension have a decreased ability to excrete a sodium load, an increase in blood pressure following salt ingestion, a reduced response of the renal vasculature to infused angiotensin II when salt loaded and a reduced responsiveness of the adrenal glomerulosa cell to angiotensin II infusion on a low sodium intake. Thus these individuals have abnormalities detectable both on a low and a high salt diet. According to Williams and Hollenberg, after salt is restricted, these so-called "non-modulators" have higher renin or angiotensin levels and a greater fall in blood pressure when given an angiotensin competitive antagonist saralasin (25). On a high salt intake, the non-modulator's renal blood supply behaves as if it is in a high angiotensin II environment and has reduced responsiveness to the infusion of AII, and a failure of the basal renal blood flow to increase the sodium loading. The administration of converting enzyme inhibitors normalizes the reduced adrenal responsiveness to angiotensin II in these individuals (26).

There is growing evidence that there is a vascular renin angiotensin system which is independent of the circulating system (27,28). For example, extrarenal renin-like enzymes, as mentioned above, have been coupled with evidence of immunoreactive angiotensin II in a variety of tissues. For instance, Swales and Thurston (29) reported that angiotensin antiserum was required to inhibit exogenous angiotensin effect in sodium loaded rats in excess of that which was predicted. The data could not be explained by alterations in AII receptor activity or sensitivity. Both vascular endothelial and smooth muscle cells appear to synthesize renin, and angiotensin converting enzyme is present in these cells. Additionally, circulating cells within the blood stream such as neutrophils have an angiotensin pathway where cathepsin G converts prorenin to renin, AI to AII and acts on substrate to produce AII (30). Such systems enable the very local interaction of the renin angiotensin system with other hormones such as prostaglandins, kinins, histamine and serotonin. This might explain how the local angiotensin system could play a role in vasospasm, hypertension, and atherogenesis.

The renin angiotensin system clearly interacts with other hormones (1-4,31). For instance, it has been shown that the administration of prostaglandin-inhibiting non-steroidal anti-inflammatories will prevent rises in plasma renin activity which might be seen by postural changes or hemorrhage. Various adrenergic agents also stimulate the production of renin as shown in a number of studies. For example, isoproterenol increases the secretion of renin tenfold, and can be blunted by a substance as propranolol. The importance of these interactions is unknown in juvenile hypertension. However, it has been shown by a number of researchers such as McCrory et al. (32), that adolescents with essential hypertension would appear to have a profile of resting norepinephrine which is higher than that of normotensive controls. Furthermore, some siblings of these individuals show a similar catecholamine pattern.

When experimental manipulations are performed such as the infusion of epinephrine, the normal autoregulatory curve where plasma renin activity increases as renal arterial pressure drops, is shifted to the right (1-4). Prostaglandins and kinins are known to be important in blood pressure regulation (1-4). For example, PGE_2, PGI_2, PGD_2, are all vasodilatory whereas thromboxane AII and PG F_2 Alpha, are vasoconstrictor in their actions (1-4). The fact that prostaglandin inhibitors will alter renin secretion suggests interaction (33,34). It is also known that prostaglandins which cause vasodilation also are involved in natriuresis and do cause renin release. The adrenergic effects of prostaglandins are important in that PGE_2 and PGI_2 are antiadrenergic. How all these factors interact is unclear. However, one obvious place for interaction is the fact that angiotensin converting enzyme is the same as kininase II. Thus, the same enzyme which forms the potent pressor AII, is that which leads to the breakdown of bradykinin. As mentioned, it is known that prostaglandin inhibitors will cause a decrease in blood pressure, and may also cause an increase in plasma renin activity.

The excretion of kallikrein has been found to vary from normal in certain sub-groups in patients with essential hypertension (34-35). Urinary excretion of kallikrein corrected for body surface area is low in early childhood and rises by age 3 to be close to adult levels (36). How this inverse pattern as compared to the findings of the renin angiotensin system is important in the development of essential hypertension is unknown. However, the level of urinary kallikrein is higher both in salt deprivation and salt loading in certain subgroups of patients with essential hypertension (34-36).

Still other hormones are known to be important in blood pressure regulation. These include ADH, serotonin (31), and natriuretic hormones such as ouabain like factors (37) and atrial natriuretic factor (38). The role of additional hormone systems in modulating blood pressure and in the interactions with the renin angiotensin system remain to be defined, especially in young people with essential hypertension.

The interactions of hormonal factors, sodium and divalent cations are no doubt important in the development and maintenance of essential hypertension in various age groups. It may be that one or more hormonal systems are abnormal, as suggested by some of the data mentioned above. Obviously this very complicated situation may require many further studies before it is elucidated.

REFERENCES

1. Vander, A.J: Renin-angiotensin systems. In: Stanley, J.C., Ernst, C.B., Fry, W.J. Renovascular Hypertension. WB Saunders Co., Philadelphia, 1984, p. 20ff.
2. Peach, M.J: The renin-angiotensin systems: Biochemistry and mechanisms of action. Physiol. Rev. 57:313, 1977.
3. Davis, J.O. (ed): Advances in our knowledge of the renin-angiotensin system. Fed. Proc. 36:1753, 1977.
4. Oparil, S. and Haber, E: The renin-angiotensin system. N. Engl. J. Med. 291:379-446, 1974.
5. Stalker, H.P., Holland, N.H., Kotchen, J.M., et al: Plasma renin activity in healthy children. J. Pediatr. 89:256, 1976.

6. Goldblatt, H., Lynch, J., Hanzel, R.F., et al: Studies on experimental hypertension. I. The production of persistent elevation of systolic blood pressure by means of renal ischemia. J. Exp. Med. 59:347, 1934.
7. Brunner, H.R., Laragh, J.H., Baer, L., et al: Essential hypertension: renin and aldosterone, heart attack and stroke. N. Engl. J. Med. 286:441, 1972.
8. Ganten, D., Schelling, P., Vecsei, P., et al: Iso: renin of extra-renal origin: The tissue angiotensinogerase systems. Am. J. Med. 60:760, 1976.
9. Ryan, J.W: Renin-like enzyme in the adrenal gland. Science. 158: 1589, 1967.
10. Re, R., Fallon, J.T., Dzau, V.J., et al:Renin synthesis by canine aortic smooth muscle cells in culture. Life Sci. 30:99, 1982.
11. Dzau, V.J., Brenner, A., Emmett, N.L: Evidence for renin in rat brain: differentiation from other renin-like enzymes. Am. J. Physiol. 242: E292, 1982.
12. Dzau, V.J. et al: Characterization of renin-like enzymes in the rabbit uterus by renin-specific antibody. Circulation. 62:III-238, 1980.
13. Ingelfinger, J.R., Pratt, R.E., Roth, T.P., et al: Androgen regulates submandibular gland (SMG) renin synthesis and secretion at multiple sites. Clin. Res. 33:362A, 1985.
14. Cohen, S, Taylor, J.M., Murakami, K., et al: Isolation and characterization of renin-like enzymes from mouse submaxillary glands. Biochemistry. 11:4286, 1972.
15. Robertson, P.W., Klidjian, A., and Harding, L.K: Hypertension due to a renin-secreting renal tumor. Am. J. Med. 43:963, 1967.
16. Pratt, R.E., and Dzau, V.J: Purification and characterization of one-chain and two-chain renins from mouse submandibular gland. Hypertension 6 (Suppl I): I-101, 1984.
17. Pratt, R.E., Ouellette, A.J., and Dzau, V.J: Biosynthesis of renin: multiplicity of active and intermediate forms. Proc. Natl. Acad. Sci. USA 80:6809, 1983.
18. Dzau, V.J., Ellison, K.E., and Ouellette, A.J: Expression and regulation of renin in the mouse heart. Clin. Res. 33:181A, 1985.
19. Ingelfinger, J.R., Pratt, R.E., Ellison, K.E., et al: Multiple sites of regulation of mouse renin expression in ontogeny. Clin. Exp. Htn. In press.
20. Piccini, N., Knopf, J.L., and Gross, K.W: A DNA polymorphism, consistent with gene duplication correlates with high renin levels in the mouse submaxillary gland. Cell. 30:205, 1982.
21. Vander, A.J: Control of renin release. Physiol. Rev. 47:359, 1967.
22. Streeten, D.H.P., Anderson, G.H., Freiberg, J.M., et al: Use of an angiotensin II antagonist (saralasin) in the recognition of "angiotensinogenic" hypertension. N. Engl. J. Med. 292:657, 1975.
23. Freeman, R.H., Davis, J.O., Watkins, B.E. et al: Effects of continuous converting enzyme blockade in renovascular hypertension in the rat. Am. J. Physiol. 236:F21, 1979.
24. Moore, T.J., Williams, G.H., Dluhy, R.G., et al: Altered renin-angiotensin-aldosterone relationship in normal renin essential hypertension. Circ. Res. 41:167, 1977.
25. Dluhy, R.G., Bavli, S.Z., Leung, F.K, et al: Abnormal adrenal responsiveness and angiotensin II dependency in high renin essential hypertension. J. Clin. Invest. 64:1270, 1979.

26. Williams, G.H. and Hollenberg, N.K: Converting enzyme inhibitors normalize the reduced adrenal responsiveness to angiotensin II in essential hypertension. J. Hypertension 2 (suppl 2): 43, 1984.
27. Lilly, S.L., Pratt, R.E., Alexander, R.W. et al: Cultured vascular endothelial cells contain the complete renin-angiotensin system.
28. Dzau, V.J: Vascular wall renin-angiotensin pathway in control of the circulation. Amer. J. Med. 77(4A):31, 1984.
29. Swales, J.D., and Thurston, H: Generation of angiotensin II antisera. Clin. Sci. Mol. Med. 45:691, 1973.
30. Dzau, V.J., Gonzalex, D., Kaempfer, C., et al: Human neutrophils release: a serine protease capable of activating inactive renin. Circulation. 68:111-385, 1983.
31. Fray, J.C.S., Lush, D.J., Valentine, A.N.D: Cellular mechanisms of renin secretion. Federation Proc. 42:3150, 1983.
32. McCrory, W.W., Klein, A.A., Rosenthal, R.A: Blood pressure, heart rate and plasma catecholamines in normal and hypertensive children and their siblings at rest and after standing. Hypertension. 4:507, 1982.
33. Lee, J.B: The renal prostaglandins and blood pressure regulation. Adv. Prostaglandin Thromboxane Res. 2:573, 1976.
34. Nasjletti, A., Malik, K.V: The renal Kallikrein-Kinin and prostaglandin systems interaction. Ann. Rev. Physiol. 43:597, 1981.
35. Margolius, H.S., Horwitz, D., Geller, R.G., et al: Urinary Kallikdrein excretion in normal man; relationships to sodium intake and sodium-retaining steroids. Circ. Res. 35:812, 1974.
36. Robillard, J.E.: The roles of Kallikrein-Kinin and prostaglandins in juvenile essential hypertension. In: Loggie, J.M.H., Horan, M.J., Gruskin, A.B. et al (eds): NHLBI Workshop on Juvenile Hypertension. BMI, NY, 1984, p. 231ff.
37. Graves, S.W., and Williams, G.H: An endogenous ouabain-like factor associated with hypertensive pregnant women. J. Clin. Endocrinol. Metab. 59:1070, 1984.
38. Currie, M.G., Geller, D.M., Cole, B.R., et al: Bioactive cardiac substances: potent vasorelaxant activity. Science. 221:71, 1983.

NUTRITIONAL ASPECTS OF HYPERTENSION AND ATHEROSCLEROSIS
CALCIUM: DOES IT HAVE A ROLE?

Russell W. Chesney, M.D.

This symposium will consider nutritional factors that contribute to the development of hypertension. Previous speakers have focused on the role of sodium and on the dietary intake of sodium as a factor in hypertension. I will limit my discussion to the role of dietary calcium as a potential contributing factor in hypertension.

Calcium is the fifth most abundant element in the body (1). It is the predominant divalent cation, although only 1% of total body calcium is found in the intra - or extracellular fluid, since fully 99% is found in bone. Calcium serves as a modulator of neuromuscular membrane function and, under conditions of hypocalcemia irritability of the neuromuscular system is universal resulting in tetany.

The suggestion that the dietary intake of calcium could influence the level of the blood pressure came from the epidemiologic observation that people drinking hard water - containing limestone or calcium carbonate - had a reduced incidence of cardiovascular disease and hypertension (2). Further studies suggested that this protective effect of water hardness was mediated through the influence of a lower blood pressure (3, 4). Although other studies have not always confirmed this association between water hardness and hypertension (5), several groups of investigators have been stimulated to examine the role of dietary calcium intake in relation to blood pressure. These studies have taken several approaches in general and each of these approaches will be discussed independently.

DIETARY CALCIUM INTAKE IN RELATION TO HYPERTENSION (TABLE I)

In the 1974 Health and Nutrition Examination Survey (HANES) carried out by the National Center for Health Statistics, it was observed that hypertensive individuals ingested a diet containing a lower amount of calcium (6-8). McCarron et al. (7) observed that, as compared to 44 normotensive controls, the calcium intake of 46 subjects with essential hypertension reported a lower intake of calcium (668 ± 55 mg/24h vs 886 ± 89 mg/24h in normotensives). The dietary intake of sodium and potassium as well as caloric intake, was similar between the two groups. He then made an extensive analysis of the HANES I data and showed that hypertensive subjects ingested 18% less calcium in their diet than normotensive individuals in HANES I - 572 ± 17 (SD) mg calcium/24h vs 695 ± 7 mg/24h in normotensive (8). When younger individuals, aged 20 to 34 years, were examined, calcium intake was not different between the normotensive and hypertensive subjects. Thus, the association between hypertension and dietary calcium intake was confined to subjects between 35 and 75 years.

In an earlier study, Langford and Watson (9) reported that women whose systolic blood pressure was under 105 mm Hg had a statistically higher intake of calcium than those whose systolic pressure exceeded 125 mm Hg. Another study from Belgium indicated a positive converse correlation between urinary calcium excretion, which can be taken to represent dietary intake, and both systolic and diastolic blood pressure (10). Finally, a cohort of subjects living in Southern California was examined and it was found that significantly lower calcium intake from milk was found in hypertensive men, but not women, and this effect was independent of obesity or age (11).

Table I. Role of Dietary Calcium in Human Hypertension

1. Atherosclerosis and hypertension are reduced in "hard" water areas (2,3); Disputed in some studies (4).

2. Dietary surveys indicate association between lower calcium intake and hypertension (6-9, 11).

3. Serum ionized calcium may be reduced and iPTH elevated in hypertensive subjects (essential hypertension) (6, 12, 15).

4. Essential hypertensive patients have a urine calcium leak (10, 14).

5. Ionized calcium reduction is present only in low renin hypertension and hypercalcemia is associated with high renin hypertension (17).

6. Provision of 1.0 gm of elemental calcium lowers BP in healthy men and women and in pregnant women (18, 19).

7. Dietary calcium lowered blood pressure in essential hypertension (20).

SERUM CALCIUM AND ITS POSSIBLE INFLUENCE

Parrott-Garcia and McCarron (12) have reviewed the evidence for abnormalities of calcium metabolism in hypertension. McCarron et al (13) found significantly higher immunoreactive PTH values in hypertensive than in normotensive subjects and the hypertensives demonstrated relative hypercalciuria. Other studies indicated a urinary calcium leak in hypertensive subjects (10, 14). McCarron et al. (15) then measured serum calcium concentration. No difference was found between normotensive and hypertensive subjects, but hypertensives had a lower serum ionized calcium content which could be responsible for the higher iPTH values. Resnick et al (16) could not confirm the finding of a lower ionized calcium level in hypertensives except in relation to plasma renin activity. When a group of pre-eclamptic women were compared to normotensive pregnant controls, the ionized calcium was reduced and iPTH was elevated, but urine calcium excretion was also reduced (17).

However, as noted in a recent review (12), not all studies have found the same changes in ionized calcium, in PTH levels and in the urinary excretion of calcium. At least 3 studies to date have not detected any abnormalities in serum calcium values, casting doubt on the universality of the findings of McCarron's group. Nonetheless, certain aspects of the data presented thus far suggest that supplementation of the diet with calcium may be warranted in clinical trials.

MODIFICATION OF CALCIUM INTAKE

Belizan et al. (18) performed a clinical trial giving a 1 gm/24h of elemental calcium to a group of healthy young men and women and compared the effects of this supplementation to a group of similar aged subjects ingesting a placebo. The calcium supplemented group showed a significant reduction in diastolic blood pressure with a fall of 5-10%. In another study, it was shown that calcium supplementation during pregnancy can reduce diastolic blood pressure in normal women between the 20th and 24th weeks of pregnancy as compared to placebo treated controls (19). This effect was lost during the third trimester when 1.0 gm of calcium was given each day, but 2.0 gm daily led to a continued reduction in blood pressure.

McCarron et al. (20) recently reported a clinical trial in which the blood pressure response to 1000 mg of elemental calcium/24h was examined in 48 subjects with essential hypertension and in 32 matched normotensive controls. During the placebo period blood pressure did not change, but the calcium period of 8 weeks resulted in a 7 mm Hg fall in systolic BP in hypertensives and a decline of > 10 mm Hg in 48% of these subjects. The response in normotensives was less marked since a decline of > 10 mm Hg in systolic BP occurred in only 18%. One feature of this trial is that few side effects were noted in accordance with the findings of Belizan et al. (18, 19). Hence, these findings suggest, but do not prove, that short term calcium supplementation may be a method of reducing blood pressure in certain patients with hypertension and is an application of the theory of "non-drug therapy in treating hypertension" (21). It is also important to recall that Kesteloot and Geboers (10) found no effect of dietary calcium supplements in their studies described previously.

ANIMAL STUDIES - CLUES TO PATHOGENESIS? (TABLE II)

Studies on dietary calcium intake and its influence on blood pressure have largely been confined to studies in rats; in particular, several of the hypertensive strains of rats have been employed. McCarron (22) examined the development of hypertension in young spontaneously hypertensive rats (SHR) and found that systolic BP was inversely correlated ($p < .001$) to calcium intake up to 20 weeks of age. Further, rats on a 4% calcium diet had a lower final BP (154 ± 7 mm Hg) than rats fed a 0.5% diet (176 ± 7 mm Hg).

Belizan (23) examined pregnant Wistar rats. He treated rats with a calcium-free or calcium-containing (control) diet. After 6 weeks the systolic BP, measured in the tail, was higher in the Ca-free rats. With pregnancy the systolic BP rose even higher in the Ca-free rats and fell in rats on the control diet. A significant increase in serum phosphate was found in rats fed the Ca-free diet.

A confirming study from France showed that a low Ca diet in juvenile SHR rats resulted in earlier and more severe hypertension than in aged matched SHR rats fed a higher Ca diet (24). In these animals, a 1.2% Ca diet was found to attenuate the development of an the long term level of hypertension.

In rats with vitamin D intoxication, SHR rats were able to tolerate the consequences of this toxicity far better than normotensive (WKY) controls (25). The authors found that SHR rats did not develop the aortic placques, and calcification of the myocardium and vessels as frequently as did WKY control animals. They suggested that an abnormality in smooth muscle calcium transport may be present in SHR animals protecting them against vitamin D toxicity.

In another study employing a high Ca:PO_4 diet, SHR rats did not develop the intimal hyaline lesions of the gonadal arterioles which were found after 45 days of feeding this diet to normotensive Sprague-Dawley rats (26). In these animals a Ca:PO_4 diet of 4.5:1 was employed. This diet was also associated with hyperlipidemia and an abnormally elevated value of corticosterone. In addition, serum calcium and phosphate fell along with the development of bloody urine suggesting that calcium-phosphate precipitates developed in the kidney. Renal stones also occurred. Although the arteries of SHR animals were protected against intimal lesions, there was no change in blood pressure, possibly since adult animals, who had already developed hypertension, were employed in this study.

This influence of calcium in the diet may relate to alterations in platelet function. In rats fed a diet of saturated fats, an increase in the level of dietary calcium resulted in a highly significant reduction in platelet reactivity and in prolongation of the clotting time (27).

A completely different mechanism has been hypothesized by Lau et al. (28). He evaluated the protective role of changes in PTH secretion, volume contraction, hypercalcemia and phosphate depletion in a group of SHR rats fed a low (0.22%), normal (1.2%) or high (4.3%) Ca diet. Since the high calcium diet prevented hypertension in normal and parathyroidectomized rats, the role of phosphate depletion was explored. Rats developed evidence of phosphate depletion with 1) hypercalciuria; 2) hypophosphatemia, 3) reduced intestinal phosphate absorption. The intravenous infusion of phosphate resulted in hypertension in these rats suggesting that the protective effect of calcium is mediated via phosphate depletion.

In normal rats, hypercalcemia results in a fall in both GFR and renal blood flow, mainly related to a vasoconstrictive effect (29). Even blocking the vasoconstrictive effect of angiotensin II and the vasodilatory effect of renal prostaglandins, which tend to offset one another, resulted in a lower GFR and RBF. It is possible that this might have a protective effect against glomerular hyperfiltration, although no change in mean arterial pressure was detected in these rats.

Garcia and McCarron (12) have postulated that the major alteration brought about by a low calcium diet is "the pivotal role of calcium ions in the regulation of vascular smooth muscle contraction and relaxation". Calcium enters the cell by a potential - dependent or receptor regulated mechanism. The calcium entering the cell complexes with calmodulin, the main intracellular calcium binding protein and also causes the release of calcium from the sarcoplasmic reticulum. These events stimulate the coupling of actin and myosin resulting in muscle contraction. Re-uptake of calcium by the sarcoplasmic reticulum results in relaxation. Some studies, reviewed by Garcia and McCarron (12), suggest that calcium fluxes are enhanced in SHR animals resulting in a state of increased vascular tone. When

Table II. Effect of a High Calcium Diet on The Development of Hypertension in Animal Models

1. Young spontaneously hypertensive rats (SHR) fed a high calcium diet (3-5%) are protected against the rapid development and full extent of hypertension (12, 22, 23, 24).

2. Pregnant SHR have less hypertension while on a high calcium diet (23).

3. Vitamin D intoxication and a high Ca:PO_4 ratio do not cause aortic calcification and intimal hyalinosis in SHR (25, 26).

4. Platelet reactivity and clotting time is prolonged by a high calcium diet (27).

5. The protective effect of a high calcium diet in young SHR relates to the extent of phosphate depletion (28).

6. Hypercalcemia results in a reduced GFR and renal blood flow (29).

7. A high calcium diet in SHR may result in greater smooth muscle vascular relaxation (vasodilatation) and less smooth muscle vascular constriction thus lowering blood pressure (12).

---

present in high amounts, calcium binds to muscle membrane sites which actually block the flux of calcium through the calcium channel. This, in turn, results in a greater state of relaxation. With a lower ionized calcium level, calcium fluxes are increased and contraction, by the mechanism described above, is favored. SHR rats also appear to requre higher levels of calcium exposure to stabilize the process and overcome contraction (12). It is also necessary for more avid binding of calcium to membranes in SHR animals to initiate the contraction process. Despite this interesting hypothesis, not all the available data fit this notion and no direct experimental proof of this hypothesis has appeared.

To summarize, a high calcium diet reduces the extent of hypertension in SHR rats under a variety of circumstances. At present, this effect may relate to a reduction in vascular tone, a lower degree of arterial intimal hyaline lesions, reduction in the formation of aortic placques, less reactive platelets, a reduction in renal blood flow or in relation to phosphate depletion. Which, if any, of these mechanisms is operative is unknown, but the effect of a high calcium diet appears to be real.

EFFECTS IN CHILDREN

Almost no data are available concerning the effect of calcium on blood pressure regulation in children. While it is known that hypercalcemia of any cause will result in hypertension, this effect is only seen at extremely high serum calcium values, usually exceeding 12.0 mg/dL (1). Perlman et al. (30) examined calcium homeostasis in

Table III. Calcium Content of Various Foods

FOOD	MILLIGRAMS of Calcium	% US RDA
8 oz. glass skim milk	296	30
8 oz. glass whole milk	288	29
1 oz. slice Swiss cheese	251	25
1 cup cottage cheese (large curd)	212	21
1 oz. slice American cheese	198	20
1 cup spinach (cooked)	167	17
1 cup fresh Broccoli (broiled, chopped)	136	14
8 oz. fish (cod, broiled, with butter)	71	7
1 fresh orange (2-5/8" diam.)	54	5
1/2 cup raisins	45	5
1/2 cup walnuts	50	5
1 cup carrots (boiled, sliced)	51	5
1 cup squash (boiled, sliced)	45	5
1 cup fresh green peas (boiled)	37	4
1 boiled egg (extra large)	31	3
8 oz. roasted chicken (light meat without skin)	25	3
8 oz. lean broiled steak, sirloin	22	2
1 cup white rice (cooked)	21	2
1 whole tomato (7 oz)	24	2
1 can tuna 3-1/4 oz. (in water)	15	2
1 slice whole wheat bread	24	2
1 slice rye bread	19	2
1 slice white bread	24	2
3 oz. lean, ground beef patty, broiled	10	1
1 cup chopped lettuce	11	1
1 baked potato (medium)	8	1
1 ear corn, boiled	2	1*

* Less than 1% RDA
** RDA = 1000 mg elemental calcium/24hr. in children > 3 years and adults

adolescents with essential hypertension. They found that hypertensive adolescents had a higher total serum calcium and phosphate than normotensive controls: calcium, 10.0 ± 0.4 mg/dL in 34 hypertensives vs 9.6 ± 0.3 in 37 controls; phosphate 4.5 ± 0.7 mg/dL vs 3.9 ± 0.7 mg/dL. Both of these differences are highly significant. No change in urinary calcium excretion or the tubular reabsorption of phosphate was found, ionized calcium and PTH were not measured.

FURTHER CONCERNS AND UNANSWERED QUESTIONS

Criticism has arisen about the role of a reduction in calcium intake in the etiology of hypertension and concerning the value of calcium supplementation in the therapy of hypertensives (31). Many of McCarron's studies are based on a 24 hour dietary recall, which has been disputed as being valid on numerous occasions. Other investigators of hypertension have cautioned that additional controlled studies are indicated. The data of Resnick et al. (16, 17) indicate that calcium intake may only be operative in low renin hypertension. The study of Perlman et al. (30) suggests that no urinary calcium leak is found in adolescent essential hypertensives. Finally, Garn and Larkin (32) have indicated that most of the world does not ingest the amounts of calcium ingested by normals and hypertensives in McCarron's studies and yet in countries where calcium intake is low, hypertension is uncommon .

Notwithstanding these criticisms, it is important to recall the information in HANES I (6, 12) that the American diet seldom contains the recommended daily allowance (RDA) for calcium. As indicated in table III, foods other than dairy products (milk, cheese, yogurt) contain little calcium. Thus, in the lactase - deficient individual or in milk intolerant subjects, it is difficult to assure adequate dietary intake of calcium. Past reviews have indicated the role of calcium deficiency in poor bone mineralization and as a contributing factor to osteoporosis (1).

Finally, hypertension is a disorder of many causes, which is the subject of this workshop on nutrition and hypertension. The need for further studies of the role of dietary calcium is incumbent. Future directions will require that careful, well designed control studies in man be performed. The role of dietary calcium intake on childhood hypertension also requires investigation. The value of calcium supplements is obviously not proven, but at least providing the RDA by dietary means and by supplements in lactase - deficient or milk - intolerant individuals may be indicated. Not only does lifelong calcium intake play a role in the development of post menopausal osteoporosis, but it may also be shown in the future to be important in hypertension.

Supported in Part by NIH Grant AM 31682 and by a Grant from Miles Laboratories

REFERENCES

1. Chesney, R.W.: Metabolic bone disease. In Behrman, R.E., Vaughn, V.C. and Nelson, W.E. (eds.): Nelson's Textbook of Pediatrics, 13th Edition, Philadelphia: W.B. Saunders, in press.

2. Schroeder, H.A.: Relation between Mortality from Cardiovascular Disease and Treated Water Supplies. J Am Med Assoc 172:1902-1908, 1960.

3. Neri, L.C. and Johansen, H.L.: Water hardness and cardiovascular mortality. Ann NY Acad Sci 304:203-219, 1978.

4. Stitt, F.W., Crawford, M.D., Clayton D.G. and Morris, J.N.: Clinical and Biochemical Indicators of Cardiovascular Disease among Men Living in Hard and Soft Water Areas. Lancet 1:122-126, 1973.

5. Comstock, G.W.: Water hardness and cardiovascular diseases. Am J Epidemiol 110:375-400, 1979.

6. McCarron, D.A.: Dietary Calcium as an Antihypertensive Agent. Nutrition Reviews Vol. 42, No. 6, June 1984.

7. McCarron, D.A., Morris, C.D. and Cole C.: Dietary Calcium in Human Hypertension. Science Vol. 217, 1982.

8. McCarron, D.A.: Calcium and Magnesium Nutrition in Human Hypertension. Annals of Internal Medicine 98:800-805, 1983.

9. From the Departments of Community and Family Medicine and Medicine, University of California, San Diego, CA and the American Heart Association, California Affiliate.

10. Kesteloot, H. and Geboers, J.: Calcium and Blood Pressure. The Lancet 4:813-815, 1982.

11. Ackley, S., Barrett-Connor, E. and Suarez, L.: Dairy products, calcium, and blood pressure. Am Journal of Clin Nutri 38:457-461, 1983.

12. Parrott-Garcia, M. and McCarron D.A.: Calcium and Hypertension. Nutrition Reviews 42:205-213, June 1984.

13. McCarron, D.A., Pingree, P.A., Rubin, R.J., Gaucher, S.M., Molitch M. and Krutzik, S.: Enhanced parathyroid function in essential hypertension: a homeostatic response to a urinary calcium leak. Hypertension 2:162-168, 1980.

14. Staessen. J. Bulpitt, C., Fagard, R., Joosens, J.V., Lijnen, P. and Amery, A.: Four urinary cations and blood pressure: a population study in two Belgian towns. Am J Epidemiol 117:676-687, 1983.

15. McCarron, D.A.: Low serum concentrations of ionized calcium in patients with hypertension. New Engl J Med 307:226-228, 1982.

16. Resnick, L.M., Laragh, J.H., Sealey, J.E. and Alderman, M.H.: Divalent cations in essential hypertension. Relations between serum ionized calcium, magnesium and plasma renin activities. New Engl J Med 309:888-891, 1983.

17. Resnick, L.M., Taufield, P.A., Ales, K., Druzin, M., Sealey, J.E. and Laragh, J.H.: Divalent cations in human hypertension. Clin Res 31:505A, 1983.

18. Belizan, J.M., Villar, J., Pineda, O., Gonzalez, A.E., Sainze, E., Garrera, G. and Sibrian R.: Reduction of Blood Pressure with Calcium Supplementation in Young Adults. JAMA 249:1161-1165, 1983.

19. Belizan, J.M., Villar, J., Zalazar, A., Rojas, L., Chan D. and Bryce, G.F.: Preliminary evidence of the effect of calcium supplementation on blood pressure in normal pregnant women. Am J Obstet Gynecol 146:175-180, 1983.

20. McCarron, D.A.: Calcium and magnesium metabolism in human hypertension. Ann Intern Med 98:800-805, 1983.

21. Kaplan, N.M.: Use of Non-Drug Therapy in Treating Hypertension. Am J Med Oct.5,pp 96-101, 1984.

22. McCarron, D.A.: Calcium, Magnesium, and Phosphorus Balance in Human and Experimental Hypertension. Hypertension 4(supp III): III-27 - III-33, 1982.

23. Belizan, J.M., Pineda, O., Sainz, E., Menendez, L.A. and Villar J.: Rise of blood pressure in calcium-deprived pregnant rats. AM J Obstet Gynecol 141:163-169, 1981.

24. Schleiffer, R., Pernot, F., Berthelot, A. and Gairard, A.: Low Calcium Diet Enhances Development Of Hypertension In The Spontaneously Hypertensive Rat. Clin and Exper Hyper-Theory and Practice, A6(4), 783-793, 1984.

25. Matthias, D., Becker, C.H. and Woossmann, H.: Different behavior of normotonous and spontaneously hypertensive rats with vitamin D intoxications. Biomed Biochim Acta 43 6, 741-748, 1984.

26. Wexler, B.C.: Susceptibility and resistance of Sprague-Dawley and spontaneously hypertensive rats to aortic calcification induced by a diet high in $CaPO_4$. Atherosclerosis, 35:471-486, 1980.

27. Renaud, S.: Risk factors for coronary heart disease and platelet functions. Adv Exp Med Biol 164:129-144, 1984.

28. Lau, K., Chen, S. and Eby, B.: Evidence for the role of PO_4 deficiency in antihypertensive action of a high-Ca diet. The American Physiological Society 0363-6135/84 pp.H324-H331.

29. Levi, M., Ellis, M.A. and Berl, T.: Control of Renal Hemodynamics and Glomerular Filtration Rate in Chronic Hypercalcemia. J Clin Invest Vol 71:1624-1632, 1983.

30. Perlman, S.A., Polinsky, M.S., Gruskin, A.B., Prebis, J.W., et al.: Calcium homeostasis in adolescents with essential hypertension. Semin Nephrol 3:149-158, 1983.

31. Kolata, G.: Does a Lack of Calcium Cause Hypertension? Science 225:705-706, 1984.

32. Garn, S.M. and Larkin F.A.: Calcium Intake and Hypertension. Science 219:112, 1982.

NUTRITION, LIPOPROTEINS AND ATHEROSCLEROSIS IN CHILDHOOD

Peter O. Kwiterovich, Jr., M.D.

DEVELOPMENT OF ATHEROSCLEROSIS

Risk factors for atherosclerosis

Epidemiologic and clinical studies. Atherosclerosis is a chronic disease process that begins early in life, progresses during young adulthood, and in middle age or later, an end-stage lesion develops that occludes the lumen of arteries, often leading to myocardial infarction, stroke, peripheral vascular disease or sudden death. A number of risk factors are associated with the development of atherosclerosis. These include age, sex (males on average develop complications of atherosclerosis 10 years younger than females), hypercholesterolemia, cigarette smoking, hypertension, diabetes mellitus, obesity, and a positive family history of premature atherosclerosis (1). An increased level of low density (beta) lipoproteins (LDL), the major carrier of plasma cholesterol, is strongly associated with coronary atherosclerosis; conversely, depressed levels of high density (alpha) lipoproteins (HDL) are independent risk factors for coronary atherosclerosis (1). Whether an increased plasma level of triglycerides, and their major carrier, very low density (prebeta) lipoproteins (VLDL) is a risk factor for atherosclerosis, independent of the other known factors, is controversial (2). In many families with premature coronary atherosclerosis, however, hypertriglyceridemia is prevalent (3).

Obesity. Results from the Health Assessment Nutritional and Educational Survey (HANES) in prepubescent American children indicate that approximately 10% of boys and 15% of girls are obese, i.e., their weight for height is greater than 120% of median. Obesity has been previously found by Frerichs and co-workers (4) to be associated with higher plasma levels of total cholesterol, total triglycerides, LDL and VLDL cholesterol, but lower levels of HDL cholesterol, a plasma lipid and lipoprotein profile that is adverse in regard to the development of atherosclerosis even in childhood (see also below). Obese children also tend to have higher blood pressure levels even after one takes into consideration the height of such individuals (5).

Hypertension. Clinically significant hypertension in childhood has been primarily associated with renal disease. However, it is now well documented that certain healthy children have higher than average blood pressure levels, for example, the 90th or 95th percentile for age and sex values, and that such values tend to track over time (5). Thus, it is likely that such children will be more prone to develop "essential hypertension" as adults. These issues have been reviewed elsewhere (5) and have also been discussed elsewhere in this symposium.

Pathologic studies. A number of human pathologic studies in children and in young soldiers killed in the Korean, Vietnam and World War II conflicts, indicate that atherosclerosis has its origins early in life in the form of fatty streaks and fibrous plaques (6). Recently, Berenson and coworkers (7), in a prospective study of autopsy specimens from children well-characterized at baseline in the Bogalusa Heart Study, found a significantly high correlation between the level of LDL cholesterol and the extent of fatty streaks and fibrous plaques; conversely, a highly significantly inverse correlation was found between the levels of HDL cholesterol and arterial lesions (7).

Positive family history. Hyperlipidemia in childhood is especially prevalent in children born in families with a history of premature atherosclerosis. A number of studies have found that about one in three children with such a history had either hypercholesterolemia, hypertriglyceridemia or both hypercholesterolemia and hypertriglyceridemia (6).

Genetic models of dyslipoproteinemia and atherosclerosis

Familial hypercholesterolemia. One of the most common recognized syndromes of familial hyperlipoproteinemia in childhood is familial hypercholesterolemia (FH) (8,9). This is an autosomal dominant disorder of LDL metabolism that has a gene dosage effect (10). Heterozygotes with one faulty gene for FH present early in life or at birth with significant elevations in plasma total and LDL cholesterol levels. The average plasma total and LDL cholesterol levels in such affected children after the age of one year is approximately 300 and 240 mg/dl, respectively. Overt clinical findings are unusual in children with heterozygous FH. Tendon xanthomas, particularly of the Achilles tendon, begin to appear in the second decade and by the third, fourth and fifth decade of life tendon xanthomas are present in approximately 50% of affected FH heterozygotes. The average age for the clinical expression of coronary atherosclerosis in FH heterozygotes is 40 years in males and 50 years in females. By the age of 65 years, 85% of FH heterozygotes have developed coronary artery disease (10).

A homozygous FH patient with two mutant alleles will have profound elevations in plasma total cholesterol, usually approaching 1,000 mg/dl. FH homozygotes develop planar xanthomas before the age of five years, and atherosclerosis of the coronary arteries, aortic valve and aorta that is expressed clinically as coronary artery disease and aortic stenosis usually between 10 and 20 years of age (10). In cultured fibroblasts from patients with homozygous FH, the high affinity binding of LDL can be absent (LDL receptor negative), or deficient (LDL receptor defective) or a defect in the uptake of LDL (internalization defect) may be present (10). Such cellular phenotypes result from a double dose of any of a number of mutant alleles at the locus for the cell surface receptor for LDL. The defect(s) in the cell surface receptor result in reduced internalization and degradation of LDL and deficient regulation of cholesterol synthesis. FH heterozygotes have a level of LDL receptor activity that falls, on average, in between that in normal cells and FH homozygous cells.

Familial combined hyperlipidemia. Another notable example of a common inherited syndrome of hyperlipidemia associated with elevated LDL levels and premature coronary atherosclerosis is familial combined hyperlipidemia (FCH) (3). FCH was initially described as a dominant phenotype that was expressed as hypercholesterolemia alone, hypertriglyceridemia alone or both hypercholesterolemia and hypertriglyceridemia (3). Tendon xanthomas are not present. Patients with FCH often have an LDL of abnormal composition (low ratio of LDL cholesterol to LDL B protein (apoB) and an elevated level of total plasma apoB) (11). Increased hepatic synthesis of apoB have been found in FCH (12). The expression of FCH is often delayed until adulthood (3), but it is not unusual to find an affected child, especially in families with premature coronary artery disease.

Familal hyperapobetalipoproteinemia. In collaboration with Sniderman from McGill University, we have identified a syndrome of dyslipoproteinemia that we have termed hyperapobetalipoproteinemia (hyperapoB), in which the LDL apoB is elevated out of proportion to LDL cholesterol, due to the presence of a species of LDL of low molecular weight and abnormal chemical composition (13-15). HyperapoB has been found in a number of patients with coronary atherosclerosis (13-15). Individuals with endogenous hypertriglyceridemia can be segregated into those who appear at risk for coronary heart disease (i.e., those with increased LDL-B) compared to hypertriglyceridemics without risk (no increase in LDL-B) (14).

Our studies in young offspring of patients who have premature myocardial infarction and hyperapoB indicate that hyperapoB is very prevalent in such children (16). We have found that mild hypercholesterolemia in children can be indicative of the presence of premature coronary artery disease in the parents, and that the use of LDL-B apoprotein assay helps in diagnosing a significantly greater proportion of these children, many of whom have normal cholesterol levels (16). Children with hyperapoB may also have mild hypertriglyceridemia (fasting plasma triglyceride levels between 100 and 200 mg/dl).

We and others (17) have postulated that, at least in some hypertriglyceridemic patients, hyperapoB may indicate the presence of FCH.

Familial hypoalphalipoproteinemia. This syndrome is defined as very low levels of HDL cholesterol levels, in the presence of normal levels of LDL cholesterol and triglycerides (18). Hypoalphalipoproteinemia is often found in families with coronary atherosclerosis (18) and has also been described in pediatric stroke victims (19).

Detection of children at risk for atherosclerosis

Screening. What is the best approach to screen selectively children at risk for atherosclerosis? After the age of two years, a blood specimen may be drawn following an overnight fast of 12 hours. The child should be on a regular diet without medication and the weight stable. Plasma is used for the determination of total cholesterol, total triglycerides, and HDL cholesterol. Electrophoresis of the plasma is not currently recommended because it is only semi-quantitative. LDL cholesterol may be estimated by the following formula: LDL cholesterol = total cholesterol - [HDL cholesterol + total triglycerides/5]. This formula is valid provided the triglyceride level is < 400 mg/dl, the patient is fasting and type III hyperlipoproteinemia (dysbetalipoproteinemia) is not present. This approach provides additional information over the measurement of plasma total cholesterol alone. It enables the pediatrician to determine whether there is an elevation of LDL cholesterol, or, a depressed level of the HDL cholesterol.

Definition of normal values. What are normal values of plasma lipids and lipoproteins in the first two decades of life? Recent results from the Lipid Research Clinics (LRC) Program Prevalence Studies have provided accurate and reasonable estimates of normal ranges (20). Using the 95th percentile for plasma total cholesterol, 200 mg/dl is a reasonable estimate to define significant hypercholesterolemia in the first two decades of life

Table 1. Normal Plasma Lipid Concentrations in the First Two Decades of Life

		Cholesterol			Triglycerides		
Age (Yr)	No.	5th	Mean	95th	5th	Mean	95th
0-4							
Males	238	114	155	203	29	56	99
Females	186	112	156	200	34	64	112
5-9							
Males	1253	121	160	203	30	56	101
Females	1118	126	164	205	32	60	105
10-14							
Males	2278	119	158	202	32	66	125
Females	2087	124	160	201	37	75	131
15-19							
Males	1980	113	150	197	37	78	148
Females	2079	120	158	203	39	75	132

Data given are from the Lipid Research Clinic Data Book (20). Lipids were determined on plasma from 11,219 fasting, white subjects (5749 males; 5470 females) who were studied in seven North American Lipid Research Clinics using common protocols and laboratory methodology. All values are expressed as mg/dl.

Table 2. Normal Plasma Lipoprotein Concentrations in the First Two Decades of Life

	HDL Cholesterol				LDL Cholesterol				VLDL Cholesterol			
Age (Yr)	No.	5th	Mean	95th	No.	5th	Mean	95th	No.	5th	Mean	95th
5-9												
Males	145	38	56	75	132	63	93	129	132	0	8	18
Females	127	36	53	73	114	68	100	140	113	1	10	24
10-14												
Males	298	37	55	74	288	64	97	133	288	1	10	22
Females	248	37	52	70	245	68	97	136	245	2	11	23
15-19												
Males	300	30	46	63	298	62	94	130	297	2	13	26
Females	297	35	52	74	295	59	96	137	295	2	12	24

Data are from the Lipid Research Clinic Data Book (20). Lipoproteins were determined from 1415 fasting, white subjects (743 males, 672 females) who were studied in seven North American Lipid Research Clinics, using common protocols and laboratory methodology. All values are expressed as mg/dl.

(Table 1). For plasma total triglycerides, approximately 100 mg/dl in the first decade of life, 125 mg/dl between ages 10-14, and 130 mg/dl for females and 150 mg/dl for males between the ages of 15-19 years (Table 1). In regard to normal ranges for the plasma lipoprotein concentrations, the approximate 95th percentile for LDL cholesterol levels is about 130-140 mg/dl in the first two decades of life (Table 2). The definition of a low HDL cholesterol level in the first two decades of life is approximately 35 mg/dl for males and females between the ages of 5 and 14 years. However, between the ages 15 and 19 years the 5th percentile is lower in males (30 mg/dl) than in females (35 mg/dl) (Table 2). These male/female differences in HDL cholesterol levels that emerge in the later part of the second decade persist throughout adult life and may explain, in part, the greater predilection of males to coronary artery disease than females.

Children with elevated levels of LDL cholesterol alone (type IIa lipoprotein pattern), elevated LDL cholesterol and plasma triglycerides (type IIb lipoprotein pattern), or normal LDL cholesterol levels with elevated plasma triglycerides (type IV lipoprotein pattern) should be treated as indicated below. Similarly, children with normal cholesterol and triglyceride levels but depressed levels of HDL cholesterol (hypoalphalipoproteinemia) should also be treated.

Secondary hyperlipidemia. Before instituting a treatment program, it is important to determine whether the hyperlipidemia or hyperlipoproteinemia is primary or secondary to other metabolic conditions. Common causes of secondary hypercholesterolemia in the pediatric age group include hypothyroidism, renal disease, dysgammaglobulinemias, porphyria and liver disease (6). Common causes of hypertriglyceridemia in pediatrics include diabetes mellitus, glycogen storage disease, pancreatitis, chronic renal failure and dysgammaglobulinemias (6). Treatment of acne with isotretinoin and the use of oral contraceptives are associated with a high prevalence of secondary hyperlipidemia.

Hyperlipidemia and renal disease. For the proceedings of this symposium, a special note is made of the association of hyperlipidemia with renal disease (Table 3). In patients with the nephrotic syndrome, profound hypercholesterolemia due to elevated LDL cholesterol levels is often present. However, it is not unusual in the nephrotic syndrome to have an accompanying hypertriglyceridemia, particularly in the later stages of the disease process. Patients undergoing hemodialysis also develop hyperlipidemia, particularly hypertriglyceridemia. A significant number of patients undergoing renal transplantation develop hyperlipidemia including both hypercholesterolemia and hypertriglyceridemia and often a combination of both. Individuals with chronic renal failure are known to have hypertriglyceridemia, and hyperlipidemia has also been associated with the hemolytic uremic syndrome.

Table 3. Association of Hyperlipidemia with Renal Disease

1. Nephrotic syndrome
2. Hemodialysis patients
3. Post-renal transplantation
4. Chronic renal failure
5. Hemolytic uremic syndrome

What is the mechanism of the hyperlipidemia associated with renal disease? Chan and coworkers (21) divided the etiology of hyperlipidemia in uremia into two categories. The first category involves decreased removal of plasma triglyceride and VLDL. Such a defect might be due to decreased levels of lipoprotein lipase. However, decreased fatty acid oxidation may also occur, particularly in hemodialysis patients in whom the blood levels are depleted of carnitine (a quaternary amine compound essential for the transport of fatty acid coenzyme A across the mitochondrial membrane for subsequent oxidation) (22). The second category concerns increased production of triglyceride in the liver. Such enhanced production may be due to dietary influences, acetate and glucose in the dialysate, hyperinsulinism, increased lipolysis of triglyceride and adipose tissue, and increased production and mobilization of free fatty acids, and drugs such as androgens and steroids. In any event, the hyperlipidemia associated with uremia and renal disease is associated with atherosclerosis and efforts should therefore be made to modify secondary hyperlipidemia associated with renal disease (23).

Treatment of hyperlipidemia

Recent evidence from the LRC Coronary Primary Prevention Trial (see below) indicates that lowering plasma total and LDL cholesterol reduces morbidity and mortality from coronary artery disease. These data, when combined with the genetic, metabolic and pathological association of elevated LDL and lipid levels with atherosclerosis (see above) provide a strong rationale for treatment.

Dietary treatment. A unified approach to the dietary treatment of hyperlipoproteinemia has been proposed by the Nutrition Committee of the American Heart Association. This diet is divided into three phases of progressive difficulty (Table 4). The nutrients as percent of total calories include a reduction in total fat, particularly in saturated fat with some enrichment in polyunsaturated fat. Plasma cholesterol is restricted to less than 300 mg/day in phase 1, progressing to 100 mg/day in phase 2. The carbohydrate is approximately 50% of the calories with an emphasis on complex carbohydrates and a decrease in simple sugars. Protein is approximately 20% of the calories.

Dietary treatment of hyperlipidemia in renal disease. Disler and coworkers (24) treated 21 renal transplant recipients who had hyperlipidemia and normal renal function for 1 year with a diet containing less than 200 mg cholesterol/day, a ratio of polyunsaturated to saturated fat of 1.2-1.4, and 125 grams carbohydrate, 75 grams of fat and 75 grams of protein. They found a significant fall in mean plasma total cholesterol, and the mean triglyceride level fell in 13 of 21 patients. Of 23 patients with post-transplant hyperlipidemia, Shen and coworkers (25) treated 12 patients for 3 months with a diet low in fat (less than 35% of calories) somewhat reduced in cholesterol (less than 500 mg/day) and less than 50% of calories as carbohydrate. The ratio of polyunsaturated to saturated fat was 1 or higher. Such treatment produced a highly significant reduction in both mean plasma cholesterol levels (313-248 mg/dl $p < .01$) and mean plasma total triglycerides (321-198 mg/dl, $p < .05$). No change occurred in the 11 hyperlipidemic patients in the untreated control group. Finally, Vacha and coworkers (22) studied 29 hemodialyzed patients with hypertriglyceridemia by giving L carnitine 20 mg/kg i.v. at the end of renal dialysis for 120 days and then followed with placebo for 120 days. They found that the blood triglyceride levels decreased if there was a

Table 4. Unified Approach to Dietary Treatment of Hyperlipidemia

Nutrients as % of total calories+	Phase 1	Phase 2	Phase 3
Fat	30-35%	<30%	20-25%
Saturated fat	<10%	8%	6%
Polyunsaturated fat	10%	10%	8%
Monounsaturated fat	10-12%	10%	8%
P/S	1.2-1.4	1.1-1.5	1.1-1.5
Cholesterol (mg/day)	<300	<200	100
Carbohydrate*	45-50%	50%	55-60%
Protein	20%	20%	20%

+ Approximate averages are provided; the percent nutrient intake will vary depending on the total daily caloric intake (e.g., 1200-2300 calories/day).

* Includes a reduction in simple sugars (10-15% of calories) and an increase in complex carbohydrates.

concomitant presence of a low level of HDL cholesterol with little change in the triglycerides if the HDL cholesterol was normal. In four of the latter nonresponders, the dose was subsequently increased to 60 mg/kg i.v., producing a decrease in the plasma level of triglycerides. Treatment of hyperlipidemia in patients with renal disease does appear to be of importance since such a condition is associated with the development of atherosclerosis. The diet in Table 4 may have to be modified in regard to protein and carbohydrate intake to accommodate the clinical condition of each patient with hyperlipidemia and renal disease (23).

Drug Treatment of Hyperlipoproteinemia. Virtually all children with hypertriglyceridemia can be managed with appropriate dietary therapy (see above). Many children with mild to moderate hypercholesterolemia will respond satisfactorily to dietary intervention (Table 4). In contrast, only about 1 in 5 of heterozygous FH children will respond to diet by lowering the total and LDL cholesterol into the normal range. The rest of the FH children will require treatment with a bile acid sequestrant. Either cholestyramine (Questran, Mead Johnson) or colestipol (Colestid, UpJohn) may be given. Both preparations come either in packets or can be given in bulk form (one scoop equals one dose). Cholestyramine is 9 grams/day, 4 grams of which is the active anion exchange resin, while colestipol is 5 grams/dose, almost all of which is active anion exchange resin. The dosage should be individualized depending on the post-dietary level of total and LDL cholesterol (Table 5) (26). This provides optimal lowering of total and LDL cholesterol without giving additional resin which is not effective, and such therapy is also expensive and difficult to take.

The major side effects of treatment with the bile acid sequestrants are constipation and some abdominal bloating or a feeling of fullness. Some children will develop low levels of serum folate, but this has not been reported to be associated with erythrocyte folate deficiency and anemia. While the potential for malabsorption of fat and fat-soluble vitamins is present, these findings are rarely if ever found using the dosages recommended (Table 5) . Nevertheless, it is prudent to check the tests of liver and kidney function, calcium, phosphorus, hematology tests, serum carotene and folate once a year while the children are on treatment. Growth and development are monitored although there is no report of any alterations in this regard. The child with homozygous FH is also treated with a combination of diet and bile acid sequestrant (up to 24-32 grams/day). It is often necessary to add nicotinic acid (up to 80 mg/kg/day in 2 to 3 divided doses) as a second agent to affect a further significant reduction in the LDL cholesterol level. FH homozygotes who have some residual LDL receptor activity, in general, tend to respond to a greater extent than FH homozygotes who do not synthesize any LDL receptor. Many FH homozygotes will require more heroic measures such as plasmapheresis, portacaval shunt and liver transplantation.

No general recommendation is made for the drug treatment of secondary hyperlipidemia of renal disease that does not respond satisfactorily to diet.

Table 5. Dosage Schedule for Treatment of Heterozygous Familial Hypercholesterolemic Children and Young Adults with a Bile Sequestrant

Daily doses of bile sequestrant	Post dietary plasma total cholesterol (TC) and low density lipoprotein (LDL) cholesterol levels (mg/dl)	
	TC	LDL-C
1	<245	<195
2	245-300	195-235
3	301-345	236-280
4	>345	>280

PREVENTION OF ATHEROSCLEROSIS

Results of the Lipid Research Clinics Coronary Primary Prevention Trial

Cholesterol hypothesis. Despite the large body of epidemiologic, pathologic, metabolic and genetic data indicating a causal role for increased levels of LDL cholesterol and the pathogenesis of atherosclerosis, definitive proof that the lowering of LDL cholesterol would prevent coronary artery disease and atherosclerosis in man was lacking. A number of previous primary and secondary prevention studies had provided tentative but not yet unequivocal evidence for the cholesterol hypothesis which can be formulated as follows. 1) The higher the plasma level of total and LDL cholesterol the greater the risk of coronary artery disease; 2) plasma levels of total and LDL cholesterol can be lowered by diet and drugs such as the bile acid sequestrant cholestyramine; but 3) does the lowering of plasma total and LDL cholesterol reduce the risk of coronary artery disease?

Study design. To answer this question, the LRC Coronary Primary Prevention Trial was designed and implemented in 1972 through 1975, at which time 3,806 men between the ages of 35 and 59 years were enrolled at 12 Lipid Research Clinics (27,28). Each of these men had primary elevations of plasma total and LDL cholesterol (type II lipoprotein patterns), had no clinical evidence of coronary artery disease at entry, diabetes, hypertension, and were otherwise healthy. The study design for this primary prevention trial involved randomization of participants into two groups: one group was given placebo, the other the bile sequestrant cholestyramine; both groups were instructed on a prudent diet low in cholesterol (< 400 mg/day) and total fat (< 35% of calories) and saturated fat (with a ratio of polyunsaturated to saturated fat of approximately 0.8). The study was double-blind, that is neither the participants nor the clinical staff knew into which of the two groups the patients had been randomized. Each participant was followed for a minimum of 7 years and some for as long as 10 years. The study ended in June of 1983 and the results were published in January of 1984 (27,28). Details of the randomization will not be reported here, but the two groups of participants were very similar in regard to their clinical and chemical characteristics. The primary endpoint was definite coronary artery disease death and/or nonfatal myocardial infarction. Secondary endpoints included all cause mortality, development of angina pectoris or positive exercise electrocardiogram, or performance of coronary artery bypass surgery.

Study Results. At the end of the study the vital status of each of the participants was ascertained (27). Both the placebo and cholestyramine groups were on similar diets, as judged with 24 hour dietary recalls, at both 1 and 7 year periods of followup. The difference between the placebo and cholestyramine groups for lowering of plasma total and LDL cholesterol levels was approximately 8.5% and 12.6%, respectively (27). The cholestyramine group experienced a 19% reduction in risk ($p < 0.05$) of the primary endpoint, reflecting a 24% reduction in definite CAD death and a 19% reduction in nonfatal myocardial infarction (27). Examination of other coronary heart disease endpoints showed a highly significant 25% reduction in risk for the development of positive exercise electrocardiograms, 20% reduction in the development of angina pectoris and a 21% reduction in the performance of coronary artery bypass surgery (27). All these differences were highly significant and of similar magnitude to the differences between the two groups in the primary endpoint. Total mortality was only 7% lower in the cholestyramine group. This was due to the fact that the drug treatment group had a higher number of deaths from suicides, accidents and homocides, which cancelled out the beneficial effect due to differences in death from coronary artery disease. The number of deaths from carcinoma were very similar in the two groups.

Because the differences between the two groups were statistically significant (using a standard clinical trial analysis) subsequent quantitative analyses were performed to examine the relation between degree of LDL lowering and CAD incidence (28). A highly significant relation was found that indicated that the greater the percent reduction in plasma total cholesterol levels in the subjects taking cholestyramine, the greater the percent reduction in coronary artery disease (Table 6). This quantitative relationship between decrease in incidence of CAD and the mass of plasma LDL cholesterol was roughly translated into the following rule of thumb: for every 1% lowering of plasma total cholesterol, there was a 2% reduction in risk for coronary artery disease (Table 6).

Table 6. Relation of Reduction in Cholesterol to Reduction in Coronary Heart Disease (CHD) Risk*

Packet Count	No.	Total Cholesterol Lowering	Reduction in CHD Risk
0-2	439	4.4%	10.9%
2-5	496	11.5%	26.1%
5-6	965	19.0%	39.3%

* Data are from 1900 male participants in the cholestyramine treatment group in the Lipid Research Clinics Coronary Prevention Trial (28).

Generalizability of study results. In summary, the major finding of the LRC Coronary Primary Prevention Trial was that this was the first study in humans to establish conclusively that lowering blood cholesterol reduced heart attacks and heart attack deaths (27,28). In regard to the generalizability of the findings (Table 7), they are strictly applicable to middle-aged men with hypercholesterolemia treated with a combination of diet and bile sequestrants. If one proposes to extend the generalizability, the results would be applicable to pediatric and geriatric patients with type II hyperlipoproteinemia, women, the top quintile of cholesterol (rather than the upper 5th percentile) and the use of diet with or without bile sequestrants (Table 7). Finally, the broadest interpretation is that the plasma cholesterol levels are too high in the population as a whole, and as a public health measure, appropriate dietary modifications (phase 1, Table 4) should be used by all Americans (in order to shift the distribution curve from a mean adult level of approximately 210 mg% closer to the mean of 150 mg% seen in adults in populations where coronary artery disease has a very low prevalence).

Table 7. Generalizability of Findings of Lipid Research Clinics Coronary Primary Prevention Trial

Generalizability	Applicable to	Estimated Number of Americans
None	Middle-aged men with a plasma total cholesterol level > 265 mg/dl treated with bile sequestrants	1-2 million
Limited	Wider age range (Pediatrics and geriatrics) Women Top quintile of plasma cholesterol level Diet $\pm$ bile sequestrants	45 million
Broad	Whole population Diet	225 million

Recommendations for Preventive Cardiology in Pediatrics

The following general recommendations are made (Table 8). A modified diet for all healthy children over the age of two years is recommended (phase 1, Table 4). Maintenance of ideal body weight and prevention of obesity are important. Blood pressure levels are monitored and the percentile followed. The patient is counseled against starting cigarette smoking. A family history for hyperlipidemia, premature cardiovascular disease before 60 years of age, and diabetes is taken and recorded for each pediatric patient. Children with such a positive family history are screened for plasma levels of total, LDL and HDL cholesterol and triglycerides and those with abnormal values are treated and followed. It is hoped that pediatrics, traditionally a specialty of prevention, will have an important role in the future prevention of premature atherosclerosis and coronary artery disease.

Table 8. Recommendations for Preventive Cardiology in Pediatrics

1. Modified diet for all healthy children over 2 years of age (American Heart Association Phase 1)
2. Maintenance of ideal body weight
3. Monitor blood pressure levels
4. Counsel against starting cigarette smoking
5. Record family history for hyperlipidemia, premature atherosclerosis (before 60 years of age) and diabetes
6. Screen children with positive family history by determining plasma levels of total, LDL and HDL cholesterol and total triglycerides

ACKNOWLEDGEMENTS

Carol McGeeney and Hazel Smith provided valuable assistance in the preparation of this manuscript. This work was supported, in part, by the General Clinical Research Centers Grant (RR-52), a contract from the Lipid Research Clinics Program (HL 2158) and a grant from the National Institutes of Health (1RO1-HL31497-01). The data from the Lipid Research Clinics Prevalence (20) and Coronary Primary Prevention Trial (27,28) studies were collected and analyzed by my colleagues in that program.

REFERENCES

1. Pearson, T.A.: Coronary arteriography in the study of the epidemiology of coronary artery disease. Epid. Rev. 6: 140-166, 1984.

2. Hulley, S.B., Rosenman, R.A., Barwal, R.D. and Brand, R.J.: Epidemiology as a guide to clinical decisions. The association between triglyceride and coronary heart disease. New Engl. J. Med. 302: 1383-1389, 1980.

3. Goldstein, J.L., Schrott, H.G., Hazzard, W.R., Bierman, E.L. and Motulsky, A.G.: Hyperlipidemia in coronary heart disease. II. Genetic analysis of lipid levels in 176 families and delineation of a new inherited disorder, combined hyperlipidemia. J. Clin. Invest. 52: 1544-1568, 1973.

4. Frerichs, R.R., Webber, L.S., Srinivasan, S.R. and Berenson, G.S.: Relation of serum lipids and lipoproteins to obesity and sexual maturity in white and black children. Am. J. Epidemiol. 108: 486-496, 1978.

5. Berenson, G.S., Cresanta, J.L. and Webber, C.S.: High blood pressure in the young. Ann. Rev. Med. 35: 535-550, 1984.

6. Kwiterovich, P.O., Jr.: Pediatric aspects of hyperlipoproteinemia. In Rifkind B.M. and Levy, R.I. (eds.): Hyperlipidemia, Diagnosis and Therapy. New York: Grune and Stratton, 1977, pp. 249-280.

7. Berenson, G.S., Voors, A.W., Gard, P., Newman, W.P., III and Tracy, R.E.: Clinical and anatomic correlates of cardiovascular disease in children from the Bogalusa Heart Study. In Schettler, F.G., Gotto, A.M., Jr. and Schlierf, G. (eds.). Atherosclerosis VI. Proceedings of the VIth International Symposium on Atherosclerosis. New York: Springer-Verlag, 1982.

8. Kwiterovich, P.O., Levy, R.I. and Fredrickson, D.S.: Neonatal diagnosis of familial type II hyperlipoproteinemia. Lancet 1: 118-122, 1973.

9. Kwiterovich, P.O., Fredrickson, D.S. and Levy, R.I.: Familial hypercholesterolemia (one form of familial type II hyperlipoproteinemia). A study of its biochemical, genetic and clinical presentation in childhood. J. Clin. Invest 53: 1237-1249, 1974.

10. Goldstein, J.L. and Brown, M.S.: The LDL receptor defect in familial hypercholesterolemia. Implications for pathogenesis and therapy. Med. Clin. North America 66: 335-362, 1982.

11. Brunzell, J.D., Albers, J.J., Chait, A., Grundy, S.M., Groszek, Z. and McDonald, G.B.: Plasma lipoproteins in familial combined hyperlipidemia and monogenic familial hypertriglyceridemia. J. Lipid Res. 24: 147-155, 1983.

12. Chait, A., Albers, J.J. and Brunzell, J.D.: Very low density lipoprotein overproduction in genetic forms of hypertriglyceridemia. Eur. J. Clin. Invest. 10: 17-22, 1980.

13. Sniderman, A.D., Shapiro, S., Marpole, D., Skinner, B., Teng, B., Kwiterovich, P.O., Jr.: Association of coronary atherosclerosis with hyperapobetalipoproteinemia (increased protein but normal cholesterol levels in human plasma low density lipoproteins). Proc. Natl. Acad. Sci. USA 77: 604-608, 1980.

14. Sniderman, A.D., Wolfson, C., Teng, B., Franklin, F.A., Bachorik, P.S. and Kwiterovich, P.O.: Association of hyperapobetalipoproteinemia with endogenous hypertriglyceridemia and atherosclerosis. Ann. Int. Med. 63: 833-838, 1982.

15. Teng, B., Thompson, G., Sniderman, A.D., Forte, T.M., Krause, R.M. and Kwiterovich, P.O.: Composition and distribution of low density lipoprotein fraction in hyperapobetalipoproteinemia, normal and familial hypercholesterolemia. Proc. Natl. Acad. Sci. USA 80: 662-666, 1983.

16. Sniderman, A.D., Teng, B., Genest, J., Cianfione, K. and Kwiterovich, P.O., Jr.: Familial aggregation and early expression of hyperapobetalipoproteinemia. Am. J. Card. 55:291-295, 1985.

17. Brunzell, J.D., Sniderman, A.D., Albers, J.J. and Kwiterovich, P.O., Jr.: Apoproteins B and A-1 and coronary artery disease in humans. Arteriosclerosis 4: 79-83, 1984.

18. Third, J.L.H.C., Montag, J., Flynn, M., Friedel, J., Laskarzewski, P. and Glueck, C.J.: Familial hypoalphalipoproteinemia. Metabolism 33: 136-146, 1984.

19. Glueck, C.J., Daniels, S.R., Bates, S., Benton, C., Tracy, T. and Third, J.L.H.C.: Pediatric victims of unexplained stroke and their families: Familial lipid and lipoprotein abnormalities. Pediatrics 69: 308-316, 1982.

20. The Lipid Research Clinics Population Studies Data Book. Volume I: The Prevalence Study. U.S. Department of Health and Human Services. Public Health Service, National Institutes of Health, NIH Publication No. 80-1527, July 1980.

21. Chan, M.K., Varghese, Z. and Moorhead, J.F.: Lipid abnormalities in uremia, dialysis, and transplantation. Kidney Int. 19: 625-637, 1981.

22. Vacha, G.M., Giorcelli, O., Siliprandi, N. and Corsi, M.: Favorable effects of L-carnitine treatment on hypertriglyceridemia in hemodialysis patients: decisive role of low levels of high-density lipoprotein-cholesterol. Am. J. Clin. Nutr. 38:532-540, 1983.

23. Krumlovsky, F.A.: Disorders of protein and lipid metabolism associated with chronic renal failure and chronic dialysis. Ann. Clin. Lab. Sci. 11: 350-360, 1981.

24. Disler, P.B., Goldberg, R.B., Kuhn, L., Meyers, A.M., Joffe, B.I. and Seftel, H.C.: The role of diet in the pathogenesis and control of hyperlipidemia after renal transplantation. Clin. Nephrol. 16: 29-34, 1981.

25. Shen, S.Y., Lukens, C.W., Alongi, S.V., Sfeir, R.E., Dagher, F.J. and Sadler, J.H.: Patient profile and effect of dietary therapy on post-transplant hyperlipidemia. Kidney Int. 24: S-147-S-152, 1983.

26. Farah, R., Kwiterovich, P.O., Jr. and Neill, C.A.: A study of the dose-effect of cholestyramine in children and young adults with familial hypercholesterolemia. Lancet 1: 59-63, 1977.

27. Lipid Research Clinics Program: The Lipid Research Clinics Coronary Primary Prevention Trial Results. I. Reduction in incidence of coronary heart disease. J.A.M.A. 251: 351-364, 1984.

28. Lipid Research Clinics Program: The Lipid Research Clinics Coronary Primary Prevention Trial Results. II. The relationship of reduction in incidence of coronary heart disease to cholesterol lowering. J.A.M.A. 251: 365-374, 1984.

DISCUSSION: HYPERTENSION AND ATHEROSCLEROSIS

PANELISTS: Sidney Blumenthal, M.D., Russell Chesney, M.D., Julie Ingelfinger, M.D. and Peter Kwiterovich, M.D.

MODERATOR: Jose Strauss, M.D.

QUESTION: Are there any data showing the possibility of detecting by non-invasive methods, evidence of premature atherosclerosis? We have been concerned with the finding of persistent hyperlipidemia in a number of children with Nephrotic Syndrome. The problem we are facing is that apart from the follow-up which will take many years, we do not have any way to determine what is the exact risk of these patients for developing premature atherosclerosis. The second question is, can you comment on the use of drugs that will increase the LDL receptors as a means of decreasing LDL cholesterol?

RESPONSE: The first question is related to the methods available to detect atherosclerosis non-invasively. Some people have done studies with digital substraction angiography of the femoral artery; several reports have been published. They have used this method to follow femoral atherosclerosis and its regression with treatment of hyperlipidemia. There are other methods which perhaps have been less tested in the pediatric group. In young adults, for example, I do not hesitate to do a stress electrocardiogram, and in some patients, a Thalium stress electrocardiogram. We recently have been doing some work with the cardiologists on computerized tomography following a stress Thalium scan; this is a sensitive indicator of the presence of occult coronary artery disease in young siblings of probands who have premature disease. Those are some of the methods that are currently available. What we really will need in the future are better non-invasive methods that do not use radioactive materials to assess the presence of coronary atherosclerosis.

The second question is related to use of drugs to increase LDL receptor activity. Cholestiramine is a bile acid secretant which binds bile in the intestine; it interrupts the entero-hepatic circulation. Since cholesterol is a C-27 steroid and it is used to make bile acids which are C-24 steroids, by interrupting the entero-hepatic circulation, more cholesterol is utilized by the liver to synthesize bile acids. This depletes the cholesterol pool in the liver, and since the synthesis of LDL receptors is regulated by the mass of cholesterol inside the cell, a greater number of LDL receptors are synthesized; they appear in the surface of the liver cells and bind LDL, which is then internalized and degraded. So, the mode of action of cholestiramine, both by cellular studies and by metabolic studies using radioactive tracer materials, indicates that this medication acts by increasing the number of LDL receptors in the liver.

MODERATOR: Would you treat the nephrotic hyperlipidemia? This is a subject we have been debating, an incredibly overlooked problem which is due to the major lipid changes that are present, as described by our group in a recent paper. After the patients go into remission these changes persist and are reflected in the blood and in the composition of subcutaneous fat; they fit the characteristics that were described earlier for patients at high risk.

COMMENT-RESPONSE: My opinion is, if the nephrotic syndrome is in remission and there are elevated levels of LDL, that should be treated. I would treat first with diet. To select a medication might be a bit trickier. I did a quick review of the literature and found some opinion that increased LDL levels in the nephrotic syndrome are related to increased synthesis of lipoproteins in the liver. If that is the mechanism and if that mechanism persists even after the syndrome is in some sort of remission, then one might have to rethink what agent one might use--perhaps some agent which would block the synthesis of lipoproteins in the liver; perhaps nicotinic acid in high doses or perhaps an inhibitor of HMG such as mevinolin would be appropriate. However, this is an experimental medication at the present time. These are important questions particularly for nephrologists. Needed are studies looking into the effects of certain drugs, whether they would be bile sequestrants or agents which would decrease the synthesis of lipids and lipoproteins in the liver.

MODERATOR: You should know that some of our patients were up to five years in remission and still showed lipid changes.

COMMENT-QUESTION: I am interested in the prudent diet which is recommended today by the American Heart Association. There are three phases. You seemed to use only the first phase in your study. I would like to discuss the distribution of calories. In some of the patients, both normal and uremic patients who have been studied, when we use a high carbohydrate concentration--especially the simple carbohydrates as opposed to the more complex ones--there seems to be a tendency to increase the cholesterol. For the new prudent diet are there specifications regarding carbohydrate type?

RESPONSE: Thank you for bringing up that point. All three phases of the diet include increase in complex carbohydrates and decrease in simple sugars. This is important because now we use these diets for hypertriglyceridemia as well as for hypercholesterolemia. Since it is known that simple sugars can lead to the so-called "carbohydrate inducibility" which will increase triglycerides, "yes" is the answer to your question. There is a decrease in the simple sugars in these diets, and an increase in the complex carbohydrates.

QUESTION: It seems to me that in the last few years in the literature there has been a switch or at least the start of a swing of the pendulum from aggressive treatment of mild hypertension to some questioning as to whether such treatment is beneficial or harmful. Several recent papers have questioned whether mild hypertension should be treated, especially with drugs. Could the panel comment on that?

RESPONSE: There are some data which suggest that the classical step therapy and the use of a thiazide diuretic are associated obviously with a lowering of blood pressure and lowering of the incidence of stroke, but not a lowering of the incidence of coronary artery disease. The explanations which have been offered have included the fact that some of the thiazides induce changes in lipid metabolism and in potassium metabolism. You are right. There is some current controversy but, in total, the mortality rate associated with the treatment of lower blood pressure is probably less. Maybe there is some trade-off. If you take it down to children, you come back with the question of the drug of choice. Should one decide to treat mild persistent hypertension starting in adolescence, one has a real problem in deciding with what to treat that patient. My personal preference is to try to obtain a renin profile in the child. If he has a high renin, use a renin blocker; if he has what looks like a low renin, maybe use a diuretic. Other people are recommending the uniform use initially of alpha blockade because one seems to get less secondary effects. I do not think that we know what to do in the pediatric population.

MODERATOR: What about the alpha and beta blockers?

RESPONSE: I am not a clinical pharmacologist. Maybe one of my colleagues can speak of it better. Of the various beta blocking agents, which I never can keep straight, some are associated with elevation in some of the "bad" lipid substances. The alpha blockers do not seem to do this; they do not seem to affect lipids and therefore are recommended.

RESPONSE: I agree with what was just said. There are no data to guide us in treating the young patient with essential hypertension. There is very little published experience using alpha blockade or centrally active alpha stimulating agents in young patients with essential hypertension. I do not want to say what the recommendation should be. What I would like to stick my neck out and say first is that given the usual age of the population we are treating, I think there is a big case to be made for using mono-therapy in the young patient with essential hypertension who requires pharmacotherapy. Second, since we do not as yet have longitudinal data showing what happens when you put people on an anti-hypertensive agent at age 13 and treat them until they are 55, or 85, or what have you, I think there is a real role for short-term treatment with anti-hypertensives clinically, to find out whether it is possible to control hypertension and perhaps, if one believes in it, "untrack" somebody from his hypertension. On the other hand, there is a need for longitudinal cooperative studies so that we can get some adequate data.

MODERATOR: One of the Guest Faculty was on the Task Force which outlined some of the initial steps to be followed in the study and treatment of hypertension in children. Those recommendations were published in 1975 in Pediatrics as a Supplement. Do you have any comments on that? Since you have been interested in "tracking", would you like to comment?

RESPONSE-COMMENT: I do not have anything to add other than the warning that I mentioned earlier in the Seminar. If one is going to treat for a limited period of time, one has to be certain that one is following these patients very carefully over a long period of time. Dr. Harriet Dustan keeps repeating this over and over again. In terms of the experience with adults, it is important to note that often those patients are controlled for short periods of time after discontinuation of therapy, and then frequently lost to follow-up. If you are going to embark on this kind of a program (and I do not see why not to), you need to be very careful. I would hope that there would be collaborative trials set up so that large numbers of patients can be observed, particularly those treated for long periods of time, in terms of the side effects.

MODERATOR: It is significant that we have cardiologists, nephrologists, and "in-between people" sitting together. I remember when the Task Force was being formed, we talked about having at least one nephrologist in that group since nephrologists believe that hypertension is a renal disease and the heart happens to get involved in the process as a bystander.

QUESTION: You mentioned the Japanese rat in your talk. Coming from an area where the main industry is the automobile, can you tell us how many of those rats you can import?

RESPONSE: That is a very good question! I do not know why these rats were discovered in Japan. I will have to get the history of them from members of the Department of Medicine at my institution who have been working with them for a long time. I can assure you that they can be obtained from local breeders. They have a whole section of spontaneously hypertensive rats of the Wistar-Kyoto strain; these are American rats fed American chow. They must have been brought over initially.

MODERATOR: I guess some people are questioning whether or not there is a difference in the way rats are bred in different countries.

QUESTION: In your review or in your general fund of information, is there a role for magnesium therapy in essential hypertension? Is there an abnormality which has been described?

RESPONSE: Very definitely there have been abnormalities described in magnesium handling, both in essential hypertensive humans and in animals. The data are the same as for calcium: they are somewhat conflicting. The levels of magnesium that have been reported to be in the serum are also conflicting: some people have reported reductions in magnesium and others have reported that the magnesium levels are normal. I think that the best reference for this (if you are interested) is the Annals of Internal Medicine of 1983, where there are reviewed a whole host of factors, including divalent minerals, in terms of hypertension. The one thing that I didn't emphasize earlier and which I want to emphasize, is that the hypertension is multifactorial. The interesting thing about the consideration of divalent minerals is that they are another part of the puzzle; it may well be that studies will show their importance in the future.

QUESTION: Has there been a role for the anions associated with sodium, which have been described independently of sodium? In other words, does chloride play a role?

RESPONSE: I honestly cannot answer that question. Maybe somebody else can.

RESPONSE: The first studies suggesting that salt is associated with hypertension, reported in the first decade of this century, actually measured chloride. There have been some experimental studies which suggest that it is chloride that is important when we are looking at salt-sensitive hypertensives, and perhaps not solely sodium. The data are a bit conflicting, but chloride is probably quite important. Obviously, chloride can be transported along with calcium, and the interaction of calcium and sodium exchanges across cells may be important in hypertension. Since there are six or seven calcium channels, there are many ways to explain some of the many findings that are now being described.

RESPONSE: Perhaps the most compelling evidence that it is related to chloride comes from studies which examined the effect of various anions. They looked at the use of sodium bicarbonate or sodium coupled with amino acids; the hypertension was really found only with sodium chloride. Using other anions, the hypertension was not found. Furthermore, there have been some studies that have looked at dietary sodium intake in infants and have reported a reduction in blood pressure in infants who were fed a low sodium diet. What was happening, actually, was that at the same time the chloride intake was being reduced to an equivalent degree. I think that there is an important role for chloride in this. A lot of data about this will be coming out in the next several years which will allow us to look into this further. If you do use sodium plus bicarbonate, you do not get the same degree of hypertension as when you use sodium plus chloride.

QUESTION: The question of non-pharmacologic management of hypertension clinically, calcium, and what not, has received some attention; yet it seems that if you encourage a high calcium diet, you may be encouraging a higher intake of cholesterol--certainly if people are increasing their intake of dietary products that we are used to. Does the calcium itself in a high quantity perhaps have other negative effects in terms of calcium excretion and so on? Would there be a higher incidence of stone disease in patients who ingest calcium even in pharmacologic forms? Has that been looked into?

RESPONSE: No, that has not been done. I guess the concern would be in people who have established hypercalciuric states, particularly of the intestinal absorptive type which can run in families. I would think, if one were advising an increase in calcium intake, that you would have to be very cautious in those individuals who have a family history of stones or a family history of hematuria in whom hypercalciuria of the hyperabsorptive type was demonstrated. In those individuals with the renal leak, there really is no influence by dietary calcium; in most individuals, dietary calcium generally is not reflected in urinary calcium excretion. One further point that you have raised regarding dairy products is that if you are taking those products in large amounts, obviously the sodium intake is going to go up and also the intake of fats is going to be higher. You can get around this by using skim milk, obviously, to reduce the fats. That is why other non-dairy products as sources of calcium may become important. I do not think that we know this at the present time; the data are not in. Actually, other calcium supplements have been used, and enhancers of calcium absorption. There is a role for milk in enhancing intestinal absorption of calcium which does not relate to the vitamin D in the milk; it really relates to the lactose in the milk. In persons who are not intolerant of lactose, it enhances intestinal calcium absorption. For that reason, if one is giving calcium supplementation, there is an advantage in giving it in the form of milk--that is, provided that the person can tolerate milk. My concern, however, is what should we be doing about children who have milk intolerance? Are they getting enough vitamin D? Are they getting enough calcium in their diet? Often they are not, unless they are eating broccoli, spinach and things of that nature.

QUESTION: Are there any differences in blood pressure among lactose tolerant and lactose intolerant individuals whom you would expect to have had a major life-long difference in calcium intake?

RESPONSE: I do not know. I do not think that has been looked at. We certainly know that blood pressure among blacks is higher than among caucasians, but I am not saying that that is the reason.

QUESTION: Can you briefly comment on the role of cigarette smoking in all of this? That is intriguing in terms of the role it may have in the modern view of atherogenesis.

RESPONSE: Most of us feel that among the risk factors that are probably causal, this is number one. It is a type of number one about which something can be done. The whole cigarette-tobacco industry and the way our country is handling it, are a national disgrace.

QUESTION: Can you give us a mechanism?

RESPONSE: I do not think that the mechanism is clearly known in terms of what it is in cigarette smoking that does the harm, but presumably it results ultimately in intimal injury. It serves as a noxious agent in terms of intimal injury which then is perpetuated.

QUESTION: My question has to do with overall mortality. I have never heard a good explanation of why there is no difference in overall mortality between the placebo group and the treated group.

RESPONSE: In the Lipid Research Clinic, the mortality from coronary artery disease was about 20-50% lower in the cholestiramine group than in the placebo group. The data on mortality were consistent with the data measuring other parameters of cardiovascular risk such as myocardial infarction, stress electrocardiogram, etc. The reason that the total mortality was not different between the two groups was that in this particular study, in the cholestiramine group, there happened to be an excess of deaths from accidents--primarily automobile accidents , suicides, and homicides. So, the difference in mortality due to coronary artery disease was cancelled out. There have been a lot of jokes made about this: "If you lower your cholesterol you are more likely to drink, or be in an automobile accident, or be killed in the street". After reviewing the autopsy material from the study, the simplest explanation in the Lipid Research Clinic study was that this was a quirk, but those men are being followed over the next five years to be sure that this may not be something important. The World Health

Organization trial, in which there are individuals who lower their cholesterol with chlofibrate, had statistically significant lower incidence of non-fatal myocardial infarctions. The reason that the mortality was not different in that study was that the chlofibrate had adverse effects such as liver disease and gall bladder disease. Also, chlofibrate being absorbed into the bloodstream has a number of systemic effects that cholestiramine does not have, since cholestiramine is not absorbed into the bloodstream. In any event, in a randomized clinical trial it is difficult to demonstrate a difference between the two groups because of differences in compliance. When you do demonstrate a difference, as in this particular study, there can be unfortunate developments which cloud the issue. My own bias is that lowering cholesterol does not enhance mortality from other causes. The epidemiologic data from some population studies on low cholesterol levels being associated with more carcinoma, have now been concluded to reveal a situation in which people with occult carcinoma happened to have lower cholesterol levels and they subsequently developed cancer, rather than the other way around. In other words, they first had the cancer which was not detected and the cholesterol levels were low; then the cancer was detected--rather than the other way around.

MODERATOR: I would like to ask the last question. It pertains to something that has been discussed in this community quite extensively and last year in Washington at a workshop that the Department of Health and Human Services called to discuss hypertension among Latins. In this community it has been found that adolescents of Latin ancestry have a higher incidence of hypertension than even blacks when matched for sex and age. I do not know how reliably that has been looked at, but apparently it is a fact. Has anyone come across this information? Is there any comment in that regard? I imagine diet and other factors may play a role, if indeed that is the case. As far as we know, Latins throughout Latin America do not have a higher incidence of hypertension.

COMMENT-QUESTION: In Philadelphia, just thinking of the populations we saw, it was quite unusual to see a hispanic who had essential hypertension. It was predominantly in the black population. Whether moving to another society has any relationship, I do not know. Are there other cities where the hispanic adolescent has more hypertension? New York City?

MODERATOR: Apparently, the group here (which has worked through the Greater Miami Chapter of the American Heart Association), so far is the only one that has come up with such data. This raises the question of validity.

COMMENT: In a study of a large number of adolescents in the New York area, the predominant group who had elevated blood pressure, as recognized by other people, was black adolescents. I do not know the data well enough in terms of how many hispanics were studied. There is a large hispanic community in New York, as you know, but I do know that in that data, it was the black population that had elevated BP's.

MODERATOR: The Latin population in New York is mainly Puerto Rican, like in Philadelphia; here it is Cuban. I wonder if that may have something to do with it. Our time is out so we will stop here. Thank you.

IV

CONGENITAL RENAL ANOMALIES

DILEMMAS CREATED BY PRENATAL DETECTION OF URINARY TRACT ANOMALIES

Warren E. Grupe, M.D.

It has been slightly more than a decade since Garrett first reported the successful in-utero diagnosis of polycystic kidneys using ultrasound (1). Advances in ultrasonographic techniques has not only allowed a rapid improvement in the ability to study fetal anatomy, but has stimulated an equally rapid expansion of routine procedures, even when there is no special indication. As might be expected, the discovery of malformations has quickly expanded. The prevalence of abnormalities approximates 1-2 per thousand ultrasound procedures, of which 20-33% are anomalies of the genitourinary tract (2,3). Over 90% of the reported prenatally detected malformations have appeared in print since 1980 (4).

The potential value of this improving capability is unquestioned. Congenital anomalies of the genitourinary tract can be detected as early as 12-15 weeks gestation (5-9). One can identify 90% of fetal kidneys by 17-20 weeks of gestation and 95% by the 22nd week (5). One can detect anomalies that require immediate postnatal treatment, many of which would not be recognized in the otherwise asymptomatic child by routine nursery examinations (8). One can also pick the time, mode, and place of delivery that will maximize postnatal care. The potential for intrauterine correction emerges. An opportunity for the parents to receive counsel and to adjust to the situation is presented. Of these possible benefits, the justification that receives the most universal support is that the postnatal management can be prospectively organized and promptly initiated.

However, before this new and expanding capability becomes a fundamental part of perinatal practice, the dilemmas created by this new technology should be examined, and its accuracy and reliability assessed (8-10). The errors in ultrasound diagnosis are few in number, but the consequences of a mistake can be considerable. Not all retroperitoneal masses, for example, are renal. The enlargement of the stomach produced by duodenal atresia can be easily confused with ureteropelvic junction abnormality (5). In like fashion, a large dilated renal pelvis has been interpreted as duodenal atresia (11). The distinction between multicystic kidneys and ureteropelvic junction obstruction is not as sharp in the fetus as it is postnatally (5). Physiologic dilatation, can appear as obstruction (3,5,6,8). In a 1982 report from the U.S.A., 8 of 13 patients (61%) with proven obstructive disease at birth had an incorrect diagnosis made at the time of prenatal ultrasound examination (12). In a 1984 study from the United Kingdom, 13 out of 32 (41%) had an incorrect diagnosis by ultrasound and three had no obstruction at all when examined postnatally (8). In another 1984 review from France, the initial prenatal diagnosis was incorrect in 10 of 44 patients (23%) (4). In three of these, the abnormality detected was mis-interpreted as nonrenal; in two others, prenatal urinary tract dilatation had disappeared after birth; in the other five, a bilateral renal lesion was thought to be unilateral (4).

Even when the accuracy of prenatal diagnosis is excellent, problems can arise. In a report from Cleveland it was noted that an experienced team was accurate 96% of the time (3). However, of 38 pregnancies terminated prior to 21 weeks, the diagnosis was incorrect in five instances. Thus, 13% of the pregnancies were terminated for the wrong reason, even in a center that had a higher than usual degree of accuracy (3). In another study from Glasgow, 18 fetuses were defined as having urinary abnormalities (13). In 16 of the 18 (89%) the original renal diagnosis was correct; the two in error were thought to be gastrointestinal in origin. However, two additional children had unrecognized abnormalities of the bowel in addition to their renal lesions and in another with a prenatal diagnosis of unilateral disease, the contralateral kidney was absent at birth (13). Five of the infants were delivered by Cesarean section because of concern that continued intrauterine obstruction would produce progressive renal damage. Seven infants died of renal or pulmonary failure (39%); for these seven, an early diagnosis was of no help (13). One conclusion made by the authors was that few fetuses with genitourinary anomalies would have been helped by intrauterine intervention (13).

It has not been easy to differentiate physiologic dilatation from high pressure obstruction (4-6,11). Transient obstruction is a normal component of the canalization of the genitourinary tract (14). A delay in canalization or a delay in the rupture of the cloacal membrane can produce transient dilatation (5). In like fashion, the close of the allantois at 16 weeks or of the urachus at 32nd weeks may be the first experience with high resistance outflow for that particular system, producing a temporary dilatation (5). Conversely, a delay in the closure of either the allantois or the urachus could produce a protracted period of decompression for an otherwise obstructed tract; by ultrasound, such a tract may seem normal at first, then become worse as pregnancy progresses. It is not surprising, therefore, that transient dilatation has been reported in as high as 10-20% of fetuses in the third trimester (3-6,8,11). Although not physiologically significant, such findings are ultrasonographically confusing. To date, the only way to define transient nonobstructive dilatation of the genitourinary tract is through serial examinations of the fetus.

The ability to assess renal function by ultrasonographic techniques is not very reliable. Currently no accurate test exists to define intrauterine renal function or to predict the potential for recovery. Oligohydramnios is the most reliable reflection of disordered function (4-6). However, the absence of oligohydramnios is no assurance of normal renal function. Two tests have been proposed to evaluate intrauterine urine production. One trial is to give furosemide to the mother to increase fetal urine output, which can then be assessed by the rate at which the bladder fills (15,16). Failure of the bladder to fill is interpreted as abnormal. A second method is to aspirate the bladder, then measure the rate at which it refills (17). Both of these methods fail on at least two counts. First, at any age, the volume of urine does not reflect the glomerular filtration rate. It is well recognized, in fact, that polyuria is the usual response to renal damage. Secondly, massive reflux, which is often present with obstruction, makes even the accurate measure of urine flow impossible; the bladder can fill quite well with the urine drained from the upper tract.

One well presented case clearly outlines how complex the problems can be (6). At 18 weeks gestation, dilatation of the posterior urethra, megacystis and minimal right hydronephrosis were diagnosed by ultrasound. The amount of amniotic fluid was normal and the bladder promptly filled at a normal rate following aspiration. A repeat ultrasonogram at 20 weeks showed the hydronephrosis to be bilateral. Again there was a normal amount of amniotic fluid and the bladder refilled once more at a normal rate. At 26 weeks, oligohydramnios was noted. However by 30 weeks the ultrasonographic examination had improved; the bladder was normal and the hydronephrophsis had resolved. At 36 weeks, the infant was vaginally delivered, but died at 16 hours of age with profound pulmonary insufficiency. A urethral valve with severe bilateral dysplasia was found at autopsy. In this particular case the resolution of urinary tract dilatation was the ominous sign of deteriorating function rather than an indication of the resolution of transient physiologic hydronephrosis.

As might be anticipated, the ability to detect urinary tract malformations in utero was almost immediately followed by efforts toward intrauterine intervention. The first attempt, reported in 1981, was considered quite successful (17). However, subsequent reports have failed to define a consistent role for the intrauterine relief of obstruction. Only three procedures have been used to any degree: 1. percutaneous needle aspiration of the bladder; 2. placement of a drain between the fetal bladder and the amniotic fluid, and 3. intrauterine surgery to decompress the urinary tract (4-7,17-19).

The reasons to attempt intrauterine intervention include preservation of renal function or prevention of pulmonary hypoplasia. There is little evidence that the intrauterine drainage of urine by any means has any influence on either of these two concerns. In several series, the number of infants with severe oligohydramnios who have been delivered with adequate renal function is very small, even after intrauterine drainage, and the benefit to the child of any intrauterine manipulation is far from obvious (4-9,17-19). The example of one report is representative (22). Intrauterine drainage was performed on eight fetuses with a rather morose outcome. Three infants died soon after delivery with Potter's syndrome; two more were lost in-utero after attempts at drainage, and two others were terminated at 13 and 17 weeks. The only viable infant with adequate renal function had bilateral ureteropelvic junction obstruction; because of the site of obstruction, it is hard to see how bladder drainage could be appropriate in the first place. It may be that the only realistic intrauterine intervention is termination of the pregnancy (23); such drastic intervention, of course, assumes that the original diagnosis is correct.

If the goal of intervention is to prevent renal dysplasia,the current evidence questions whether dysplasia can be avoided at any stage of gestation (4,5,7). That dysplasia is commonly associated with obstructive uropathy is not firm evidence that they are causally related or that relief of obstruction will alter the abnormal development of the kidney (24,25). If, on the other hand, dysplasia evolves from a primary abnormality in the origin of the ureteric duct, then the relief of obstruction would not be expected to change the pattern of nephron development (26,27). The presence of irreversible dysplasia at 15 weeks gestation in one case report suggests that at least for some, even successful intervention does not alter the course of abnormal embryogenesis (7).

The second reason for intervention is an attempt to prevent the development of pulmonary hypoplasia. When the amount of amniotic fluid is reduced by uterine aspiration in the rat, pulmonary hypoplasia develops (28). Such data suggest that oligohydramnios from genitourinary obstruction could produce pulmonary hypoplasia, a suggestion that has some support in human experience (20,29,30). If the release of obstruction could lessen the degree of pulmonary dysfunction, then intrauterine drainage could have value. Unfortunately the human experience is not that clear; the degree of oligohydramnios may have no relationship to the amount of subsequent pulmonary involvement. For example, in one case report, the successful relief of intrauterine obstruction at 32 weeks of age resulted in an infant born with the prune belly syndrome and adequate renal function who at four months of age was using a home respirator for his pulmonary disease (6).

The risks of intervention are not miniscule and include hemorrhage, sepsis, abortion, premature labor, fetal and maternal death. These must be seriously considered in any program of intrauterine intervention. At the moment, none of the therapeutic manipulations currently undertaken in utero can be considered to have benefit. Nevertheless, the availability of fetal intervention tends to encourage an unrealistic attitude towards its role and importance.

One aspect not frequently discussed is the effect that intrauterine diagnosis has on the parent(9,10,13). By the very nature of the ultrasonographic studies, it is impossible to conceal that a diagnositic problem exists. Even though the average time of detection is about 30 weeks gestation, there are increasing instances of diagnoses made much earlier. Thus, the parents could have more than five months to wonder and worry. Feelings of inadequacy, guilt, fear, and anger; a refusal to bond to the infant or a refusal to anticipate delivery are not surprising. It is impossible to reassure a parent when the accuracy of the diagnosis may be open to question. A parents quest for precise answers, therefore, must often be met by a facade of uncertainty and equivocation. It is exceedingly difficult to counsel patients when the diagnosis has a reasonable chance to be either incorrect or incomplete. An incorrect diagnosis can produce inappropriate antenatal advice. The consequences of a mistake in diagnosis can be quite considerable in some instances; that termination might be advised for the wrong reasons could even qualify as a disaster (3).

Since the dilemmas are poorly resolved, guidelines for management that protect the fetus and parents as much as possible would be helpful. Several protocols have been offered (4,5,8,17,18). First, a single examination is never enough to either include or exclude fetal abnormalities. Second, early delivery is rarely necessary. One must avoid the natural urge "to do something", and resist those same pressures from the family. Prematurity generally worsens the prognosis of postnatal surgery. It is probably a more valuable use of time to carefully arrange and plan the postnatal management of the infant.

Third, fetal surgery, so far, is limited to drainage only (19). Unilateral disease rarely needs intrauterine intervention. If there is bilateral dilatation with adequate amniotic fluid, intervention is probably not required until after delivery. If obstruction is bilateral with severe oligohydramnios, current evidence suggests that interventions are futile. More difficult are the small number of fetuses where bilateral obstruction is present with equivocal amounts of amniotic fluid; there is still no evidence that intrauterine manipulation clearly alters the course for these children. In no circumstance is there clear evidence that early drainage avoids dysplasia, improves renal function, avoids a pulmonary complication, or offers any advantage over appropriate postnatal surgery following a term delivery. Finally, studies must be repeated post delivery no matter how convincing the prenatal evidence is. What existed in-utero may no longer exist.

Intrauterine diagnosis identifies the child at risk and in need of further, more reliable, evaluation. Over half of these children would have remained unknown (8). A system should be in place to support the parents extensively (9,10,13). Early knowledge of an anomaly, even with counseling, is not an assurance that the parents will adjust to the situation calmly, gradually, or successfully. Communication between all providers of care becomes essential if an appropriate postnatal plan is to be formulated. This includes coordination between the obstetrician, the ultrasonographer, the pediatrician, the neonatologist, the nephrologist and the urologist.

REFERENCES

1. Garret, W.J., Grunwald, G. and Robinson, D.E. Aust. New Zeal. Obstet. Gynaec. 10:7-9, 1970.
2. King, L.R. J. Urol 133:155, 1985.
3. Gauderer, M.W.L., Jassani, M.N. and Izant, R.J. J. Ped. Surg. 19:404-407, 1984.
4. Broyer, M., Guest, G., Lestage, F. et al. Adv. in Nephrology 14:21-38, 1985.
5. Kramer, S.A. J. Urol. 130:641-646, 1983.
6. Diamond, D.A., Sanders, R., and Jeffs, R.D. J. Urol. 131:1155-1159, 1984.
7. Bellinger, M.F., Comstock, C.H., Grosso, D. and Zaino, R. J. Urol. 129:1238-1239, 1983.
8. Turnock, R.R. and Shawis, R. Arch. Dis. Child 59:962-965, 1984.
9. Editorial: When ultrasound shows fetal abnormality. Lancet 1:618-619, 1985.
10. Mervyn Griffiths, D. and Gough, M.H. Lancet 1:623-624, 1985.
11. Sanders, R. and Graham, D. J. Ultrasound Med. 1:341-348, 1982.
12. Mahan, J., Gonzales, R., Godec, C.J. and Vernier, R.L.: Intrauterine obstructive uropathy: is early detection and intervention beneficial? Proceedings of the Northwestern Pediatric Society, 1982.
13. Hutson, J.M., McNay, M.B., MacKenzie, J.R. et al. Lancet 1:621-623,1985.
14. Ruano-Gil, D., Coca-Payeras, A. and Tejedo-Mateu, A. Eur. Urol. 1:287-293, 1975.
15. Wladimiroff, J.W. Brit. J. Obst. Gynaec. 82:221-224, 1975.
16. Waldimiroff, J.W. and Campbell, S. Lancet 1:151-154, 1974.
17. Harrison, M.R., Filly, R.A., Parer, J.T., et al. JAMA 246:635-639, 1981.
18. Harrison, M.R., Golbus, M.S. and Filly, R.A. JAMA 246774-777, 1981.
19. Harrison, M.R., Golbus, M.S., Filly, R.A., et al. N. Eng. J. Med. 306:591-593, 1982.
20. Duckett, J.W., Harrison, M.R., de Lorimer, A.A., et al. Dialogues Pediat. Urol. 5:1-8, 1982.
21. Blane, C.E., Koff, S.A., Bowerman, R.A. and Barr, M., Jr. Radiology 147:95-99, 1983.
22. Golbus, M.S., Harrison, M.R. and Filly, R.A. Sem. in Perinatology 7:102-108, 1983.
23. Campbell, S. and Pearce, J.M. Clin. Obstet. Gynecol. 10:475-506, 1983.
24. Beck, A.D. J. Urol. 105:784-789, 1971.
25. Bernstein, J. Ped. Clin. N. Amer. 18:395-407, 1971.
26. Schwarz, R.D., Stephens, F.D. and Cussen, L. J. Invest. Urol. 19:97-100, 1981.
27. Mackie, G.G. and Stephens, F.D. J. Urol. 114:274-280, 1975.
28. Symchych, P.S. and Winchester, P. Amer. J. Path. 90:779-782, 1978.
29. Harrison, M.R., Nakayama, D.K., Noall, R. and de Lorimier, A.A.: J. Pediatr. Surg. 17:965-974, 1982.
30. Mauer, S., Dobrin, R. and Vernier, R. J. Pediatr. 84:236-238, 1984.

NUTRITIONAL ASPECTS OF GROWTH IN CHILDREN WITH CONGENITAL RENAL ANOMALIES

Carolyn Abitbol, M.D., Michael Freundlich, M.D., Gaston Zilleruelo, M.D. and Jose Strauss, M.D.

The problem of the uremic dwarf is of primary concern to the pediatric nephrologist. The ultimate rehabilitation of the pediatric patient with progressive renal failure will depend on our ability to solve this dilemma. It is undoubtedly a multifaceted problem, since growth, normal and abnormal, is influenced by genetic, humoral, and nutritional factors.

When one examines normal patterns of growth by growth velocity curves, it is apparent that maximum growth occurs in the first two years of life and doubles during adolescence. These are the periods when the physiologic system is primed for maximum growth response to the various stimuli imposed upon it. Logically speaking, therefore, growth loss would be maximal when growth potential is maximal. Hence, those patients with significant physiologic stress from birth appear to be most affected with height loss. This is the circumstance frequently imposed by congenital renal disease. Most observers report near normal growth rates in these same patients in the interims between infancy and adolescence (1). Hence, it appears that relatively speaking, a temporary growth delay in infancy is potentially more damaging than a similar delay in later childhood.

Humoral-genetic factors appear to predominate during adolescence, while nutritional-genetic factors may be most influential on growth during infancy (2). The potential for catch-up growth, that is, the regaining of lost linear growth, may also be limited to the prime times of infancy and adolescence. The prototype of this statement is the infant born small for gestational age from intrauterine malnutrition who fails to regain linear percentiles during the first year of life, rarely achieving normal adult stature (3).

Clinical workers in the field have long recognized some influence of protein and energy malnutrition on growth in children with renal failure. A brief review of these experimental and clinical data is necessary to present an appropriate perspective of the problem. Even though the influence on growth by uremic anorexia and poor nutritional intake was recognized many years ago (4), it was difficult to demonstrate absolute malnutrition since frequently those were obese uremic children.

Nevertheless, Simmons et al. (5) demonstrated increased growth velocity in dialyzed children provided daily non-protein energy supplements for a period of six months. Although the benefit of increased energy intake on linear growth was indisputable, the problem in practical clinical terms was that patients too often found the diet unpalatable and were unable to maintain the supplements for prolonged periods. Moreover, in those that did continue calorie supplementation, the benefits were short-lived and obesity became the trade-off.

In the classical laboratory model of rats rendered chronically uremic by sub-total nephrectomy (6), the sub-normal growth which results are mirrored in paired, control animals fed an identical quantity of rations. A small differential in linear growth between the uremic and pair fed animals has been attributed to osteodystrophy which is partially treated by calcium, phosphorus, and vitamin D supplementation (7). Some studies have indicated that, in the uremic animal, there is suppression of protein synthetic rates (8) as well as increased catabolism (9-10). Either circumstance would result in increased requirements for maintenance as well as growth. Since dietary supplementation in the uremic rat model is extremely difficult, no long-term prospective laboratory study has been performed. A study on rats who have congenital lesions of the hypothalamus and excessive appetite (hyperphagic rats), showed that these rats ate a quantity similar to that of normal controls (11). They also had similar linear growth rates suggesting that the uremic animal has a potentially normal growth response to adequate intake.

The influence on growth by other factors such as metabolic acidosis, metabolic bone disease, and hormones remains controversial. At this point, it seems safe to say that uremic hypophagia with inadequate nutrient intake presents a potentially remediable problem. The therapeutic theorem would be that appropriate nutrition administered during the period of maximum linear growth velocity could result in normal growth. We have yet to determine whether the uremic infant or child is capable of normal growth; and, if so, what the nutritional requirements would be for that growth. In an holistic sense, our clinical approach has been to formulate a program of nutritional management directed towards early intervention (first two years of life) in infants and children with congenital renal insufficiency. In so doing, we have selected a small population of patients who might prospectively answer some of the questions posed.

To date, we have provided early nutritional intervention to seven children with chronic renal insufficiency secondary to congenital renal diseases. In each case poor appetite was considered to be an ominous sign when associated with weight loss or maintenance below the tenth percentile for age. When the infant was first encountered, a program of nutritional surveillance was begun and the caretaker was encouraged to maintain a dietary diary on daily short term bases. If the infant's intake fell below 100 percent of that recommended for age, progressive steps were taken to supplement to the appropriate level. The basic infant formula feeding was provided through the low solute formula Similac PM 60/40® and nutritional supplements were provided by non-protein sources of glucose polymers or corn oil. When oral supplements were refused, enteral feedings were implemented at home. Other factors were monitored on a monthly basis by laboratory studies to recognize and treat problems of acidosis or bone disease as necessary.

Naso-gastric and gastrostomy feedings have been necessary in four of the seven patients. Technical complications have centered around the naso-gastric tube. Some parents have been frustrated by the need to insert this tube and the child has also frequently been resistant to its insertion. Moreover, the patients seem to experience more discomfort and otitis when they develop upper respiratory infections with the naso-gastric tube in place. Some parents have also expressed reticence to take their children in public with the unsightliness of the tube. In all, the gastrostomy has proved to be better tolerated and managed on a long term basis. One patient was tried for six months on naso-gastric feedings with continued weight loss and poor growth. After placement of the gastrostomy, her growth and development improved markedly.

In evaluating the patient's response to the controlled feeding regimens, growth was measured on a monthly basis. Length was measured by the same observer with an infantometer; weight was measured on a standard balance scale. Linear growth was evaluated according to variations in linear growth velocity and absolute progression along standard growth channels corrected for mid-parental heights. Standards for weight over height were also used to evaluate gross accumulation of body mass and excessive linear growth. Mid-arm circumference and triceps skin-fold measurements were performed but proved to be too variable in infants.

Genetic influence on growth seems to be especially important to consider during the first year of life. We are currently using the mid-parental height adjustment according to the tables of Himes et al. (12) for U.S. children relative to the growth charts of the National Center for Health Statistics. This adjustment in two of our patients proved to be quite important in their clinical management. Patient ML of short lineage increased to normal growth channels with mid-parental height adjustment and then began to accumulate excess weight for height suggesting that she had had a maximum response to nutritional supplementation. She would have simply become obese if we had persisted with forced high calorie intakes. Patient DT, on the other hand, was of tall lineage. When his length was adjusted for mid-parental height, he was noted to have fallen significantly below appropriate growth channels, suggesting the need for increased nutritional supplementation.

Normal growth, as defined by linear growth within two standard deviations of the mean, adjusted for mid-parental height was maintained normal for five of the seven infants. Maximum growth velocity appeared to be better in those infants who did not have clinical bone disease. However, the presence of bone disease did not prevent an apparent response to the nutritional supplementation. This statement must be made with the understanding that bone disease was being monitored and treated as clinically feasible within the limits of drug toxicity. Obesity, as defined by a weight:length ratio in excess of 75th percentile, occurred in two patients who had low mid-parental height suggesting a genetic limitation to their linear growth potential. A disturbing finding was the consistent presence of hyperlipidemia in response to the non-protein calorie supplementation.

In analyzing growth velocity response to controlled feeding regimens, one must consider the reference standard used for nutrient intake which is the recommended dietary allowance (RDA). It is important, at this point, to review the absolute definition of the RDA (13, 14). RDA is derived from observation of a defined population and recommendations are intended to be broadly based and cannot easily be extrapolated to patients with undefined needs. For all nutrients, the Gaussian distribution of the intake for that defined population is determined. In order to avoid making a potentially inappropriate recommendation, most recommended nutrient allowances (including those for protein) are defined at the level to include 95 percent of the population or two standard deviations above the mean. The exception is the energy RDA which is placed at the mean energy intake of the population to avoid the propensity for obesity. Philosophically, then, the protein allowance could be decreased to 50 percent of the RDA and still be within the 95 percent confidence limits for defined requirements for growth and maintenance. In contrast, a decrease of only 25 percent of the RDA for energy intake would result in an energy intake below the confidence limits for projected requirements for growth.

With this in mind, we have expressed the correlation of linear growth velocity to energy intake as the percent of RDA for energy as well as the percent of minimum dietary allowance or MDA, defined as two standard deviations below the mean. Protein intake ranged from 65 to 160 percent of RDA, with a mean of 84 percent. Energy intake ranged from 57 percent to 135 percent RDA with a mean of 85 percent. Linear growth velocity did not correlate with protein intake ($R = 0.4$, $n = 26$, p was not significant). However, linear growth velocity did correlate positively with energy intake.

In summary, this is a complex and perplexing problem. To attempt to reduce it to a simplistic clinical approach does not seem justifiable. It does appear from our early observations that a normal growth response to recommended nutrient intakes is possible in some patients with congenital renal insufficiency. Early intervention, particularly in the first year of life, appears to offer some advantage. Careful clinical monitoring, particularly as pertains to relative toxicities of this treatment including obesity and hyperlipidemia, is of paramount importance. It is our hope that continued diligence in this clinical field will ultimately make some impact on the problem of uremic dwarfism.

REFERENCES

1. Mehls, O., Ritz, E., Gilli, G. et al.: Growth in renal failure. Nephron 21: 237-247, 1978.

2. McCance, R. and Widdowson, E.: Nutrition and growth. Proc. R. Soc. 156:326-334, 1962.

3. Fitzhardine, P. and Steven, E.M.: The small for date infant. Later growth patterns. Pediatrics 49:671- 1972.

4. West, C. and Smith, W.: An attempt to elucidate the cause of growth retardation in renal disease. Am. J. Dis. Child. 91:460-476, 1956.

5. Simmons, J.M., Wilson, C.J., Potter, D.E. et al.: Relation of calorie deficiency to growth failure in children on hemodialysis and the growth response to calorie supplementation. New Engl. J. Med. 285:653-656, 1971.

6. Chantler, C., Lieberman, E., and Holliday, M.A.: A rat model for the study of growth failure in uremia. Pediatr. Res. 8:109-113, 1974.

7. Mehls, O., Ritz, E., Gilli, G. et al.: Effect of vitamin D on growth in experimental uremia. Am. J. Clin. Nutr. 31:1927-1931, 1978.

8. Holliday, M.A., Chantler, C., MacDonell, R. et al.: Effect of uremia on nutritionally induced variation in protein metabolism. Kidney Inter. 11:236-245, 1977.

9. Clark, A.S. and Mitch, W.E.: Muscle protein turnover and glucose uptake in acutely uremic rats. J. Clin. Invest. 72:836-845, 1983.

10. Hoil, W.H. and Heidland, A.: Enhanced proteolytic activity--cause of protein catabolism in acute renal failure. Am. J. Clin. Nutr. 33:1423-1427, 1980.

11. Kleinknecht, C., Gros, F., Jean, G. et al.: Growth and free amino acids levels in uremic hyperphagic rats. Am. J. Clin. Nutr. 33:1690-1695, 1980.

12. Himes, J.H., Roche, A.F., Thissen, D. et al.: Parent-specific adjustments for evaluation of recumbent length and stature of children. Pediatrics 75:304-312,

13. National Research Council, Food and Nutrition Board: Recommended Dietary Allowances. Ninth Edition. Washington, D.C. National Academy of Sciences, 1980.

14. Beaton, G. H.: Uses and limits of the use of the Recommended Dietary Allowances for evaluating dietary intake data. Am. J. Clin. Nutr. 41:155-164, 1985.

DISCUSSION: CONGENITAL RENAL ANOMALIES

PANELISTS: Carolyn Abitbol, M.D., Joan Chesney, M.D., Warren Grupe, M.D., Abdollah Iravani, M.D., Catherine Poole, M.D., George Sfakianakis, M.D. and Norman Siegel, M.D.

MODERATOR: Jose Strauss, M.D.

QUESTION: The question at this point is, what should be the universal approach to evaluating the kidneys of the neonate? Of course, with all my respect to views already analyzed here, I believe that there is still a place for the nuclear scan. We have to consider probably a comparative study to finalize this question.

COMMENT: There is no question that the advantage of the nuclear scan is that you can evaluate function. I think, however, that in the routine child with uro-sepsis, abnormal renal function is really not a problem. The advantages of ultrasound are that it's very easy to do, it's noninvasive, there is no ionizing radiation, and it's cheaper. So, I still would prefer, in the routine approach, to go first to renal ultrasound. Certainly, if there is a question about abnormal renal function, the nuclear scan is the premier modality to use.

QUESTION: How long do you have to hold still for an NMR (MRI) Scan? Is that a problem in pediatrics?

RESPONSE: Motion, in general, right up to the moment is a problem with abdominal imaging. It depends on what sequence you use. You can take a few to several seconds to obtain each one. You do get degradation of the image with respiratory motion, peristalsis of the gastro-intestinal tract, and that sort of thing. Improvements are being made, primarily with instituting gating procedures. Both cardiac and respiratory gating are now available with most MR. So, motion is becoming less of a problem. As we sophisticate our techniques, if you will, scanning time is going to decrease. It is a temporary inconvenience--one that will be rapidly overcome with improved technology.

QUESTION: There was a recent abstract indicating promise for the use of MRI in distinguishing between allograft rejection and cyclosporine A nephrotoxicity. Early experience at our institution with a relatively small number of patients has not been as good as the abstract. I am wondering if you or any one else has had experience in this area?

RESPONSE: Your experience is 100% more than mine. I would be interested to know if anybody else has had any? The answer is: "nobody".

QUESTION: Would you please comment on the indications and the techniques of the antigrade pyelography?

RESPONSE: Antigrade pyelography is a percutaneous puncture of the kidney, basically. You can use it for diagnostic purposes to localize the level of obstruction in the urinary tract if you are not able to do so with less invasive procedures. One step further is with the use of a trocar and the introduction of nephrostomy tubes; I think it is the procedure of choice for temporary drainage of such obstructed collecting systems. For example, a baby who had meningitis and possibly AIDS, was certainly not a candidate for surgery at the time we picked up his GU obstruction. He was an ideal candidate for a temporary urinary diversion by that technique.

QUESTION: We did a collaborative study with the Dallas group; the results were recently presented elsewhere. We treated three groups of children, randomized, and gave them antibiotics in one dose versus three days versus seven days. Rate of recurrence at one month and rates of success or failure were not statistically different. However, we chose the children among the ones who had the first urinary tract infection. We have in our population of children around 40% of proteus mirabilis in boys. Do you have an explanation for those findings and results?

QUESTION: What drug did you use?

RESPONSE: Sulfamethoxazole-trimethoprim.

RESPONSE: That is encouraging. There are a number of papers written about proteus mirabilis in young boys, one in particular from Australia where they commented that in their first UTI in young boys, 30-40% were due to proteus mirabilis. They had no explanation for that. I thought it was interesting to look at the fimbriae issue. Proteus mirabilis does not have fimbriae that adhere. This has been looked at in the monkey. There are some monkeys who have the same receptor that humans have for the fimbriae. The proteus not only don't have it but they don't adhere well to the uro-epithelial cells in the monkey; so, I really don't have an explanation. It is an observation others have made but I don't know why males should select proteus mirabilis out of that whole flora.

COMMENT: I have mentioned that bacterial adhesions to the uro-genital area are a complex phenomenon. This is due not only to the bacterial specie, but also to the host mechanism. When there is a decrease in the host's immune mechanism, that is the time when these bacteria can colonize and adhere to the epithelial cells in the vagina or urethra. Some of the organisms such as proteus which you mentioned do have the fimbriae, but the mechanism is not known. I think the host is the main factor in developing urinary tract infection.

QUESTION: One of the speakers made the comment that we should be concerned with healthy newborns who develop spontaneous pneumothorax since there is increased incidence or possibility of renal hypoplasia. The question is, are you doing ultrasounds on all these children? How are you evaluating them? What has been the result of this evaluation?

RESPONSE: That possibility needs to be taken into account when you see a newborn with this particular problem. I cannot really advise you with regard to how to go about evaluating him because with all of the imaging techniques, it really depends upon the local expertise. So, I can't tell you whether or not ultrasound will be equally as good as an IVP versus a radionucleotide scan. You have to evaluate that on a local basis. I would make one plea with regard to the imaging techniques in the fetus and the newborn, especially with regard to the renal system: we critically lack studies of sensitivity and accuracy of diagnosis. This is true not only in the fetus, as was elegantly described here, but also in the newborn infant. The pictures that were presented are very pretty and frequently demonstrate things that are very dramatic, but a study of the long-term accumulated results of either ultrasound, IVP, or nucleotide scanning has not been done with any type of systematic approach to evaluating the different techniques and their diagnostic capabilities in the urinary tract. We really need to make a plea for our colleagues to begin to look at this problem in a much more critical way.

RESPONSE: As a radiologist, I entirely agree with you. There are no large studies which have documented any advantages of one method versus another. Of course, this is partly due to the fact of changing modalities. Ultrasound has not been around for long. Nuclear studies, it has been only about 10 to 12 years since we started using them for everyday pediatric work. Our experience favors radionuclide studies because in addition to the morphological information, they provide functional information and many times detect lesions which are not detectable by ultrasound. As an example, renal vein thrombosis would give us an absolutely normal study on an ultrasound. A radionuclide study would show nearly total absence of activity in the acute phase; in the absence of obstruction, this is diagnostic of renal vein thrombosis. As far as infection is concerned, I happen to have here an abstract from a hospital in Chicago. They say they studied 38 children with clinical diagnosis of urinary tract infection, and 26 of the patients demonstrated abnormal renal parenchyma findings with radionuclide studies. So, there are some papers but I agree with you that we need to do extensive, thorough studies with the current modalities to determine what is the best modality for each individual problem.

COMMENT: What happens to the child who has had that kind of problem in the nursery, reflects on how you handle children who have been diagnosed by ultrasound in utero. I would like to put out a plea for something which happens to the human. You will notice in what has been presented here that in those infants with dysplasia and obstruction, renal function improved. That was not a function of the nutrition, but the nutrition allowed it to happen. Had they been poorly nourished, it would not have happened. Compensatory hypertrophy in the fetus does not begin really until that cord is clamped. So, an infant who looks absolutely atrocious in the nursery, still requires effort and programs of support. With correction of the anatomic abnormalities, if they exist, and the nutritional programs which have been pointed out here, those kids now have a chance; don't give up on them too soon.

COMMENT: I absolutely agree.

QUESTION: I want to get back to the proteus issue. As we were talking about the 40 to 60% incidence of proteus in males in Australia, I remembered hearing an infectious disease specialist at Mass General mentioning at one point that he sees this most often in uncircumcised males. Does anybody know if this is true, and if this has been reported?

MODERATOR: Let me add something here, as part of the question, before the question is answered. There is a good friend of ours in Sao Paulo, Brazil who did a study of UTI in boys and cultured the smegma of the prepuce; he found a lot of proteus under those conditions, but there was not a good correlation with UTI. In other words, the patients who had proteus in the smegma did not necessarily have proteus also in the urine. As you answer the question, you may want to touch upon the relationship of infections that may be located in proximity to the urethra.

RESPONSE: That is a very interesting observation. It was not addressed in the papers I saw which focus on the issue of the incidence of proteus. That may be an obvious explanation, because these were males who had acute uncomplicated UTI's, which are so unusual anyway and proteus should be involved. I don't think that was looked into. That may be a prospective study to be done.

QUESTION: Data have been presented elsewhere suggesting that it is uncircumcised males who are predisposed to infections; I don't know whether proteus were looked specifically into or not. One of the Dallas groups also sees proteus under those conditions. In addition, another group reviewed retrospective data on males with UTI and found proteus predominant among uncircumcised males though the predominant approach to males was to circumcise. So, there are a lot of data suggesting that lack of circumcision does predispose males under three months of age to UTI.

QUESTION: You stated that you would not do radiological investigations on a girl after the first UTI over the age of five years. Of what is that age a cut-off?

RESPONSE: That age is not a cut-off. The incidence of urinary tract abnormalities decreases with age; before two years of age it is significantly high; after then, there is a 10% incidence of urinary tract abnormalities in male children and about five percent in females. That is why, during that age, it is best and most rewarding to do those studies. After five years of age, if the child is normal, there are less chances of having abnormalities. That cut-off is arbitrary and some people will consider doing these studies in children who are less than two years of age, and some may do them up to 12 years of age. Another thing that I did not mention is ultrasound. I think that in patients who have acute infection we may go ahead and do an ultrasound study during the acute phase, and if it is normal, we may do a voiding cystogram after six to eight weeks; but if the ultrasound is abnormal, then we may do an IVP. So, a combination of ultrasonography and voiding cystourethrogram or IVP would delineate most urinary abnormalities. I do not know if you agree with that approach.

MODERATOR: This is an important question about which I would like to ask for opinions. What should be the recommendation? Would you like to tell us what is the routine that you follow in terms of studies after the first UTI?

COMMENT-RESPONSE: Yes. In terms of girls, it is different than in terms of boys. I am always worried about boys. In girls, I think that it is true, once you get above five years of age, the prevalence of abnormalities, progression of abnormalities, etc., begin to go down; this is the age at which covert bacteria become a much more common thing. So, I am much more inclined to do the studies if I see evidence of systemic involvement such as fever, something that makes me think of pyelonephritis; also, if there is an organism other than E. coli--that is, their first known infection is by an unusual organism; if there is a concentrating defect, or if there is an inability to clear the organism with an antibiotic.

MODERATOR: Anybody else? My good friend over there, what do you do? What is your routine? Do you have a routine?

COMMENT-RESPONSE: I guess that the honest answer is that we do not. I think that it is one of the things in pediatrics which should not be cookbooked. There is no question that in the young child, especially in the first one to two years of life, one wants to pick up the underlying congenital anomaly because of the combination of infection and obstruction (or partial obstruction) of the urinary tract. Beyond that, I think that one has to evaluate each case on a very individual basis. The more ill the patient the more likely it is that the patient is presenting with an upper tract or tissue infection and the more likely it is that we are going to study that patient early whether a male or a female; the less systemic symptoms present, the less likely we are going to study that patient.

MODERATOR: My concern is that we have gone a little bit too far in not studying girls. It happens less frequently, but still, if it happens at all, now that we have non-invasive tools, should we not be more aggressive? If we miss even one patient who has some congenital anomaly, we may be in trouble. Identification of an anomaly does not need to lead to surgery; we cannot say that by fixing the congenital anomaly we are going to solve the problem, because we know that the patient may continue to have problems after surgical correction, even after properly indicated and performed surgery. Also, a study can be important for medico-legal purposes, and just to know so that you can make your decision more intelligently or better-informed. Are you scientifically correct or legally protected if you do not study a patient simply because it is not statistically likely to occur?

COMMENT-RESPONSE: I feel compelled to respond to that. You are saying, "Let's go for a 100%, because maybe we will miss something". My concern with that is that you have to show me that the morbidity of going for 100% is likewise low. One child who dies from some reaction to the study, the morbidity of going through those studies, all that has to be put into it. We did a sort of a minor cost analysis on a study of girls who were over five years of age in which no difference was seen between those who had covert bacteria who were treated and those who had covert bacteria and were not treated. Something hidden in that data is that in order to find those patients and follow them in what would be a reasonable medical plan, they were talking about high costs. If we paid for modest costs for only the studies, not for physician and not for morbidity, the cost per positive was something like $6,000. This was per positive IVP or VCUG. That is horrendous!

MODERATOR: Yes, but you are talking about IVPs with reactions. Now, we have ultrasonography.

COMMENT: But ultrasound also costs!

MODERATOR: The late John Askin reviewed the IVPs that were done prior to the time when voiding cystourethrograms became frequently done and he found significant numbers, in the 10-15-20% range, of anomalies present. Obviously, it all depends on what was defined as an anomaly; maybe it included duplication of a ureter or something of that sort. I am not so sure that if my daughter, age seven, had a UTI, that I would not study her, at least with an ultrasound.

COMMENT-RESPONSE: I think you are making a classical error in the assumption that the ultrasound is close to 100% diagnostic, and I challenge you to find one study in the Pediatric Radiologic literature in which the accuracy, the diagnostic precision of the ultrasound of the kidney in pre-pubertal children, has been looked at in a systematic way. It is not there! The studies are not there! So, you are putting a lot of faith into a particular technique because we say it is non-invasive; I am not yet convinced that it is also diagnostic frequently enough to put that much faith in it. I think that that makes a big difference; we just don't have that kind of precision! If the Clinical Chemistry Laboratory told you that a test was diagnostic for reflux nephropathy because they can find it in the serum, you'd ask them immediately for the number of false positives and the number of false negatives in children screened who had other diseases. We never get that information from our radiological colleagues. I think that you are putting a lot of faith into a study without knowing its accuracy and its dependability of diagnosis.

MODERATOR: In practice, we actually go to the renal scan, but I think that we are talking about a yes or a no. I think it is risky to say that I would not study a girl simply because the frequency of problems is less than in boys. Conceptually it bothers me. I have been involved in some legal problems of general pediatricians. When general pediatricians ask me, "Should we study that first urinary tract infection?", my answer is "yes" because we can do studies with today's safe type of techniques. Ultrasound may not be the most revealing but it will give you some information and is non-invasive. With the renal scan, there are no complications. What you were referring to were the IVPs and it scares me to do an IVP for screening purposes. I absolutely agree with you. I saw a girl die from an IVP that was questionably indicated. So we know that can happen. At least if it's going to happen, it should happen because we had a specific purpose in mind like doing some corrective surgery. Therefore, my emphasis is: if we want to evaluate the GU tract, let's put emphasis on something like the renal scan, somehow combine it with the ultrasound. I have the feeling that ultrasound has not been properly utilized. That comparative study should be done since good people put a lot of emphasis on its accuracy.

COMMENT: In the past two or three issues of Radiology, there was a paper on children with possible upper urinary tract infection who were screened with ultrasound. They also did cystograms. With those two approaches, they said that if both studies were normal, they were acceptable as criteria for not having upper urinary tract problems. That's one side of the coin. The other side comes from a hospital in Chicago, where ultrasound had more than 50% false negative in children. I do not think that ultrasound alone can give answers. Before scars and morphological changes occur, there may be infection going on in the kidney without having a positive ultrasound study. Of course, this is part of the issue of screening. If there is a cystic structure, yes, the ultrasound will pick it up or if there is an obstruction it may not be able to say what is the level of obstruction but it will pick it up. I agree with you that ultrasound is not the panacea for everything, but considering the trauma which a child goes through with the cystogram, particularly the little girls, ultrasound may be all that is needed in addition to a renal scan or IVP. I believe that unless there is a real need for the study, the cystogram should not be done.

COMMENT: I think that in early childhood, since the incidence of urinary tract abnormalities is very high, we have to evaluate immediately children who develop urinary tract infections, even during the acute infection. But the incidence of these abnormalities decreases especially after five years of age. Also, considering the clinical presentation, in a child who develops infection with a high fever, you know that that is an indication for doing radiological studies. However, I think a child who is over five years of age, who develops a urinary tract infection and responds well to a reasonable course of antibiotic therapy such as seven days or three days, and remains free of infection after that acute phase, does not need any other studies done. Now that semi-quantitative cultures are available, the parents can even do the cultures at home, one week after therapy, four weeks after therapy, and continue for a couple of months; if that child remains free of infection, I do not think we need to do any further studies to exhaust our radiological availability.

COMMENT: I just want to support the previous comment. Some time ago I was doing all the procedures myself, even though I was not a radiologist, the contrast cystogram and radionucleotide cystogram. Even though the latter is less noxious than the other and the parent can be with the child, it seems to be pretty traumatic; accordingly, I limited my use of them to essentially what we are saying here.

COMMENT: I am against the ultrasound as the mode of evaluating the child with a urinary tract infection because I think that for the most part, what we are looking for is reflux and we do not have a non-invasive way of finding reflux. This is especially true in the one to two year old child where obstructive or major GU anomalies could be a problem. If you decide to evaluate the child, you are fooling yourself if you think ultrasound is adequate evaluation without some form of cystogram to look for reflux.

COMMENT: When you do these evaluations, actually you are looking for obstructions with a high pressure in the urinary tract. So, if an ultrasound is done and there is no evidence of any hydronephrosis, even if there is a mild grade of reflux, I do not know what the significance of it is because the reflux should be intrarenal in order to cause any renal scarring or damage. That is why ultrasound early in the phase of infection of a small child may be helpful to some extent to rule out significant anomalies.

COMMENT: In a similar vein, some English authors, in a classical paper in the Quarterly Journal of Medicine in 1977, followed a huge number of patients and their postulate was that they felt comfortable with doing exclusively IVPs (in those times they only did IVPs) if the upper tracts were normal. What if the patient had reflux Grade I? Assessment of the integrity of the upper tracts seems like the main priority and if the upper tracts are intact, so what if we have reflux grade I since most of them improve spontaneously anyway? If we could find a compromise in a renal scan and ultrasound, maybe, just maybe, rather than an IVP to assess the upper tracts in a reliable way, that is the way to go in an uncomplicated UTI.

COMMENT: I do not agree because in the past six months I had two girls who never had any history of documented urinary tract infection and they came with high fever, no dysuria, but urine analysis was abnormal, culture proved that they had UTI, and on radiological studies (which included scan and VCU) they both had VU reflux. One was 15 and the other 17, and if I believe that their urine culture will remain normal because they were never picked up before this age group, I will miss the diagnosis of reflux. I agree with the other comment that if they have upper tract signs, one should investigate any age group whether it's the first or second infection, whether it's male or female.

COMMENT: I agree with you and perhaps I did not make myself clear. I mentioned that if the patients are symptomatic and have symptoms of upper tract, especially fever, and I showed the slides of children who had fever with urinary tract infections, in whom there were suggestions of upper tract involvement and even presence of urinary tract anomalies. So, at any age, if the patient presents with acute pyelonephritis with high fever, I go ahead and study the patient. We are talking about patients who develop a urinary tract infection and clinically do not have symptoms of upper tract involvement. What we want to know is: do we really have to go ahead and study these children?

COMMENT: Everybody seems to be very scared about the business of doing IVPs in studying children with urinary tract infections. Apparently, this seems to be the only way to assess correctly the anatomy of a UTI. I wonder what is the incidence of complications of IVP. During the last 10 years we have never seen a patient with an acute episode of complications due to an IVP. Since everybody seems to be so scared about doing an IVP and it is the only way, anatomically speaking, to assess the urinary tract, I would like to know what is the incidence of complications?

MODERATOR: Does anybody have the information? The answer seems to be "no".

COMMENT: I do not think that we are afraid of doing an IVP. The main question is, when is it indicated? When should we do it? A lot of patients with urinary tract infections remain under treated, under evaluated. On the other hand, some individuals who do not need evaluations are fully evaluated. So, actually we should consider the age group, the clinical findings, and if the patient has recurrences or not.

COMMENT: On clinical grounds, it is very difficult to put a patient in one or the other group, talking about complicated or uncomplicated urinary tract infections. We are clinicians, and we are seeing many patients as clinicians. On clinical grounds, we usually make a lot of errors trying to group patients in one or the other side. The only way to say that the patient is having an uncomplicated urinary tract infection is to be sure that the urinary tract is normal. Not on clinical grounds.

COMMENT: Just a short comment about your question, and I would like to say that I am afraid to do IVPs. I asked a radiologist once how often there were allergic reactions to the IVP dye; this is again just on a single encounter, I was continuously being called by the radiologist because these kids were having hives. He said that this occurred in one in three, or even one in two of the patients, but it was dismissed usually as a transient or insignificant complication; in fact, it was not considered a contra-indication to doing another IVP. Well, frankly, I am deathly afraid of anaphylaxis; I would never subject my child to a one time IVP if she tended to be allergic and, I certainly would never do it twice if there developed a systemic allergic reaction such as hives.

COMMENT: I usually treat adolescents with urinary tract infections--about several thousand adolescents a year. The criteria that I have chosen for doing these studies in these patients are: 1) If they have recurrent UTIs, more than three or four in 12 months; 2) If they present infections with upper tract symptoms like fever; or 3) If the bacteria are unusual or resistant. In the hundreds of IVPs and renal scans that I have done, the yield has been less than two percent. The yield is not very high; that is why I do not do them in every patient.

COMMENT: I understand the concern about this problem, especially legal. I feel very comfortable to do a sonogram in a patient that I admit for UTI especially if this patient has not had radiological studies prior to admission. If it is a baby without sepsis problems, I feel comfortable doing a sonogram even if I might not detect dysplasia or pyelonephritis. The other thing is that if the patient does not show up for follow-up, at least I will have some information from the sonogram obtained during admission. This is a legal concern because once you talk with the mother about doing a VCU and IVP and you explain the procedure and possible complications, she might not come back. So, I think that it is a good step to do a sonogram in a patient with all the characteristics mentioned--fever, less than five years old, no previous radiological studies. I think it is very useful to take a look at the kidneys.

MODERATOR: I am scared about the IVPs too. In one of those cases for which I was asked to be an expert witness when a pediatrician was being sued, my point in defending his not getting an IVP was that if every child with a fever of unknown origin were subjected to an IVP (which was the situation in this case, the child was discovered at age five to have basically end stage renal disease from obstructive uropathy that had been overlooked), we probably would have more complications from the IVPs than findings, since the yield is so low. Subsequently, my position has been that that statement cannot be made today because we have ultrasonography. In order words, if I had to appear in court for a similar problem today, I would have a hard time defending the pediatrician who did not study that child at least by ultrasound.

QUESTION: A very short question regarding the patients with recurrent UTIs, especially girls. What is the best approach, to treat every infection separately or to keep the patient on long-term prophylactic therapy?

RESPONSE: In girls with the first but uncomplicated UTI, those that have normal urinary tracts and then recur, it depends on the frequency of the recurrence. If they are isolated cases happening every three or four months, I think each isolated case should be treated separately. I do not think that those patients should be exposed to long-term antimicrobal therapy. However, if the patient develops more frequent recurrences, and if there is no reflux or any other anomaly, low-dose, long-term, prophylactic therapy is indicated.

QUESTION-RESPONSE: I have two questions here that were handed to me on a sheet of paper. The first question is, "what is the experience with children who have UTI and malnutrition with short course therapy?" I don't think that has been studied. I don't have any information on that issue. The second question is, "can you separate by laboratory tests or clinical presentation an upper tract infection from a lower tract infection?" A Swedish investigator compared sedimentation rate, CRP, fever and symptoms to see if he could identify those with upper tract versus lower tract infections. Although his results looked very good, subsequent studies that have actually compared bladder wash out to determine if there was or was not renal bacteriuria have not really supported his findings. You can have a high CRP with a lower tract infection, you can have a low CRP and no fever or other upper tract symptoms with renal bacteriuria. And, in fact, to me this is the biggest black box of all. I wonder if finding renal bacteriuria in a bladder wash-out really does indicate renal infection or whether it just indicates upper tract colonization.

MODERATOR: What about CRP quantitated? Were you referring to a high or low with an accurate method?

RESPONSE: Yes. They have quantitated values. They used values of over 30 and under 30. But even when more rigid criteria are applied, it does not turn out to be helpful.

QUESTION: My question to the group relates to single dose or short-term therapy. Most of those studies have been in older girls with minimal, if you would, urinary tract involvement. That is the group that the Cardiff study has found to have covert bacteriuria, that maybe does not need treatment at all. I am wondering if there is any success with single dose therapy. Does that mean that we should not compare it to 10 day therapy but should compare it to no therapy?

RESPONSE: The patient population that I treated with single-dose or short-term therapy was randomized. They were identical to those who were treated for seven days or 10 days. They had positive urine cultures and were symptomatic. So, therefore, I did not treat a patient who had a history of recurrent UTIs within the past 12 months. For example, if the patient had three, four or five infections, I did not go ahead and treat her with single dose. If she had no history of UTI or history of UTI one or two times in the past 12 months, I treated her with single dose and the response was good.

QUESTION: My question is not whether your results were good or not. I am saying that if your results were good, were they better than no treatment at all?

RESPONSE: I think that it is a risk that we may take, not treating the patients. In a young adolescent girl with symptoms of acute renal tract infection, in most cases the symptoms may resolve regardless of whether you treat the patient or not. But this does not mean that the urine becomes sterile also. And sometimes they develop severe renal involvement although they have uncomplicated infections. That is why I do not know if it is ethical or not, not to treat the patient but wait and see what happens. I do not know if I answered the question or not, but I cannot compare those patients who were treated with single dose with a group which is not treated. I do see occasionally patients who have self limited infections.

COMMENT: I think that is an excellent point. It is a question with which I have wrestled. There are two things I could say. One is that in this day and age of people working and having to get back to work and children in day care centers, any time you can reduce the morbidity of an infection, that may be important. I do not know if we are clear about that in terms of treating lower urinary tract infections. I think that the point made was a good one. We need to look at a group that was not treated and see if they get better just as fast as with the antibiotic. The second issue is that an article was published earlier this year in which there were three women of a series who got one dose therapy. One of the women went on to have fairly severe acute pyelonephritis with fever and flank pain; the other two continued to have bacteriuria with positive antibody coated bacteria. That was of concern enough to them that they are not quite so positive about recommending one dose therapy any more.

COMMENT: I just want to share with the group our own experience with single dose therapy with gentamicin. Our group included children over six months of age with no azotemia up to the age of 12. There was no differentiation between initial UTI or recurrent UTI. All the children coming to the clinic were included; this was only an out-patient study. We did all the blood tests to differentiate between upper and lower tract infections and the success rate was as good as 10 days therapy in the lower tract infection. We isolated bacteria from the urine in upper tract infection patients in those who later on turned out to be complicated urinary tract infections. The relapse rate was very high. As regards the costs of treating a single infection, we did not find much difference because in every patient, whether it was conventional therapy or protocol patient, we did urine cultures 48 hours after the therapy.

MODERATOR: It is obvious that there is no simple, single answer to all those questions and it is good to have diversity of opinions. Thank you very much. We will see you at the next session.

V

RENAL REPLACEMENT THERAPY

DIALYSIS

FOUR YEARS EXPERIENCE - CAPD and CCPD IN CHILDREN

H.E. Leichter, M.D., I.B. Salusky, M.D. and R.N. Fine, M.D.

Since the introduction of CAPD in 1976 by Popovich et al. (1) and its modification by Oreopoulos et al. (2), peritoneal dialysis has been used with increasing frequency as the dialytic treatment of choice for adults (3-5) as well as for children (6-8). In order to decrease the peritonitis rate which was presumed to be related to the multiple connections and disconnections, continuous cycling peritoneal dialysis (CCPD) was introduced (9). In contrast to CAPD where the exchange is performed by the patient every 4-5 hours during the day, CCPD utilizes an automated cycler to deliver dialysis exchanges at night. There is usually only one daytime dwell. With this approach, no dialysis procedures are necessary during the day. In this report, we present our 4 years experience with home peritoneal dialysis (CAPD/CCPD) in children.

MATERIALS AND METHODS

Over a four year period (August 1980 - August 1984), 80 pediatric patients (45 males, 35 females) aged 0.5 - 21.2 years, mean 11.0 $\pm$ 5.5 (SD) years have been trained for CAPD and/or CCPD. Prior to starting dialysis a permanent dialysis catheter was inserted and a partial omentectomy performed. Single-cuff, double-cuffed Tenckhoff and column disc (Life Cath) catheters were used. After catheter insertion, continuous lavage with low dialysate volumes and more frequent exchanges were performed over a period of 48 to 72 hours. Cefazolin 250 mg/l and Heparin, 250 U/l were added to the dialysate. After the catheter insertion, training for CAPD or CCPD was initiated. Patients who required immediate dialysis were placed on intermittent peritoneal diaysis (IPD) for 8 hours three times a week until their training for CAPD/CCPD was completed. If the child was older than 12 years, he or she was trained to perform the CAPD/CCPD procedure; in younger patients, a parent(s) was trained. Training for CAPD and/or CCPD was usually accomplished in 10 training sessions; if the patient had been on CAPD and was switched to CCPD, only two training sessions were required. CAPD was performed with four or five daily exchanges with a volume of 30-50 ml/Kg body weight per exchange. The CCPD regimen consisted of five two hour nocturnal cycles (American Medical Products 80/2 Cycler, Freehold, N.J.) and a single diurnal dwell at half the nocturnal volume or no daytime dwell. The dialysate glucose concentration (1.5%, 2.5%, 4.25% Dianeal® Travenol, Deerfield, Ill.) was adjusted to the patient's needs which was determined by body weight and blood pressure. According to the degree of acidosis, either PD1 or PD2 dialysate solution was used to maintain the serum bicarbonate level within normal limits.

The diagnosis of peritonitis was based upon clinical findings (i.e. abdominal pain, nausea, vomiting, fever) and an increased dialysate cell count (> 100 cells/mm^3). Recurrent peritonitis was defined as the presence of the same organism within two weeks after discontinuing antibiotic therapy. Exit site infections were defined as the presence of erythema and exudate. A tunnel infection was considered present if there was tenderness along the subcutaneous catheter tract with swelling or warmth.

RESULTS

Patient data

Sixty-six patients (80%) were trained primarily for CAPD and 14 patients (19%) for CCPD. The reason for primary CCPD training was patient preference (6), young patient age and other young children at home (4), single working parent (2), psychotic mother (1) and inability to perform CAPD (1). Twenty-four (36%) of the 66 patients who were initially trained for CAPD were switched to CCPD, whereas only one (2.6%) of the 38 patients trained for CCPD was converted back to CAPD. Transfer to hemodialysis because of membrane failure in relationship to an episode of peritonitis was necessary in 5 (6%) of the 80 patients.

As of September 1, 1985, a total of 43 patients were undergoing home peritoneal dialysis; 18 (42%) on CAPD and 25 (58%) on CCPD. The total experience with home peritoneal dialysis in the 80 patients was 1274 patient months; CAPD - 850 patient months (67%), CCPD - 424 patient months (33%).

Twenty-nine patients received 32 transplants (21 cadaver donor, 11 live-related donor). As of September 1, 1985, 22 patients (76%) had a functioning graft. Nine patients (13%) transferred care to either other units in the United States (5 patients) or returned to their country of origin (4 patients). Two patients (2.5%) died, one because of a cardiomyopathy, the other because of severe gastrointestinal and retroperitoneal hemorrhage in the immediate post-transplant period.

Clinical data

Biochemical and hematologic parameters. Control of the biochemical and hematologic parameters associated with uremia were evaluated in 10 patients who were on CAPD for at least 5 months and then were transferred to CCPD for at least a 5 month period. There was no significant difference in serum electrolytes, calcium, phosphorus, alkaline phosphatase, albumin, total protein and BUN between the period of CAPD and the period of CCPD. Only the mean serum creatinine level was significantly higher during the period on CCPD (10.8 ± 0.9(SEM)mg/dl, $p<0.01$) as compared to that on CAPD (9.7 ± 1.0mg/dl). Hematocrit and hemoglobin values were stable on both dialysis modalities; CAPD (24.0 ± 1.0%, 8.2 ± 1.9g/dl), CCPD (23.6 ± 1.4%, 8.1 ± 1.5g/dl).

Hypertension. At the beginning of CAPD and/or CCPD almost 50% of the patients were receiving anti-hypertensive medication. Following the initiation of dialysis, no additional blood pressure medication was necessary. Only 2 (5%) of the 43 patients who are currently on peritoneal dialysis require regular antihypertensive medication; 10 patients (23%) require occasional anti-hypertensive drugs. Captopril therapy is usually effective in these patients. No patient who was normotensive prior to CAPD and/or CCPD became hypertensive following initiation of dialysis. An occasional patient required intravenous fluid administration because of hypotension.

Transfusion requirements. It is difficult to assess the transfusion requirements in our patient population because all patients are enrolled in a pre-transplant blood transfusion protocol. In general, the transfusion rate was higher in anephric patients (1 unit every 2 months) as compared to patients with their native kidneys in place (1 unit every 4 months). However, a number of patients did not require any transfusions during two to three years of CAPD and/or CCPD. One patient had a rise in the hematocrit value to 40% following initiation of peritoneal dialysis.

Renal osteodystrophy. Renal bone disease was retrospectively evaluated in 14 children undergoing CAPD. In 9 of these 14 children who were treated with low doses of 1,25 dihydroxycholecalciferol (calcitriol) or dihydrotachysterol, as well as phosphate binders, renal osteodystrophy could not be controlled. Their calcium levels were lower and serum alkaline phosphatase and iPTH activity were higher than in the group of patients in whom clinical and radiologic signs of secondary hyperparathyroidism improved. We, therefore, evaluated prospectively the use of high doses of calcitriol in 17 pediatric patients who had been on CAPD for a mean of 24 ± 9.5

months. They were followed over 14.7 + 3 months and the dose of calcitriol was increased by 0.25 µg/day each month to maintain the serum calcium level above 10.5 mg/dl. At the end of the study period, serum calcium levels significantly increased from 10.1 ± 0.9 mg/dl to 10.8 ± 0.7 mg/dl ($p<0.01$), whereas the phosphorus levels remained stable. Serum alkaline phosphatase decreased from 433 ± 300 U/l to 210 ± 60 U/l. Serum iPTH levels decreased significantly in 11 patients whereas in 4 patients elevated values persisted. In 2 of these 4 patients aluminum related bone disease was diagnosed. Bone X-rays showed improvement of secondary hyperparathyroidism in 16 of the 17 patients. Calcitriol doses ranged from 0.25 to 2.25 µg/day (mean 0.6 ± 0.4 µg/day). In conclusion, with "high" doses of calcitriol, improvement of renal osteodystrophy occurs. A dynamic approach with regard to calcitriol dosage is necessary to maintain the serum calcium level above 10.5 mg/dl. These findings are consistent with in vitro studies which show an abnormal "set point" of the parathyroid glands in the suppression of PTH release.

Growth. Sixteen prepubertal children who were maintained on CAPD and/or CCPD for more than 1 year were evaluated. All patients were growth-retarded prior to the evaluation. Over a one year period, 4 children (25%) showed accelerated growth (more than 6-7cm/year), four (25%) revealed normal growth (5-6cm/year) and eight children (50%) had retarded growth (3.5-4cm/year).

Complications

Peritonitis. In the 80 patients, a total of 113 peritonitis episodes occurred over a period of 1274 patient months, leading to an overall peritonitis rate of 1 episode every 11.3 patient months. The rates for CAPD and CCPD were 1 per 11.8 patient months and 1 per 10.3 patient months, respectively. Cloudy bags, abdominal pain, nausea, vomiting or fever were present in most of the patients with peritonitis, although some patients presented with only one of these symptoms. Of these 113 episodes, 44 cultures (39%) showed no growth, 37 (32%) revealed gram positive and 26 (25%) gram negative bacteria. One culture grew anerobes, whereas 3 episodes (3%) showed 2 organisms. The incidence of fungal peritonitis was low (2%) with only 2 cases seen; however, both episodes necessitated catheter removal and transfer to hemodialysis. A total of 5 patients had to be switched to hemodialysis because of membrane failure. Sixteen recurrent peritonitis episodes (16/113 - 14%) occurred in 15 patients (15/80 - 19%). In Table 1, the organisms which caused complications are listed.

Table 1. Peritonitis - Organisms Associated with Complications

Organism	Total No.	No. Recurrent	No. Catheter Replaced	No. Modality Failure
No growth	44	0	1	0
Staph. aureus	17	8	9	1
Coag.neg.staph.	14	3	2	0
Pseudomonas	8	1	5	1
Strep. viridans	6	1	1	0
Enterobacter	4	1	0	0
Serratia	3	1	1	0
E. coli	2	1	1	0
Candida	2	0	2	2
Corynebacterium	1	0	1	1

Catheter-Related Problems. A total of 137 catheters were inserted in 80 patients; 92 (67%) were double-cuffed Tenckhoff, 21 (15%) were single-cuff Tenckhoff, and 24 (18%) were column disc (Life-cath) catheters. Forty-one patients (51%) received one catheter, whereas 39 had 2 or more catheters (25 patients - 2 catheters, 10 patients - 3 catheters and 4 patients - 4 catheters). The reason for catheter replacement is shown in Table 2.

Table 2. Reason for Catheter Replacement (57 Catheters)

1.	Peritonitis	24
2.	Tunnel infection	16
3.	Persistent exit site infection	5
4.	Obstruction	3
5.	Cuff erosion	2
6.	Peritoneal fluid leak	2
7.	Hernia	2
8.	Reinsertion following failed transplant	3

Exit-site and tunnel infections were frequent infectious complications. Oral antibiotic therapy was usually successful in preventing the progression of exit site to tunnel infections; however, in 5 instances, the catheter had to be replaced because of persistent infection. If tunnel infections were present, incision and drainage of the abscess together with antibiotic therapy was at times curative; however, in 16 cases, the catheter had to be replaced because of persistent infection.

Mechanical Complications. Hernia was the most frequent non-infectious procedure related complication, followed by dialysate leaks and hydrothorax. Twenty-eight patients (35%) developed 47 herniae; 30 (64%) ventral, 11 (23%) inguinal and 6 (13%) umbilical herniae. All herniae presented as a painless swelling. Only one patient developed an incarceration. There was a predominance of younger patients with herniae; 2 of the 3 patients who were less than 1 year of age developed a hernia, whereas none of the 4 patients who were older than 20 years presented with a hernia. Surgical repair was required in 31 (66%) of the 47 herniae, whereas conservative treatment like switching to CCPD (2), decrease or elimination of the CCPD daytime dwell (7) and decrease of the dialysate volume (2) led to improvement. In 5 instances, no specific treatment was necessary because of the small size of the herniae.

Dialysate leaks occurred in 11 (14%) patients. Most occurred spontaneously, although some developed immediately after catheter insertion or concomitantly with an abdominal hernia. Reduction of the dialysate volume or transfer to CCPD in order to reduce the intra-abdominal pressure was successful in 4 patients, whereas in 2 patients, elimination of the daytime dwell or an abdominal binder led to resolution. Nevertheless, surgical repair was required in 5 (45%) patients.

Hydrothorax developed in 2 patients (3%); one patient was on CAPD and one on CCPD. The CAPD patient was temporarily switched to IPD and dialyzed with lower volumes until she was trained for CCPD. The patient on CCPD was transferred to hemodialysis for 3 weeks and then switched back to CCPD with reduced dialysate volumes.

DISCUSSION

Our experience with CAPD and CCPD indicates that peritoneal dialysis is an acceptable dialytic treatment modality for infants, children and adolescents awaiting renal transplantation. When compared to hemodialysis, several medical and psychological advantages can be seen. Medically, stabilization of the biochemical milieu, better control of hypertension, improvement of renal osteodystrophy; minimal fluid restriction and a more liberal diet are significant benefits. The possibility to attend school regularly and the minimal need for contact with the medical personnel has a salutary effect in children. Psychologically, especially in the adolescent patients, the possibility to undertake the dialytic procedure leads to higher self-esteem.

Despite these advantages, there are several medical and psychological problems which are disadvantages of these dialysis modalities. Repetitive exchange procedures, especially with CAPD, can lead to patient and/or parent burn-out. Transfer to CCPD can alleviate or at least delay such symptoms. Close communication between the patient care team and the patients and/or parents is necessary to detect early symptoms of fatigue. Psychosocial intervention often can prevent further deterioration. Infectious complications like peritonitis and catheter related problems such as exit-site and tunnel infections are the major medical disadvantages.

The overall incidence of peritonitis in our patient population is comparable to other pediatric dialysis centers, where the rates range from 1 episode every 13.1 patient months (10) to 1 every 6.1 months (11). Gram positive bacteria are the dominant organisms, accounting for most of the recurrent peritonitis episodes. The use of CCPD did not lead to a reduction in the peritonitis rate, as reported in adult patients (9), which indicates that fewer connections and disconnections are not necessarily associated with a lower infection rate. Other factors, such as the cellular and humoral defense system may also play an important role.

Modality failure after peritonitis necessitating transfer to hemodialysis occurred in 5 patients. Recurrent or severe peritonitis may lead to peritoneal membrane failure and thereby limit the long-term use of these peritoneal dialysis modalities. In a recent prospective study (3) where the membrane function in 19 adult patients was studied, no deterioration in the peritoneal membrane characteristics could be found after 1 year. The follow-up period of 1 year is a short time and further experience is necessary. Efforts to decrease the incidence of peritonitis by using in-line filters (12), ultraviolet radiation (13) or sterile connection devices (14) have not as yet proven effective in reducing the incidence of peritonitis in controlled studies.

For access to the peritoneal cavity, Tenckhoff catheters are reliable. Column disc catheters, which were transiently used in our unit, caused problems in small children because of the predominance of the spike elbow, which often protruded through the skin and caused a hematoma or skin erosion. Procedure related mechanical problems like herniae, dialysate leaks and the development of a potentially dangerous hydrothorax were managed without difficulty. In cases of mild herniae formation or leaks, conservative treatment, such as reducing the dialysate volume or switching to CCPD, was successful, whereas in more severe cases surgery was required.

In conclusion, CAPD and/or CCPD are effective dialysis modalities for children with ESRD. Despite the infectious and mechanical, as well as access related problems, these dialysis modalities have become the modality of choice in our pediatric population. Additional follow-up of patients undergoing CAPD/CCPD is needed to evaluate the long-term efficacy of the peritoneal membrane, as well as the metabolic side effects (hypertriglyceridemia) of the constant glucose absorption. Psychosocially, the rehabiliation is easier with CAPD/CCPD with increased freedom and improved quality of life of children with ESRD.

REFERENCES

1. Popovich, R.P., Moncrief, J.W., Decherd, J.B. et al.: The definition of a novel portable/wearable equilibrium peritoneal dialysis technique. Abstract, Trans. ASAIO 5:64, 1976.

2. Oreopoulos, D.G., Robson, M., Izatt, H.S. et al.: A simple and safe technique for continuous ambulatory peritoneal dialysis (CAPD). Trans. ASAIO 24:484, 1978.

3. Rubin, J., Kirchner, K., Barnes, T. et al.: Evaluation of continuous ambulatory peritoneal dialysis. Am. J. Kid. Dis. 3:199, 1983.

4. Ramos, J.M., Gokal, R., Siamopolous, K. et al.: Continuous ambulatory peritoneal dialysis: Three years experience. Quart. J. Med. 206:165, 1983.

5. Steinberg, S.M., Cutler, S.J., Nolph, K.D. et al.: A comprehensive report on the experience of patients on continuous ambulatory peritoneal dialysis for the treatment of end-stage renal disease. Am. J. Kid. Dis. 3:233, 1984.

6. Balfe, J.W., Irwin, M.A.: Continuous ambulatory peritoneal dialysis in pediatrics. In Legrain, M., (ed.): Continuous ambulatory peritoneal dialysis. Amsterdam: Excerpta Medica, 1980, p. 131.

7. Baum, M., Powell, D., Calvin, S. et al.: Continuous ambulatory peritoneal dialysis in children. Comparison with hemodialysis. N. Engl. J. Med. 307:1537, 1982.

8. Salusky, I.B., Kopple, J.D., Fine, R.N.: Continuous ambulatory peritoneal dialysis in pediatric patients: A 20-month experience. Kidney Int. 24, Suppl 15:101, 1983.

9. Diaz-Buxo, J.A., Walker, P.J., Farmer, C.D. et al.: Continuous cyclic peritoneal dialysis. Abstract, Kidney Int. 19:145, 1981.

10. Balfe, J.W., Vigneux, A., Williamsen, J.: The use of CAPD in the treatment of children with end-stage renal disease. Perit. Dial. Bull. 1:35, 1981.

11. Warady, B.A., Campoy, S.F., Gross, S.P. et al.: Peritonitis with continuous ambulatory peritoneal dialysis and continuous cycling peritoneal dialysis. J. Ped. 105:726, 1984.

12. Ash, S.R., Horswell, R. Jr., Heeter, E.M. et al.: Effect of the peridex filter on peritonitis rates in a CAPD population. Perit. Dial. Bull. 3:89, 1983.

13. Eisinger, A.J., Bending, M.R., Goodwin, S. et al.: Ultraviolet light sterilization in CAPD. Preliminary experience in the U.K. Abstract, Perit. Dial. Bull. Suppl 4:21, 1984.

14. Ogden, D.A.: Multi-center field evaluation of the sterile connection device (SCD) in CAPD in the prevention of peritonitis. Abstract, Perit. Dial. Bull. Suppl 4:46, 1984.

LIPID CHANGES IN CHILDREN ON DIALYSIS

Gaston Zilleruelo, M.D., Milan Novak, Ph.D., Michael Freundlich, M.D., Carolyn Abitbol, M.D. and Jose Strauss, M.D.

Hyperlipidemia (mainly with elevated triglyceride levels) is a frequent finding in uremic patients on dialysis. The reported incidence of hypertriglyceridemia in adults with end stage renal disease (ESRD), as well as in those patients undergoing chronic hemodialysis, varies from 30 to 70 percent (1). The predominant pattern of this hyperlipidemia is Type IV, consistent with an increase in total triglycerides (TG) and very low density lipoproteins (VLDL) with near normal total cholesterol (TC). Prospective epidemiologic studies in patients with and without renal disease indicate that the Type IV pattern is associated with an increased incidence of ischemic heart disease (2-3). The hyperlipidemia associated with uremia may begin in adults when creatinine clearance falls under 50 ml/min (4). It has been reported that hyperlipidemia in children also occur early in the course of chronic renal failure (CRF) when creatinine clearance falls below 40 $ml/min/1.73m^2$ (5). As renal function deteriorates serum triglyceride levels become significantly elevated and HDL levels markedly decrease, while serum total cholesterol, phospholipids and LDL remain essentially unchanged. These lipid abnormalities worsen further with the onset of hemodialysis (5).

In addition to the elevated fasting triglyceride rich VLDL and decrease in HDL, increased formation of lipoprotein remnants has been demonstrated in adults with CRF (6). It appears that there are qualitative and quantitative changes in the lipoproteins of patients undergoing maintenance hemodialysis, including an enrichment of intermediate density lipoproteins (IDL) and low density lipoproteins (LDL) with triglycerides. This lipoprotein remnant formation has been proposed as a high risk factor for the development of premature or accelerated atherosclerosis (7).

The pathogenesis of disturbances of lipid metabolism in patients on dialysis remains unclear. Studies in adults and children have postulated that the decreased catabolism of triglyceride rich lipoproteins, due to a selective decrease in either lipoprotein lipase or hepatic triglyceride lipase or both, is a contributing factor to the hypertriglyceridemia in patients with CRF (8a, 8b). On the other hand, several reports suggest that overproduction of triglycerides may also contribute to uremic hypertriglyceridemia (9). Moreover, the

This study was funded in part by FDA Grant No. FD-R-000118-01 and by the State of Florida, Department of Health and Rehabilitative Services, Children's Medical Services.

pathogenesis of abnormal increase in lipoprotein remnants derived from the catabolism of triglyceride rich lipoproteins has not been elucidated in these patients.

The concentration of circulating serum triglycerides is determined by the balance between the synthesis of hepatic triglyceride and its removal by peripheral lipoprotein lipase. After heparin, there was reduced peripheral lipoprotein lipase activity in both non-dialyzed and dialyzed uremic patients (10). Uremic non-nephrotic patients had reduced levels of adipose tissue lipoprotein lipase (11). The findings described above suggest that the uremic and hemodialysis hypertriglyceridemia may be, at least in part, the result of decreased peripheral triglyceride clearance. In addition to the quantitative decrease in lipoprotein lipase activity, some evidence suggests that uremic plasma contains agents that have an inhibitory effect on lipoprotein lipase activity (12). This inhibitor may be a protein that accumulates early in the course of uremia. Some studies suggested that increased hepatic TG synthesis contributed to hemodialysis hypertriglyceridemia and hyperinsulinemia; however, subsequent studies have not always shown the expected rise in either insulin or serum growth hormone (13). Even more, patients with ESRD and poor nutritional status often have low serum TG which usually rises after hemodialysis and improved diets are instituted (14).

Hemodialysis patients have important differences between the sexes in both serum cholesterol and triglycerides levels (10). The quantitative frequencies of percentage curve for serum triglycerides and cholesterol in adult patients are shown in Figure 1. Male patients showed higher triglycerides than females, while females showed higher serum cholesterol than males. In other studies, dietary and hormonal factors did not appear to play a significant role in the pathogenesis of the hyperlipidemia. Hemodialysis itself includes exposure to factors contributing to abnormal lipid metabolism such as heparin, glucose and acetate. Glucose and acetate have not appeared to contribute as much to abnormal lipid patterns in patients on hemodialysis as in patients on CAPD (15).

Acute changes in serum lipids and lipoproteins induced during hemodialysis are mainly caused by heparin; these changes have been evaluated by comparing dialysis with heparin and dialysis without heparin (16). Gabexate mesilate (GM), a synthetic proteinase inhibitor, was used as an anticoagulant during dialysis without heparin (16). In dialysis with heparin, there was a significant increase in free fatty acids, high density lipoprotein cholesterol and plasma lipolytic activity; triglycerides were decreased reciprocally. In contrast, in dialysis without heparin, no significant changes were observed in any of the parameters of lipid metabolism (16). It is likely that the decrease in lipoprotein lipase activity in hemodialysis patients is due to the metabolic derangement of uremia rather than heparin induced depletion. These changes can be partially reversed by renal transplantation. In patients with advanced renal failure, decrease of lipase activity may contribute to hypertriglyceridemia; in contrast, overproduction of triglycerides due to hyperinsulinemia may be the mechanism of the hyperlipidemia associated with transplant recipients. Hyperlipidemia in mild renal failure in the absence of detectable anomalies in lipase activities or insulin levels, suggests other pathogenetic factors in this group of patients.

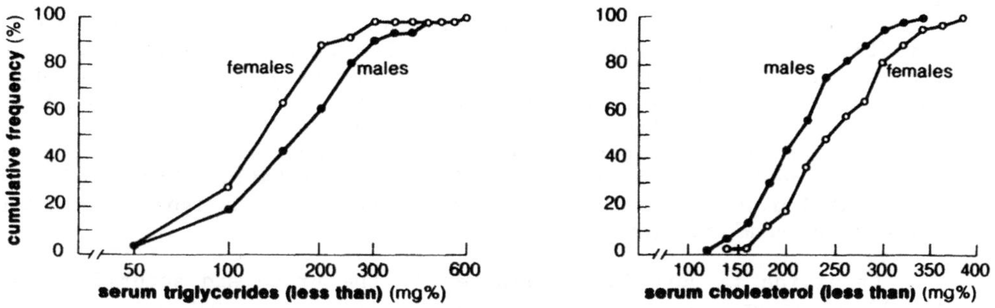

Figure 1: Differences by sex in serum lipids in adult patients on hemodialysis. Reproduced with permission from: Pierides, A.M., Weightman, D., Goldfinch, M., et al.: Hyperlipidemia of regular hemodialysis and successful renal transplantation. Cardiovascular Medicine 3:185, 1978.

Several studies have implicated the loss of carnitine into the dialysis effluent and subsequent decrease of carnitine in plasma and tissues as a factor in the reduced capacity for fatty acid oxidation and, thus, impaired utilization of fat found in ESRD patients (17-20). L-carnitine is a natural substance present in skeletal muscle, liver, kidneys and many other organs as well as in plasma and interstitial fluid. It has an important role in the normal metabolism of fats as a source of energy for muscle contraction. Muscle weakness, myocardiopathy and lipid abnormalities are frequent findings in primary or secondary carnitine deficiency syndromes (21-23). Cardiac enlargement, accompanied by congestive heart failure, has been noted in occasional patients with either systemic carnitine deficiency (low plasma and tissue carnitine concentration with multisystem involvement) or myopathic carnitine deficiency (normal plasma concentration but low skeletal muscle carnitine concentration) with progressive muscle weakness. Since the aerobically working cardiac muscle uses long-chain fatty acids as a primary and preferred substrate, it is highly sensitive to carnitine depletion.

Carnitine has a recognized function in the transfer of acyl residues from the activated fatty acids (AcylCoA) across the mitochondrial membrane into the mitochondrial matrix for oxidation (Figure 2). It is noteworthy that patients on long-term maintenance hemodialysis complain frequently of muscle related symptoms including limitation of activity; muscle weakness occurs in up to 52% of adult patients, muscle cramps in 32% and tremors in 10% (24). Also, ESRD patients tend to develop various types of myocardial involvement with decrease in left ventricular performance (25). Echocardiographic studies in adults and children with chronic renal failure have confirmed left ventricular dysfunction in the majority of the patients undergoing chronic hemodialysis (26, 27).

Carnitine is normally eliminated in the urine and accumulates in the blood of uremic patients (28). After the uremic patient is placed on long-term maintenance hemodialysis, the serum levels of carnitine decrease rapidly since carnitine readily crosses the dialysis membranes. At the end of a six hour dialysis session, serum levels of carnitine declined to 22% of values before dialysis (29). We and others have found that the average amount of carnitine lost during each dialysis session is about 600 nmoles (30, 31); this amount is greater than the estimated total amount of carnitine in serum and interstitial fluid and suggests losses from tissues (mainly skeletal muscles). Shortly after a hemodialysis session, serum carnitine rises rapidly, suggesting transfer of carnitine from tissues. The more gradual increase observed after several hours is considered to be due to carnitine synthesis and carnitine intake with food. Serum carnitine reaches again normal levels one day after dialysis and pre-dialysis levels (usually higher than normal) in approximately two days. Consequently, patients on long-term maintenance dialysis have low average levels of carnitine, both in serum and in skeletal muscles (32).

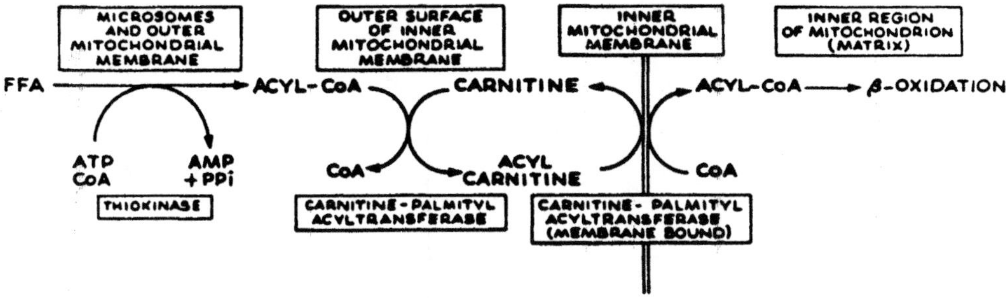

Figure 2: Schematic representation of carnitine shuttle process for free fatty acid (FFA) oxidation.

In a preliminary study to assess plasma carnitine concentration in children on hemodialysis and CAPD, we also documented carnitine losses in the dialysis effluent (33). We confirmed that there was a significant removal of carnitine during dialysis; it was greater on hemodialysis than on CAPD (Table). In addition, there was a significant decrease of carnitine, both free and total, immediately following hemodialysis (Table). There was a significant increase in free fatty acids pre-hemodialysis with further increases post-hemodialysis (Figure 3) and a significant hypertriglyceridemia in both hemodialysis and CAPD (Figure 3). Thus, it is tempting to speculate that despite normal pre-dialysis plasma carnitine concentrations, cumulative carnitine losses during dialysis may lead to carnitine body depletion and aggravate hyperlipidemia.

TABLE

FREE CARNITINE (FC) AND TOTAL CARNITINE (TC) CONCENTRATION IN PLASMA AND DIALYSIS EFFLUENT (x+SD)

Dialysis Modality		Plasma mol/L FC	Plasma mol/L TC	Dialysis TC losses mol/week	%Plasma TC removed per dialysis session
HD	PRE	35+12	61+14	2,316+636	631+288
	POST	13+6†	25+11†		
CAPD		43+7	76+18	567+595	108+114
CONTROLS		43+10	55+12		

† = P < 0.01 compared to controls

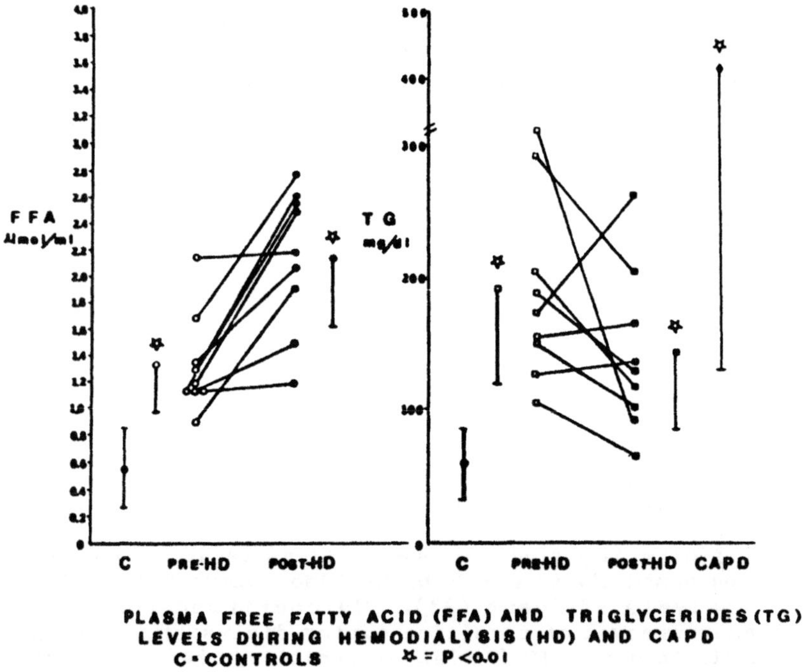

Figure 3: Changes in plasma free fatty acids (FFA) and triglycerides (TG) during hemodialysis (HD) in 10 uremic children. Normal values (C) and TG during CAPD are also given for comparison.

Although the loss of carnitine into the dialysis fluid leading to reduced plasma and tissue carnitine levels have been well documented, the subsequent administration of carnitine has generated conflicting results. Some investigators have observed a reduction in plasma lipids but this has not been confirmed by others (34, 35). A recent study has suggested that the presence of low HDL levels was associated with a decrease in triglycerides after carnitine administration (36). Still, the long-term beneficial effects of L-carnitine supplementation in children on dialysis needs to be assessed. In addition, the different factors affecting uremic hyperlipidemia should be identified in each particular patient and corrected if feasible.

The therapy of uremic hyperlipidemia should be directed to the different factors involved in its pathogenesis; however, in general, the achievement of ideal body weight, graded exercise and adequate diet may play a crucial role (37). In addition, the physician taking care of these patients should identify any drugs to be avoided such as beta blockers, androgens, estrogens, glucocorticoids, ethyl alcohol and diuretics. Finally, specific lipid lowering agents, such as clofibrate, nicotinic acid, activated charcoal and L- carnitine, all could be considered as therapies with potential but unproven benefits.

REFERENCES

1. Chan, M.K., Varghese Z. and Moorhead, J.F.: Lipid abnormalities in uremia, dialysis and transplantation. Kidney Int. 19:625-637, 1981.

2. Lindner, A., Chana B., Sherrard, D.J. et al.: Accelerated atherosclerosis in prolonged maintenance hemodialysis. New Engl. J. Med. 299:1326-1329, 1978.

3. Bagdade, J.D.: Atherosclerosis in patients undergoing maintenance hemodialysis. Kidney Int. 8(Suppl), S-370, 1975.

4. Frank, W.M., Rao, T.K.S., Manis, T. et al.: Relationship of plasma lipids to renal function and length of time on maintenance hemodialysis. Am. J. Clin. Nutr. 31:1886-1892, 1978.

5. Papadopoulou, Z.L., Sandler, P., Tina, L.U. et al.: Hyperlipidemia in children with chronic renal insufficiency. Pediatr. Res. 15:887-891, 1981.

6. Nestel, P.J., Fidge, N.H. and Tan, M.H.: Increased lipoprotein-remnant formation in chronic renal failure. New Engl. J. Med. 307:329-333, 1982.

7. Chait, A., Brunzell, J.D., Albers, J.J. et al.: Type-III hyperlipoproteinaemia (remnant removal disease): insight into the pathogenetic mechanism. Lancet 1:1176-1178, 1977.

8a. Savdie, E., Gibson, J.C., Crawford, G.A. et al.: Impaired plasma triglyceride clearance as a feature of both uremic and posttransplant triglyceridemia. Kidney Int. 18:774-782, 1980.

8b. Asayama, K., Ito, H., Nakahara, C. et al.: Lipid profiles and lipase activities in children and adolescents with chronic renal failure treated conservatively or with hemodialysis or transplantation. Pediatric Res. 18(8):783-788, 1984.

9. Cramp, D.G., Tickner, T.R., Beale, D.J. et al.: Plasma triglyceride secretion and metabolism in chronic renal failure. Clin. Chim. Acta 76:237-243, 1977.

10. Pierides, A.M., Weightman, D., Goldfinch, M. et al.: Hyperlipidemia of regular hemodialysis and successful renal transplantation. Cardiovascular Medicine 3:185, 1978.

11. Person, B.: Lipoprotein lipase activity of human adipose tissue in health and in some diseases with hyperlipidaemia as a common feature. Acta Med. Scand. 193:457-462, 1973.

12. Murase, T., Cattran, D.C., Rubenstein, B. et al.: Inhibition of lipoprotein lipase by plasma, a possible case of hypertriglyceridemia. Metabolism 24:1279-1284, 1975.

13. Cramp, D.G., Beale, D.J., Moorhead, J.F. et al.: Triglyceride turnover in chronic renal failure. Clin. Sci. Mol. Med. 50:80-85, 1976.

14. Gutman, R.A., Uy, A., Shalhoub, R.J. et al.: Hypertriglyceridemia in chronic nonnephrotic renal failure. Am. J. Clin. Nutr. 26:165-172, 1973.

15. Swamy, A.P., Cestero R.V.M., Campbell, R.G. et al.: Long-term effect of dialysate glucose on the lipid levels of maintenance hemodialysis patients. Trans. Am. Soc. Artif. Intern. Organs 22:54-59, 1976.

16. Teraoka, J., Matsui, N., Nagakawa, S. et al.: The role of heparin in the changes of lipid patterns during a single hemodialysis. Clinical Nephrol. 17(2):96-99, 1982.

17. Bohmer, T., Bergrem, H. and Eiklid, K.: Carnitine deficiency induced during intermittent hemodialysis for renal failure. Lancet 3:126-128, 1978.

18. Bartel, L.L., Hussey, J.L. and Shrago, E.: Perturbation of serum carnitine levels in human adults by chronic renal disease and dialysis therapy. Am. J. Clin. Nutr. 34:1314-1320, 1981.

19. Moorthy, A.V., Rosenblum, M., Rajaram, R. et al.: A comparison of plasma and muscle carnitine levels in patients on peritoneal or hemodialysis for chronic renal failure. Am. J. Nephrol. 3:205-208, 1983.

20. Bartel, L.L., Hussey, J.L., Elson, C. et al.: Depletion of heart and skeletal muscle carnitine in the normal rat by peritoneal dialysis. Nutr. Res. 1:261-266, 1981.

21. Rebouche, C.J. and Engel, A.G.: Carnitine metabolism and deficiency syndromes. Mayo Clin. Proc. 58:533-540, 1983.

22. Tripp, M.E., Katcher, M.L., Peters, H.A. et al: Systemic carnitine deficiency presenting as familial endocardial fibroblastosis. New Engl. J. Med. 305:385-390, 1981.

23. Bieber, L.L., Emaus, R., Valkner, K. et al.: Possible functions of short-chain and medium-chain carnitine acyltransferases. Fed Proc. 41:2858-2862, 1982.

24. Anderson, W.W. and Mann, J.B.: Kiil versus coil dialysis - A comparative clinical study. In Bailey G.L. (ed.), Hemodialysis Principles and Practices. New York: Academic Press 373-381, 1982.

25. Schott, C.R., LeSar, J.F., Kotler, M.N. et al.: The spectrum of echocardiographic findings in chronic renal failure. Cardiovas. Med. 3:217-227, 1978.

26. D'Cruz, I.A., Bhatt, G.R., Cohen, H.C. et al.: Echocardiographic detection of cardiac involvement in patients with chronic renal failure. Arch. Intern. Med. 138:720-725, 1978.

27. Soler, P., Zilleruelo, G., Bennett, V. et al.: Left ventricular function in children on chronic dialysis. Pediatr. Res. 16:106A, 1982.

28. Bartel, L., Hussey, J.L. and Shrago, E.: Perturbation of serum carnitine levels in human adults by chronic renal disease and dialysis therapy. Am. J. Clin. Nutr. 34:1314-1320, 1981.

29. Bartel, L., Hussey J., Ewart, R. et al.: (Abstract) Serum carnitine (CAR) and free fatty acid (FFA) levels during hemodialysis. Fed. Proc. 37:445, 1978.

30. Zilleruelo, G., Freundlich, M., Novak, M. et al.: Carnitine losses and free fatty acid (FFA) changes in children on hemodialysis (HD). Proceedings, IX International Congress of Nephrology, Los Angeles, June 1984.

31. Bartel, L.L., Hussey, J.L. and Shrago, E.: Effect of dialysis on serum carnitine, free fatty acids, and triglyceride levels in man and the rat. Metabolism 31:944-949, 1982.

32. Battistella, P.A., Angelini, C., Vergani, L. et al.: (Letter) Carnitine deficiency induced during haemodialysis. Lancet 2:939, 1978.

33. Zilleruelo, G., Freundlich, M., Novak, M. et al.: Carnitine losses in children on hemodialysis (HD) and continuous ambulatory peritoneal dialysis (CAPD). Pediatr. Res. 18:373A, 1984.

34. Bertoli, M., Battistella, P.A., Vergani, L. et al.: Carnitine deficiency induced during hemodialysis and hyperlipidemia: effect of replacement therapy. Amer. J. Clin. Nutr. 34:1496-1500, 1981.

35. Weschler, A., Aviram, M., Levin, M. et al.: High dose of L-carnitine increases platelet aggregation and plasma triglyceride levels in uremic patients on hemodialysis. Nephron 38:120-124, 1984.

36. Vacha, G.M., Giorcelli, G., Siliprand, N. et al.: Favorable effects of L-carnitine treatment of hypertriglyceridemia in hemodialysis patients: decisive role of low levels of high density lipoprotein-cholesterol. Am. J. Clin. Nutr. 38:532-540, 1983.

37. Golper, T.A.: Therapy for uremic hyperlipidemia. Nephron 38:217-225, 1984.

MINERAL METABOLISM IN PATIENTS ON CONTINUOUS AMBULATORY PERITONEAL DIALYSIS

Michael Freundlich, M.D., Gaston Zilleruelo, M.D., Carolyn Abitbol, M.D. and Jose Strauss, M.D.

Since the pioneering reports describing continuous ambulatory peritoneal dialysis (CAPD) as a novel dialytic therapy (1, 2), it has become an accepted therapeutic modality for patients with end stage renal disease (ESRD). Because of its relative technical simplicity and compatibility with home dialysis, CAPD rapidly has become a suitable therapy for children, particularly small infants (3). Aspects pertaining to mineral metabolism and renal osteodystrophy (ROD) are of particular interest in the pediatric population, and require careful scrutiny in order to fully assess the potential benefits of CAPD.

The established ESRD is associated with a series of derangements of mineral metabolism that eventually lead to the development of ROD. The latter includes several skeletal disorders such as osteitis fibrosa cystica, osteomalacia, osteosclerosis, osteoporosis, and growth retardation (4). Osteitis fibrosa, characterized by the presence of marrow fibrosis and immature woven bone, is the predominant form of ROD in North American adults (5). Osteomalacia (rickets), characterized by excess osteoid and a diminished calcification front, seems to be the predominant lesion in children, probably related to their high rate of bone modeling (6). Hyperparathyroidism secondary to chronic renal failure (CRF) and diminished vitamin D synthesis accompanying decreased functional renal mass, are the main pathogenetic events leading to ROD (4, 7-9). Thus, amelioration of these events constitutes one of the chief goals of dialytic therapies.

With the institution of chronic dialysis, further changes in bone and mineral metabolism occur. Approximately 700 to 1100 mg of calcium enter the patient during 10 hours of hemodialysis when the dialysate calcium level exceeds the diffusable concentration in plasma by 1.5 to 2.0 mg/dl (10). Parathyroid hormone (PTH) or its fragments are not removed from the circulation by hemodialysis (11) and serum levels of 1,25-dihydroxyvitamin D [$1,25(OH)_2D$] are usually low in patients on chronic hemodialysis (12). Since CAPD leads to substantial losses of middle and large molecular weight protein fractions, important changes in mineral, vitamin D, and PTH metabolism are expected to take place.

Serum calcium (total or ionized) has been found to be low (11, 13), normal (11, 13-19), or elevated (20) during CAPD. Calcium mass transfer (MT) studies in adults have also revealed variable information, ranging from positive (absorption from dialysate to patient) to negative balances (5, 19, 21) (Table). In children, most MT determinations have revealed negative (or near zero) daily calcium balances (losses of

This project is funded in part under an agreement with the Department of Health and Rehabilitative Services, State of Florida Children's Medical Services.

calcium into the peritoneal effluent) (Figure) (22, 23). As expected, calcium MT correlated inversely with serum calcium concentration (23). Since peritoneal losses of calcium are most pronounced during high-dextrose dialysate exchanges (24), the frequent utilization of these solutions, particularly in small infants (25), may result in important calcium losses. Conceivably, selected patients may benefit from the use of higher than standard calcium-containing dialysate solutions (26).

REPORTED STUDIES ON CALCIUM MASS TRANSFER

STUDY REFERENCE #	PERITONEAL CALCIUM BALANCE mg/day
11	9.8
14	-50
19	84
21	300
23 (children)	-18

Modified from Freundlich, M., Zilleruelo, G., Strauss, J. Mineral metabolism in children and adults receiving continuous ambulatory peritoneal dialysis. Seminars in Nephrol. 3:159-165, 1983.

While the mean amount of phosphorus removed daily (175 $\pm$ 112 mg) (Figure) was substantial, most patients required oral phosphate binders to control hyperphosphatemia. Hypermagnesemia, a frequent finding in ESRD patients, tends to ameliorate during CAPD, but in most patients serum magnesium remains elevated during CAPD (23). This is partly explained by the fact that daily peritoneal removal rates of magnesium (18 $\pm$ 6 mg) (Figure) are below its net daily intestinal absorption (16, 23).

Blood levels of 25(OH)D, the vitamin D metabolite generated in the liver, are mostly normal at the start of CAPD (11, 13, 14, 20) but have been occasionally reported to be low in some children (23). These differences may be the result of different original disease processes, duration of CRF and state of nutrition preceding the initiation of CAPD. Both 25(OH)D and its carrier protein, D-binding protein, are lost into peritoneal effluents (23, 27); thus, progressively diminishing blood concentrations while on CAPD are expected (23). This situation, analogous to that of patients with nephrotic syndrome in which urinary losses of vitamin D metabolites are considerable, conceivably may affect adversely bone mineralization (28). In addition, peritoneal losses of $1,25(OH)_2D$ albeit small (1% of the daily oral intake) were noted in some children (23).

FIGURE

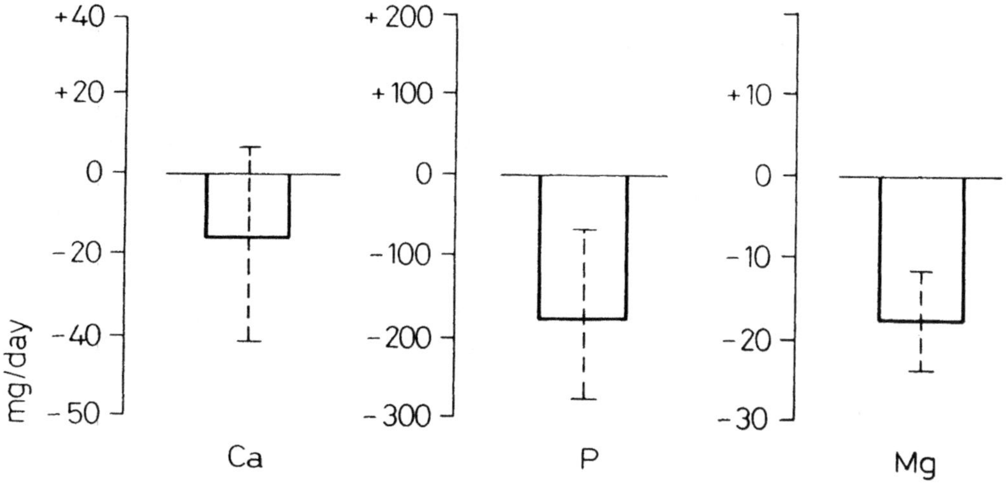

Recently reported studies on peritoneal MT of PTH in children demonstrated readily detectable immunereactive PTH (iPTH) in peritoneal effluents (23). These losses were associated with mean declines of 30% and 23% in serum iPTH and alkaline phosphatase concentrations, respectively. Although elevated serum PTH has not consistently fallen in children treated with CAPD (18), some have demonstrated improvement in hyperparathyroidism and its beneficial effect on somatic growth (29).

More recent preliminary data demonstrated effective suppression of circulating iPTH to nearly half of control values with intraperitoneal administration of $1,25(OH)_2D$ in adults on CAPD (30).

Data concerning the impact of CAPD on bone mineralization and structure are beginning to emerge. Conventional radiographs have shown deterioration of previously existent or emergence of new bone lesions in some children on CAPD (31). On the other hand, another study in which sequential densitometric determinations were obtained, demonstrated either stabilization or remineralization in most patients tested (23). In a controlled study comparing the effects of hemodialysis and CAPD on bone histomorphometry, the authors found overall more favorable effects of CAPD on ROD with a marked improvement in the osteomalacic component as compared to hemodialysis (32).

Based on the above reviewed considerations, it seems that most CAPD patients requiring phosphate binding agents, may experience overall salutary effects on the existing disturbances of mineral metabolism, and may benefit from the use of different calcium dialysate concentrations and the judicious administration of active vitamin D metabolites.

REFERENCES

1. Popovich, R.P., Moncrief, J.W., Dechard, J.B. et al.: The definition of a novel portable/wearable equilibrium peritoneal dialysis technique. Am Soc Artif Intern Organs 5:64, 1976 (abstr).

2. Oreopoulus, D.G., Robson, M., Izatt, S. et al.: A simple and safe technique for continuous peritoneal dialysis (CAPD). Trans Am Soc Artif Organs 24:484-487, 1978.

3. Alexander, S.R., Tseng, C.H., Maksym, K.A. et al.: Clinical parameters in continuous ambulatory peritoneal dialysis for infants and children. In Moncrief, J.W., Popovich, R.P. (eds.): CAPD update. New York, Masson, 1981, pp 195-207.

4. Norman, M.E.: Vitamin D in bone diseases. Pediat Clin N America 29:947-971, 1982.

5. Agus, Z.S., Goldfarb, S. and Wasserstein, A.: Renal osteodystrophy, In Klahr, S., Massry, S.G. (eds.): Contemporary Nephrology, Vol 1. New York, Plenum, 1981, pp 282-290.

6. Norman, M.E., Mazur, A.T., Bordeu, S.B. et al.: Early diagnosis of juvenile renal osteodystrophy. J Pediatr 97:226-232, 1980.

7. Bricker, N.S.: On the pathogenesis of the uremic state. An exposition of the "trade-off" hypothesis. N Engl J Med 286:1093-1098, 1972.

8. Slatopolsky, E., Rutherford, E., Hruska, K. et al.: How important is phosphate in the pathogenesis of renal osteodystrophy. Arch Intern Med 128:848-852, 1978.

9. Massry, S.G., Ritz, E. and Verbeckmoes, R.: Role of phosphate in the genesis of secondary hyperparathyroidism. Nephron 18:77-81, 1977.

10. Mirahmadi, K.S., Duffy, B.S., Shimaberger, J.H. et al.: A controlled evaluation of clinical and metabolic effects of dialysate calcium levels during regular hemodialysis. Trans Am Soc Artif Intern Organs 17:118-124, 1971.

11. Delmez, J.A., Slatopolsky, E., Martin, K. et al.: Minerals, vitamin D, and parathyroid hormone in continuous ambulatory peritoneal dialysis. Kidney Int 21:862-867, 1982.

12. Eisman, J.A., Hamstra, A.J., Kream, B.E. et al.: 1,25-dihydroxyvitamin D in biological fluids: A simplified and sensitive assay. Science 193:1021-1023, 1976.

13. Gokal, R., Ellis, H.A., Ramos, J.M. et al.: Improvement in secondary hyperparathyroidism in patients on continuous ambulatory peritoneal dialysis. In Gahl, G.M., Kessel, M., Nolph, K.D. (eds.): Advances in Peritoneal Dialysis: Proceedings of the Second International Symposium on Peritoneal Dialysis, Berlin (-West), June 16-19, 1981. Amsterdam, Excerpta Medica, 1981, pp 461-466, (International Congress Series no 567).

14. Calderaro, V., Oreopoulus, D.G., Meema, E.H. et al.: Renal osteodystrophy in patients on continuous ambulatory peritoneal dialysis: A biochemical and radiologic study. In Moncrief, J.W., Popovich, R.P. (eds.): CAPD Update. New York, Masson, 1981, pp 243-247.

15. Balfe, J.W., Vigneus, A., Willumsen, J. et al.: The use of CAPD in the treatment of children with end-stage renal disease. Perit Dial Bull 1:35-38, 1981.

16. Alexander, S.R., Tseng, C.H., Maksym, K.A. et al.: Clinical parameters in continuous ambulatory peritoneal dialysis for infants and children. In Moncrief, J.W., Popovich, R.P. (eds.): CAPD Update, New York, Masson, 1981, pp 195-207.

17. Guillot, M., Clermont, M.J., Gagnadoux, M.F. et al.: Nineteen months' experience with CAPD in children: Main clinical and biological results. In Gahl, G.M., Kessel, M., Nolph, K.D. (eds.): Advances in Peritoneal Dialysis: Proceedings of the Second International Symposium of Peritoneal Dialysis, Berlin (-West), June 16-19, 1981. Amsterdam, Excerpta Medica, 1981, pp 203-207 (International Congress Series no 567).

18. Baum, M., Powell, D., Calvin, S. et al.: Continuous ambulatory peritoneal dialysis in children. Comparison with hemodialysis. N Engl J Med 307:1537-1542, 1982.

19. Blumenkrantz, J.K., Kopple, J.D., Moran, J.K. et al.: Metabolic balance studies and dietary protein requirements in patients undergoing continuous ambulatory peritoneal dialysis. Kidney Int 21:849-861, 1982.

20. Kurtz, S.B., McCarthy, J.T. and Kumar, R.: Hypercalcemia in continuous ambulatory peritoneal dialysis patients: Observations on parameters of calcium metabolism. In Gahl, G.M., Kessel, M., Nolph, K.D. (eds.): Advances in Peritoneal Dialysis: Proceedings of the Second International Symposium on Peritoneal Dialysis Berlin (-West), June 16-19, 1981. Amsterdam, Excerpta Medica, 1981, pp 467-472 (International Congress Series no 567).

21. Parker, A. and Nolph, K.D.: Magnesium and calcium mass transfer during continuous ambulatory peritoneal dialysis. Trans Am Soc Artif Intern Organs 26:194-196, 1980.

22. Nolph, K.D., Popovich, R.P. and Moncrief, J.W.: Theoretical and practical implications of continuous ambulatory peritoneal dialysis. Nephron 21:117-120, 1978.

23. Freundlich, M., Zilleruelo, G, Abitbol, C. et al.: Minerals and bone-modulating hormones in children on continuous ambulatory peritoneal dialysis. Nephron 41:267-272, 1985.

24. Freundlich, M., Zilleruelo, G., Canterbury, J.M. et al.: Calcium, phosphorus, uric acid, vitamin D and parathyroid hormone metabolism in children on continuous ambulatory peritoneal dialysis. Pediatr Res 17:349, 1983 (abstr).

25. Kohaut, E.D. and Alexander, S.R.: Ultrafiltration in the young patient on CAPD. In Moncrief, J.W., Popovich, R.P. (eds.): CAPD Update. New York, Masson, 1981, pp 221-226.

26. Bingswanger, T.: Personal communication to Kogal R: Renal osteodystrophy in continuous ambulatory peritoneal dialysis. Perit Dial Bull 2:111-115, 1982.

27. Guillot, M., Garabedian, M., Lavocat, C. et al.: Evaluation of 25-hydroxyvitamin D and vitamin D-binding protein losses of thirteen children on continuous ambulatory peritoneal dialysis. Int J Pediatr Nephrol 4:99-102, 1983.

28. Freundlich, M., Bourgoignie, J.J., Zilleruelo, G. et al.: Bone modulating factors in nephrotic children with normal glomerular filtration rate. Pediatrics 76:280-284, 1985.

29. Kohaut, E.C.: Growth in children treated with continuous ambulatory peritoneal dialysis. Int J Pediat Nephrol 4:93-98, 1983.

30. Delmez, J., Dougan, S., Gearing, B. et al.: The effects of high dialysate calcium and intraperitoneal $1,25(OH)_2D$ on PTH levels and calcium mass transfer during CAPD. Proceedings, 18th Annual Meeting, American Society of Nephrology, 1985. Abstr. 82A.

31. Hewitt, I.K., Stefanidis, C., Reilly, B.J. et al.: Renal osteodystrophy in children undergoing continuous ambulatory peritoneal dialysis. J Pediatr 103:729-734, 1983.

32. Shusterman, N., Fallon, M., Kaplan, F. et al.: Favorable response of renal osteodystrophy in CAPD patients. Proceedings, 18th Annual Meeting, American Society of Nephrology, 1985. Abstr. 88A.

DISCUSSION: RENAL REPLACEMENT THERAPY
DIALYSIS

PANELISTS: Richard Fine, M.D., Michael Freundlich, M.D. and Gaston Zilleruelo, M.D.

MODERATOR: Jose Strauss, M.D.

QUESTION: Plasma level of 1,25 Vitamin D in these children who were undergoing CAPD was 58, which is very reasonable, in fact, a perfectly normal level. What Vitamin D metabolite were they on? If they had been given anything other than 1,25 initially, one could interpret this in a different way.

RESPONSE: Five of the patients were on calcitriol in varying doses, 0.25 up to 1.25 mcg/day, except the infant who was on DHT towards the latter part of the clinical course and one patient was on no medication. The data on the six initial patients include a mean of 59. The initial calcitriol level might represent an adequate dosing of calcitriol for those patients or an interference with the DHT since the assay cannot discriminate between the two of them.

COMMENTS: Let me make several comments about the levels of 1,25D. First, I do not think these measurements are absolutely essential in following patients. It is an expensive and difficult assay. However, if you do measure 1,25D levels in patients who are on DHT, you are going to get very high values in the range of 2-3 times normal. We have found values as high as 600 pg/ml. The DHT has a pseudo one alpha activity, and this fools the receptor assay. When we looked at this in our own CAPD patients, some had been on DHT and we had very similar findings in them. The second thing is that when you are measuring the levels of 1,25D in patients with renal failure after dosing, <u>when</u> you obtain the sample is very critical because the peak serum sample is going to be achieved somewhere between two and a half to four hours after the dose, and then it rapidly falls. By the next day, it is back down to base line. I am assuming that you measured these about the same time each day. If you do not do that, then you are going to be fooled. The third thing and I think perhaps the most critical, is that the plasma level of 1,25D after a dose of 1,25D may not be terribly important because I believe that there is a first pass phenomenon as the 1,25D goes across the intestine; it is bound to the receptor in the intestine, and it increases intestinal calcium absorption. We certainly saw this ourselves where we measured 1,25D levels in a number of patients and there was not a tremendous increase in them; they were increased only into the normal range. But, at the same time, we could demonstrate a tremendous increase in intestinal calcium absorption. We looked at this in rats; and, indeed, at least in rats, there was evidence of this first pass phenomenon.

QUESTION: Would you define CCPD? Is this seven days a week, five days a week? Do you use the same time schedule, same glucose concentration?

RESPONSE: Seven days a week, ten hours at night, five two- hour exchanges, and generally a half-volume during the day. Except in the very young children, to improve appetite we try to avoid doing anything during the day. The glucose concentration is dependent upon how much fluid one needs to remove, and it is adjusted. The number of 1.5, 2.5, and 4.25 bags are adjusted according to how much fluid needs to be removed.

QUESTION: Do you have any peritonitis data looking at the relationship to age or the amount of glucose used?

RESPONSE-QUESTION: I do not have any specific data but I am sure I could get some. Why do you ask the question?

RESPONSE: My reason for asking is, if you use more glucose you should have more ultrafiltration in more convected transport, more loss of IgG. Similarly, if the younger membrane is more permeable, you might expect more IgG losses.

RESPONSE: That is an excellent idea. The problem is that we looked at IgG levels at the beginning of dialysis (just as it started), and then a year or two later we looked at them again. The patients who had low IgG levels at the beginning, had persistently low levels at the end. Those that were high at the beginning were high at the end. So, there did not appear to be any change over time, any excessive losses if you will. This is something that one could look at.

QUESTION: Do you have any thoughts on why one starts with a low IgG level? Were these children malnourished, cachectic, and so on?

RESPONSE: Those are all potential reasons; I do not have any specific reasons why some patients have low IgG levels at the beginning in comparison with other groups. Certainly, some of the patients with lower levels post-transplantation had a period of chronic rejection with catabolism induced by corticosteroids; this may have contributed to the low levels at the initiation of dialysis. For instance, the patient who had seven episodes of peritonitis was a patient who started CAPD after having rejected a transplant that had lasted roughly three to four years. His level was low at the beginning, and I think potentially low because of the immunosuppressive and steroid therapy.

COMMENT-QUESTION: Conversely, if they start with a low IgG and do well, why don't the levels go up? Any thoughts?

RESPONSE: No.

COMMENT: Relative to the infants that you have on PD, I notice that they had increased infection (peritonitis) relative to the rest of the patients. Am I correct?

RESPONSE: No, not at all.

QUESTION: It does not really matter. Is there any particular reason that you chose CCPD over CAPD for those patients?

RESPONSE: One of the problems one gets into with long dwell dialysis is that there is more protein loss with long dwell than with shorter dwell dialysis. In the very young child, that is one advantage of CCPD over CAPD: the difference in the potential for a lot of protein losses. The primary reason we chose CCPD over CAPD was not because of that; it was because the parent only had to do two exchanges a day--when the patient went on dialysis in the evening and when he came off in the morning. With CAPD, the patient needed four or five; sometimes in a young child, if he is oliguric, even more than five exchanges a day are needed to be able to lower and maintain the potassium level and also remove sufficient fluid. You can use CCPD in infants up to nine to twelve months of age. It is not that difficult to put them on 12, 14 or 16 hours of dialysis a day with no added inconvenience to either the parents or the children. Once they start crawling around, then it becomes a problem. At more than a year of age or anytime after they start walking, they do not like to be connected to the machine for prolonged periods of time. But, they sleep for at least 10 or 12 hours and then, CCPD is not a major problem; it is much more convenient for the parent. In addition, we felt that if we were able to dialyze them just at night and leave no dialysate in during the day, we would improve their intake. Indeed, we have had one who ultimately had to go to a half-volume exchange during the day; the mother told us that when there was something in the abdomen during the day, the appetite was certainly diminished. Whether their reduced desire to eat is related to the glucose and the hyperglycemia turning off the appetite or the sense of fullness, I do not know. It has been our impression that the reduction in fluid volume during the day to some extent has been associated with improved oral intake; conversely, there was some appetite reduction in patients in whom we had to resort to fluid instillation during the day. Thus, the major reasons for putting these patients on CCPD were parental psychosocial reasons which predominated, and the improved oral intake potential with either limited or no exchanges during the day.

COMMENT: Do you have the same impression as we do that the young child's ultrafiltration does not seem to be as good as in older patients and, therefore, that we are essentially obligated to use the high dextrose in infants? Is that your experience?

RESPONSE: If you look at it on an ml/kg basis and look at what you want to do, you are going to have to get more fluid out; plus, if you do the long dwell exchanges, the one thing that you are going to find is that the younger the children, the more glucose they are going to absorb, which means that longer dwells also are going to be less efficient. One of the Guest Faculty found this in work with animal models. I think that is why you may need to use a higher glucose concentration in younger children.

QUESTION: Do you have any hard data on protein losses in CCPD versus CAPD?

RESPONSE: Yes, but not available to discuss today. We have a study of about 14 patients. We put them in the Clinical Research Center for four studies each, on three exchanges at night or five exchanges at night with or without a daytime dwell, measuring the protein losses. I do not have the data at my fingertips to give you.

QUESTION: That would be CCPD?

RESPONSE: Right. We have the data from CAPD on the same patients. If you look at the initial studies, more than 50% of the protein loss with CCPD, occurs during the long daytime dwell. The real question is: if you have nothing in during the day or a smaller amount in during the day, will you lose less protein? Or, when you put the first dwell in for CCPD, will you have an enormous amount of protein lost at that time? I cannot give you an answer to that yet; that is what our study was designed to answer. I agree with you; as of now there are no data to answer the real question.

QUESTION: I am interested in the patients who had a positive, so to speak, Desferal test. Did they have more severe anemia than the rest of the patients?

RESPONSE: Not to my knowledge.

QUESTION: On Desferal treatment you have not seen an improvement in their transfusion requirement or anything like that?

RESPONSE: The patients that we have had on Desferal have been on really for too short a period of time for us to be able to make an evaluation as to whether it influences anything other than the serum aluminum levels. Initially, the aluminum levels go up; I really cannot give you any data yet.

QUESTION: With regard to loss of ultrafiltration, have you had any problems with it?

RESPONSE: The major problem with ultrafiltration has been in patients who have lost their membrane function secondary to peritonitis. Of the five patients, two were with candida, one with pseudomonas, one with corinebacterium, and I think the other was with serratia. Of these patients, in two it was more a loss of ultrafiltration; in three there was such a fibrotic peritoneum that we could not get a catheter to work at all. But in two, from a biochemical standpoint, we could maintain their BUNs and creatinines at a reasonable value, but it was impossible to remove any fluid despite going up to six percent glucose concentration. So, that has been the main problem.

Someone handed me the following question: "It was once suggested that placement of the catheter be done about four to six weeks before initiation of CAPD to prevent formation of the hernia which often appears later on. What is you opinion?" I think it is a good idea to place the catheters in as long as possible prior to when you actually need them; this allows the tissues time to heal. Sometimes we do not have that luxury. However, I do not think that it is as much related to hernia development, at least in our experience, as it is to dialysate leak. If you have to start with large volumes immediately, I think the potential for a dialysate leak is greater than the potential for a hernia.

COMMENT-QUESTION: Out of your 30 patients that were transplanted, I noted that 16 required dialysis in the post-operative period. Is that different from other patients? Do you think CAPD patients have a higher incidence of dialysis requirement post-transplant?

RESPONSE: No. I think that if we looked at it in comparison to those that had hemodialysis, we would find similar results. It is a reflection of the fact that we have many more patients awaiting transplantation following rejection of a previous kidney who have high levels of antibodies and, therefore, the kidneys we get that are cross-matched negative are kidneys which frequently come from longer distances and have prolonged perfusion times. We do not have the impression that there is any relationship between CAPD and the post-transplant need for dialysis. Although we think the patients may be dryer because we manage their fluids better on CAPD than we do on hemo, they are not really dryer because if you have a patient on CAPD who then gets a kidney and it is a good diuresing kidney, in 24 to 48 hours you are amazed to see how much fluid-overloaded the patients really were. That is intimated by your question that maybe with CAPD we dry out the patients too much, and that may have some hemodynamic effect on the ATN that occurs. I really do not believe that the patients are that dry.

QUESTION: I noticed that in the "Non-infectious Complications", you did not mention one-way obstruction. Do you do omentectomy as a routine? Have you noticed higher peritonitis incidence in adolescent patients? Presumably, adolescents might think they are more independent, versatile, and start to improvise.

RESPONSE: We have had three instances of obstruction. In all three the obstruction occurred within the first 24 to 48 hours. The problem was technical, and we routinely do omentectomy on all our patients. We have had no late obstructions and only these three patients had early obstructions. They were all older adolescents, not young patients. With regard to non-compliance and experimentation in the adolescent, these do occur to some extent. When I looked at peritonitis by age groups, it was not my impression that the adolescent patient had a higher incidence of peritonitis. We routinely have all patients over 12 trained to dialyze themselves; under 12, the parents do it. It has not been our impression that the adolescent's behavior had any detrimental effect. Of course, it depends upon whom you are comparing. In our general population, if you look at the one parent and the two parent family, there is a dramatic difference between those two groups. In the adolescent, the incidence of peritonitis would probably be similar to that of a child with one parent.

QUESTION: I am worried about peritonitis in CAPD patients after a kidney transplant. You stated that you had one patient who had peritonitis; what organism was that? Did it grow anything else?

RESPONSE: It was a staph aureus and it responded immediately to therapy.

COMMENT-QUESTION: We had one patient who developed peritonitis the night prior to the transplant, and the living related donor backed out; the transplant had to be rescheduled with a cadaver kidney. We have gotten more conservative; we put some patients who have had peritonitis on hemodialysis (instead of CAPD) a week or so before the transplant. Do you have any thoughts on that?

RESPONSE: I think it is a risk. We had it happen on one occasion. A patient came in for a cadaver transplant; he had peritonitis and we cancelled it. We also had a patient who came in for a transplant with an abscess at the site of the old transplant; we had to cancel it. I personally do not feel that those are circumstances which would indicate the need to initiate hemodialysis from a prophylactic standpoint. We also have had the circumstance of a patient, an older adolescent, who had two episodes of peritonitis immediately before a live-related donor transplant. We began to wonder whether this patient was telling us that she really did not want to go through this procedure; but ultimately, she did. I personally have not seen that as a major problem; we do not usually switch from CAPD to hemo beforehand. We have done transplants within a week to ten days of stopping antibiotic therapy for a previous episode of peritonitis. The incidence post-transplant has been relatively small.

COMMENT: In regard to that last point, as a guide we have used the return of the cell count to normal as an indication that it is safe to proceed with the transplant.

RESPONSE: I think that is probably quite reasonable. If the culture is negative, I would agree.

MODERATOR: If there are no pressing further questions, we will stop here.

VI

RENAL REPLACEMENT THERAPY

PROGRESSSION OF RENAL DISEASES AND TRANSPLANTATION

EFFECTS OF PROTEIN ON RENAL FUNCTION AND DISEASE

J. J. Bourgoignie, M.D.

The current inability to prevent, let alone to reverse, the progressive deterioration of renal function in patients with chronic renal disease remains an important challenge. Recent observations correlate the progressive and inexorable loss of glomerular filtration rate (GFR) that accompanies chronic renal disease with excess dietary protein. This brief review will assess the impact of protein on renal function and disease.

EFFECTS OF PROTEIN ON RENAL FUNCTION IN RODENTS

The adverse effects of high protein diets on renal function and survival have been noted for more than 60 years in laboratory rats. These observations led to advocate restriction of dietary protein in humans with chronic renal insufficiency. However, acceptance of protein restriction has been sporadic except to achieve temporary relief of symptoms in patients with advanced disease and uremia. Even this was largely abandoned with the advent of dialysis.

Recent revival of interest in the adverse role of protein on renal function is the result of a series of rigorous studies in rats by Brenner et al. (1,2) which led to a concept of hemodynamic glomerulopathy. This concept, illustrated in Fig. 1, stems from the correlation observed between measurements of intrarenal hemodynamics, proteinuria, renal morphology and survival of rats fed different amounts of protein.

In brief, when renal mass is reduced, intrarenal vascular resistances decrease; there is a two to threefold increase in single nephron plasma flow and single nephron glomerular filtration rate; and intraglomerular hypertension ensues. These adaptive intrarenal hemodynamic changes are immediately beneficial in terms of overall

GFR; however, in the long run, they may have adverse effects on single

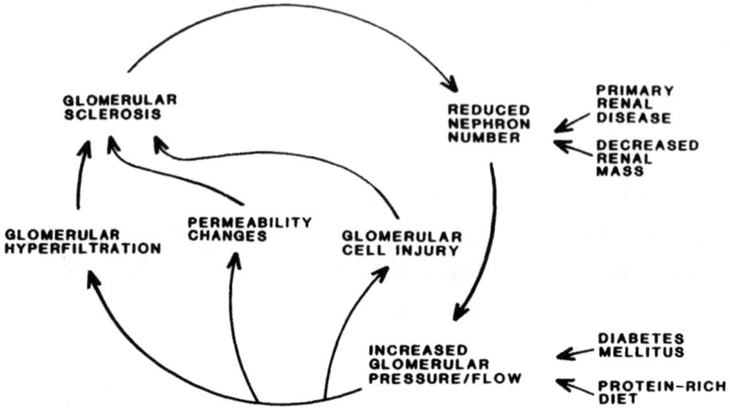

Fig. 1. The concept of hemodynamic glomerulopathy.

nephron function resulting in progressive proteinuria, mesangial expansion, and glomerular sclerosis leading, ultimately, to glomerular obsolescence of the surviving nephrons with progressive decrease in total GFR and death in uremia. A high protein intake accelerates this process; whereas dietary protein restriction reverses the intrarenal hemodynamic changes, prevents the proteinuria and limits the glomerular sclerosis. Thus, survival of rats with a remnant kidney is prolonged by a low protein intake. The severity of the glomerulopathy is directly proportional to the amount of renal mass removed and to the amount of protein in the diet.

These events, originally described in rats with a remnant kidney, are not limited to this experimental model of renal disease. A high protein diet induces disease in the remaining kidney after unilateral nephrectomy. Uninephrectomy accelerates the nephropathy associated in rodents with experimental diabetes, hypertension, systemic lupus, nephritic serum nephritis, puromycin nucleoside nephrosis, and renal irradiation. Again, reduction of dietary protein limits the progressive loss of renal function in these various experimental models (2).

Moreover, the nephrotoxicity of a relative excess of dietary protein has been extended to conditions where renal mass is originally intact but where primary changes in the kidney may be hemodynamic as in diabetes or hypertension. In these conditions again, a low protein diet decreases proteinuria and glomerular sclerosis and increases survival. The concept also applies to the progressive loss of GFR and focal glomerular sclerosis that occur in aging rats (2). Intermittent feeding of rats over a lifetime period, rather than feeding ad libitum, has been shown to attenuate the development of renal insufficiency and glomerular sclerosis (3).

ROLE OF FACTORS OTHER THAN PROTEIN

Excess phosphorus intake has been incriminated in the progression of renal disease. Low phosphorus intake maintains GFR and prolongs survival in rats with a remnant kidney and in rats with nephrotic serum nephritis (4-6). However, unlike the glomerulopathy associated with protein feeding, the renal pathology of high phosphorus intake is characterized primarily by renal interstitial lesions. Although hyperphosphatemia is clearly nephrotoxic in chronic renal disease, several studies in rats have dissociated in rats the adverse effects on GFR of dietary phosphorus and protein (7-9).

Others view systemic hypertension as the major offender to explain the progressive decline in GFR in rats with a remnant kidney. Hypertension, often severe, regularly occurs in rats after renal ablation. Hypertension, by damaging the capillary endothelium, may result in platelet aggregation and intraglomerular thrombosis, leading to proteinuria, glomerular sclerosis and more severe hypertension. A vicious circle ensues resulting in progressive nephron loss and uremia. Support for this sequence of events in rats is found in the beneficial effects of agents that inhibit platelet aggregation or thromboxane release and decrease blood pressure (10).

Hypertension, without a doubt, is an important factor of progressive renal dysfunction. However, the effects of hypertension appear to differ from those of excess protein since protein restriction may be protective without changes in blood pressure in rats with a remnant kidney and in rats with DOCA-salt hypertension (11,12). Moreover, an adverse effect of hypertension does not conflict with but merely complements the hypothesis of Brenner since intraglomerular hypertension, rather than glomerular hyperfiltration, appears to be the culprit in protein-rich diets.

EFFECTS OF RENAL MASS REDUCTION AND DIETARY PROTEIN IN OTHER ANIMAL SPECIES

Whereas the evidence that protein may have adverse effects on renal function in rats is convincing, similar data are scanty and less compelling in other species.

Rabbits with renal mass reduction develop interstitial nephritis and obstructive nephropathy (13).

Dogs, like rats, increase GFR after a protein load and develop a striking anatomic hypertrophy and functional increase in single nephron GFR after renal mass reduction. Few studies, however, report on the outcome of GFR as a function of time after renal mass ablation in dogs. Robertson et al.(14) found no decrease in GFR 48 months after ablation of renal tissue, even in dogs fed a 56 percent protein diet. However, total GFR in these animals was only decreased 34 to 42 percent. Polzin et al.(15) observed dogs with a remnant kidney fed a 44% protein diet to maintain GFR constant during a 40 week follow-up. In the former study, renal mass ablation may not have been severe enough and, in the latter, follow-up may have been too short. Thus, neither study demonstrated progressive renal dysfunction in terms of GFR and proteinuria, and each showed only modest structural changes in the remnant glomeruli.

Our own experience in dogs with a remnant kidney and a 70% decrease in GFR indicates that although GFR may remain stable for years after renal ablation, progressive proteinuria and progressive structural changes develop in the remnant kidney. Proteinuria and changes in glomerular morphology were evident 3 to 6 months after 7/8 reduction in renal mass. In all dogs in which protein excretion was measured, abnormal proteinuria developed; and in animals studied repetitively, the proteinuria was progressive (Fig.2). The proteinuria was associated with morphological changes of glomerular mesangial hyperplasia or sclerosis in the remaining glomeruli. And, in dogs

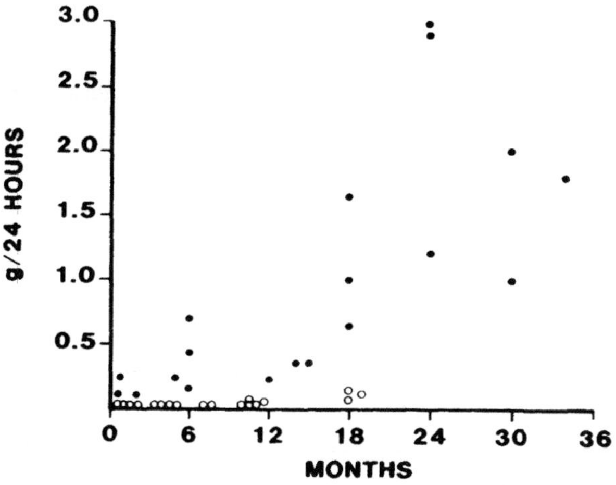

Fig.2. Proteinuria (g/24 hours) as a function of time in normal dogs (O) and in dogs with a remnant kidney (●). Each point is the average of 2 to 7 measurements.

studied sequentially, the histologic alterations progressed from focal mesangial hyperplasia to focal and segmental glomerular sclerosis or diffuse glomerular obsolescence.

EFFECT OF PROTEIN ON RENAL FUNCTION IN PRIMATES

Glomerular sclerosis is a common pathologic manifestation of many seemingly unrelated renal diseases, including sickle cell anemia and diabetes (16). Glomerular sclerosis has been reported in patients with unilateral renal agenesis (17), after uninephrectomy (18,19), or after kidney donation for renal transplantation (20). Whether these isolated observations represent a trend that may, ultimately, commonly develop with longer follow-up is presently unclear.

Thus, the concept that progressive glomerular sclerosis may result from a hemodynamic glomerulopathy secondary to excessive protein intake has broad implications for humans. An enormous population is potentially at risk, including patients with various degrees of renal insufficiency, patients with a single kidney, and patients with diabetes or other pathology associated with early renal hyperemia. The decline in GFR with age may also be the consequence of a lifetime of eating too much protein (10).

Whereas the data in rats provide a powerful argument to restrict protein intake in patients with chronic renal disease and in those individuals potentially at risk, it is well to remember that differences exist between various species. For instance, rats and dogs subjected to renal mass ablation rapidly develop a striking anatomic hypertrophy of the remnant renal tissue; and the development of glomerular sclerosis in rats is associated with hypertrophy of the remnant kidney. Such renal hypertrophy does not occur in primates. In baboons, Dicker and Morris (21) found little evidence of anatomic hypertrophy in the remaining kidney 17 weeks after uninephrectomy (Fig.3). We observed a 20% difference in kidney weight in adult baboon subjected to uninephrectomy 8 weeks earlier. The same observation applies to human adults. After kidney donation for transplantation,

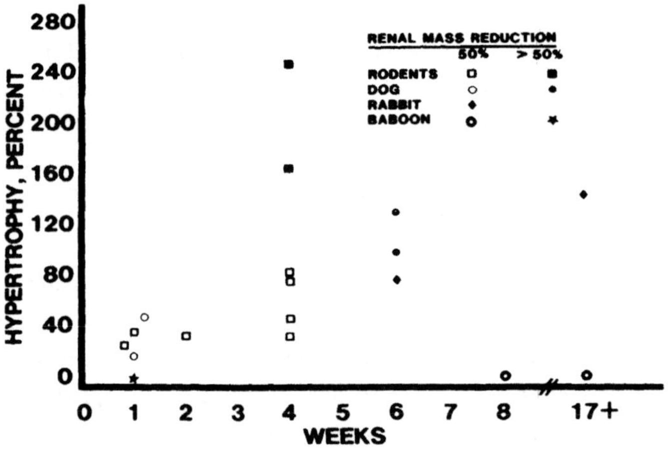

Fig. 3. Renal hypertrophy after renal mass ablation in different animal species. Own data and data from the literature.

increase in size of the remaining kidney has been estimated at 10-20% in adults (22,23). Nevertheless, in human and non-human primates, functional hyperfiltration and hyperemia develop, and single kidney

GFR and renal blood flow may double after uninephrectomy (Table 1).

Renal hemodynamics increase dramatically in fasting rats after protein ingestion or after infusion of amino acids (24). Renal hyperemia also occurs in primates. In baboon and in man, GFR and renal blood flow may increase 20 to 60% over fasting values with infusion of amino acids or ingestion of a protein meal (25-27). These changes are rapidly and readily reversible. In uninephrectomized baboon (Table I), or in patients with renal disease, such a renal hemodynamic reserve may no longer be apparent but may be restored after administration of a diet low in protein (25,28).

Table 1. Effect of glucagon (8.3 ng/min/kg iv) on single kidney hemodynamics in baboon before and 8 weeks after uninephrectomy.

	Intact baboon*	After uninephrectomy
Kidney wt, g	31.2	38.0
Inulin clearance		
Control, ml/min	21.0	43.5
Glucagon	30.5	37.0
Control, ml/min/gKw	0.67	1.14
Glucagon	0.98	0.97
PAH clearance		
Control, ml/min	98.5	238.0
Glucagon	178.0	231.0
Control, ml/min/gKw	3.16	6.26
Glucagon	5.71	6.08

* Single kidney clearances were estimated at 50% of two kidney values.

Long term effects of protein rich diets have also been recognized to affect renal hemodynamics in man (29). Whereas the normal GFR for healthy vegetarians may average 60 ml/min or less, values in adults ingesting a protein rich diet may exceed 120 ml/min

(25). It is therefore important when GFR is measured to evaluate renal function under similar conditions of fast and with a knowledge of the type of diet an individual may be eating. It is likely that the notorious variability in GFR measurements may result from a lack of appreciation of the effects of dietary protein on renal hemodynamics.

There is no study in humans that evaluates the potential benefit of protein restriction alone on the progressive loss of GFR in chronic renal disease. The data on protein restriction in humans are usually uncontrolled and do not distinguish between the effects of protein vs phosphorus restriction; nor do they account for the concomitant administration of keto-acid supplements. Nevertheless, protein restriction (combined with phosphorus restriction and/or keto-acids administration) has been shown to delay the progression of renal failure in patients with a serum creatinine greater than 6 mg/dl (30-36). However, at this advanced stage of disease, restriction of protein intake results only in a limited time gain before institution of dialysis is needed. Retrospectively, Masschio et al.(37,38) in Italy and, prospectively, Rosman et al.(39) in Holland have presented evidence that protein (and phosphorus) restriction significantly retards the decline in GFR in patients with a serum creatinine of 2 to 4 mg/dl (GFR 30 to 60 ml/min). The importance of the issue is reflected in an NIH call for a prospectively controlled clinical trial to evaluate the effects of protein restriction on progressive renal dysfunction in patients with early renal insufficiency. Were protein restriction to prevent progressive loss of GFR, the impact on society would be enormous in terms of preservation of well-being and economic savings.

The mechanism whereby proteins increase GFR and renal blood flow has not been elucidated. Since proteins are absorbed as amino acids, the increase in renal hemodynamics after protein ingestion results from an amino acid load. Intravenous administration of amino acids increases GFR in rat (24), dog (40), baboon and in man (26). The specificity of individual amino acids in stimulating GFR is unknown. The effect is independent of renal denervation (40) and is blocked by simultaneous administration of somatostatin, suggesting the existence of a humoral mediator (24,26). It may depend on an intact pituitary gland but is independent of male hormones (24). It may also be prostaglandin dependent since prostaglandin blockade with indomethacin prevents the rise in GFR induced by amino acids in man (41). On the other hand, the constancy of prostaglandin E excretion after ingestion of meat speaks against a role for prostaglandin production in postprandial renal hyperemia (27). Glucagon and growth hormone are potential humoral candidates since both are capable of inducing renal vasodilation. Glucagon reproduces the effects of amino acids on GFR in baboons (Fig.4). The existence of a glomerulopressin released from the liver as a result of amino acid stimulation of glucagon has been recently proposed as a mechanism to explain the renal vasodilation after protein ingestion (42,43).

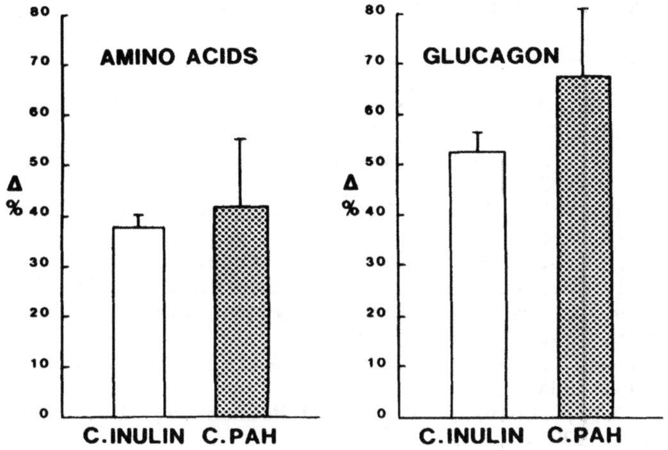

Fig. 4. Relative increases, in percent of control, in inulin and PAH clearances in adult male baboons (N=5) during intravenous infusion of amino acids (Travasol 10% at 8.3 mg/min/kg) or glucagon (8.3 ng/min/kg). All changes were statistically significant ($p < 0.01$).

ACKNOWLEDGMENTS

Mrs. Gilda Manicourt provided expert secretarial assistance. The author was supported by Public Health Service Grant AM 19822 and acknowledges the help of the Mannheimer Primatological Foundation in baboon studies.

REFERENCES

1. Brenner, B.M., Meyer, T.W., and Hostetter, T.H. New Engl. J. Med 307:652-659, 1982.
2. Brenner, B.M. Am. J. Physiol 249:F324-F337, 1985.
3. Gehrig, J.J., Jr., Rose, J.C. and Jamison, R.L. Clin. Res. 34:729, 1986 (Abstract).
4. Ibels, L.S., Alfrey, A.C., Haut, L., and Huffler, W.E. New Engl. J. Med. 298:122-126, 1978.
5. Tomford, R.C., Karlinsky, M.L., Buddington, B., and Alfrey, C. J. Clin. Invest. 68:655-664, 1981.
6. Alfrey, A.C., and Tomford, R.C. In: Controverses in Nephrology and Hypertension (Ed. R.G. Narins) Churchill-Livingstone, New York, 1984, pp. 557-566.
7. El-Nahas, A.M., Paraskevakou, H., Zoob, S., Rees, A.J. and Evans, D.J. Clin. Sci. 65:399-406, 1983.
8. Laouari, D., Kleinknecht, C., Gubler, M.C., and Broyer, M. Kidney Int. 24:S248-S253, 1983.
9. Lumlergul, D., Burke, T.J., Gillum, D.M., Alfrey, A.C., Harris, D.C., Hammond, W.S., and Schrier, R.W. Kidney Int. 29:658-666, 1986.
10. Purkerson, M.L., Joist, J.H., Yates, J., and Klahr, S. Proc. Natl. Acad. Sci. USA 82:193-197, 1985.
11. Dworkin, L.D., Hostetter, T.H., Rennke, H.G. and Brenner, B.M. J. Clin. Invest. 73:1448-1461, 1984.
12. Meyer, T.W., Anderson, S., and Brenner, B.M. Ann. Int. Med. 98:832-838, 1983.
13. Eddy, A.A., Falk, R.J., Sibley, R.K., and Hostetter, T.H. Kidney Int. 25:243, 1984 (Abstract).
14. Robertson, J.L., Goldschmidt, M., Kronfeld, D.S., Tomaszewski, J.E., Hill, G.S. and Bovee, K.C. Kidney Int. 29:511-520, 1986.
15. Polzin, D.J., Osborne, C.A., Hayden, D.W., and Stevens, J.B. Am. J. Vet. Res. 45:506-517, 1984.
16. Goldszer, R.C., Sweet, J., and Cotran, R.S. Ann. Rev. Med. 35:429-449, 1984.
17. Kiprov, D.D., Colvin, R.B. and McCluskey, R.T. Lab. Invest. 46:275-281, 1982.
18. Zucchelli, P., Gagnoli, L., Casanova, S., Donini, U., and Pasquali, S. Kidney Int. 24:649-655, 1983.
19. Guttierez-Millet, V., Nieto, J., Praga, M., Usera, G., Martinez, M.A. and Morales, J.M. Arch. Int. Med. 146:705-709, 1986.
20. Brenner, B.H., and Meyer, T.W. In: Nephrology II (Ed. R.R. Robinson), Springer-Verlag, New York, 1984, pp.1233-1247.
21. Dicker, S.E., and Morris, C.A. J. Physiol. 223:365-373, 1972.
22. Heideman, H.D. and Rosenbaum, H.D. Radiology 94:599-601, 1970.
23. Orecklin, J.R., Craven, J.D. and Lecky, J.W.J. Urology 109:952-954, 1973.
24. Meyer, T.W., Ichikawa, I., Zatz, R., and Brenner, B.M. Trans. Assoc. Amer. Phys. 96:76-83, 1983.
25. Bosch, J.P., Saccaggi, A., Lauer, A., Ronco, C., Beleldonne, M., and Glabman, S. Am. J. Med. 75:943-950, 1983.
26. Castellino, P., Cada, B., and DeFronzo, R.A. Kidney Int. 27:243, 1985 (Abstract).
27. Hostetter, T.H. Amer. J. Physiol. 250:F613-F618, 1986.

28. Pena, J.C., Romero, E., Fernandez, M., Moscoso, J., Gabbai, F., and Herrera-Acosta, J. Proc. 9th. Int. Congr. Nephrology, Los Angeles 1984, p.358A (Abstract).
29. Pullman, T.N., Alving, A.S., Dern, R.J. and Landowne, M. J. Lab. Clin. Med. 44:320-332, 1954.
30. Mitch, W.E. Ann. Rev. Medicine 35:249-264, 1984.
31. Giordano C. Kidney Int. 22:401-408, 1982.
32. Mitch, W.E., Walser, Mc., Steinman, T.I., Hill, S., Zeger, S. and Tungsanga, K. New Engl. J. Med. 311:623-629, 1984.
33. Walser, M.D. Lancet 1:340-342, 1983.
34. Alvestrand, A., Ahlberg, M. and Bergstrom, J. Kidney Int. 24:S268-S272, 1983.
35. Gretz, N., Korb, E., and Strauch, M. Kidney Int. 24:S263-S267, 1983.
36. Ando A., Orita, Y., Nakata, K., Fukuhara, Y., Mikami, H., Fujii, N., Nakafima, Y., Veda, N., Abe, H. Med. J. Osaka Univ. 32:31-37, 1981.
37. Maschio, G., Oldrizzi, L., Tessitore, N., D'Angelo, A., Valvo, E., Lupo, A., Loschiavo, C., Fabris, A., Gammaro, L., Rugiu, C., and Panzetta, G. Kidney Int. 22:371-376, 1982.
38. Maschio, G., Oldrizzi, L., Tessitore, N., D'Angelo, A., Valvo, E., Lupo, A., Loschiavo, C., Fabris, A., Gammaro, L., Rugiu, C., and Panzetta G. Kidney Int. 24:S273-S277, 1983.
39. Rosman, J.B., Meyer, S., Slutter, W.J., Terwee, P.M., Priers-Brecht, T., Donker, A.J.M. Lançet 2:1291-1295, 1984.
40. Smith, H.W. In: The Kidney: Structure and Function in Health and Disease. Oxford Univ. Press, New York, 1951, pp. 470-476.
41. Ruilope, L., Rodicio, J., Garcia Robles, R., Sancho-Rof, J., Hammonde, T.G., Knox, F.G. and Romero, J.C. Proc. 9th. Int. Cong. Nephrology, Los Angeles 1984, p.399A (Abstract).
42. Uranga, J., Fuenzalida, R., Rapoport, A.L., and del Castillo, E. Horm. Metab. Res. 11: 275-279, 1979.
43. Alvestrand, A. and Bergstrom, J. Lancet 1:195-197, 1984.

PROTEIN AND ENERGY REQUIREMENTS IN RENAL INSUFFICIENCY

W. Grupe, M.D., N. Spinozzi, R.D. and W. Harmon, M.D.

Manipulations of nutrient intake have always been a significant component in the management of children with renal diseases, usually to reduce that which the kidney must excrete or to replace that which the kidney cannot retain. Most clinical recommendations have evolved empirically or theoretically without firm experimental data. This is particularly true for the child with chronic renal failure where reliable data have not been available to define the precise requirements. Although clear recommendations for the amount of dietary protein have been limited by a lack of dependable information, it has been common practice to reduce protein intake in children with renal insufficiency. In the absence of data, many have suggested that protein and energy intakes approximate the recommended dietary allowances (RDA) made by the National Academy of Science for children of either the same weight, the same height, or the same bone age (1,2). This practice has evolved from a generally accepted impression that children with renal insufficiency have protein and energy needs that are very similar to normal children. It must be realized, however, that RDA amounts were devised for groups, not individuals; for normal children undergoing normal growth, not for those with chronic diseases; and seem to change regularly as more information becomes available to the Board.

The goal of all management strategies should be to maintain adequate nutrition within the limits imposed by an altered renal excretory and regulatory capacity, while at the same time avoiding excesses of nitrogen, hydrogen ion, phosphate, sodium, potassium and fluid. Unfortunately, the limits of such a goal are ill defined. Nutritional management has been further complicated by the emergence of multiple therapeutic modalities including prolonged conservative management, hemodialysis, peritoneal dialysis and transplantation (2-4). Nutrients that must be restricted at one point in therapy might require supplementation later on. The child with cachexia must be approached very differently from the child with equally poor renal function but a normal or elevated weight for height. The nutritional needs during continuous peritoneal dialysis differ from those during intermittent hemodialysis. Thus, a routine "renal failure" diet is not applicable to all situations. In addition, each nutritional prescription must be individualized to the emotional, metabolic and functional limitations of the child and adjusted during each therapeutic phase (5,6).

Attempts to estimate the requirements for energy and protein have inate problems when applied to children with chronic renal failure. For example, nutritional standards which have been derived from metabolically normal children with normal body composition, normal activity and normal growth may not be applicable to children with renal failure (1,7,8). Growth may not be an appropriate outcome variable even though it is an appropriate goal of therapy; growth changes are not regularly related to energy or protein intake (9-12). In fact, the height deficit seems to be more related to the duration of renal disease than to the current degree of nutritional deficit; for many children, weights are actually higher than expected for their height (9,10,13,14). Some outcome variables may be quite insensitive. Body weight, for example, can be maintained, or even increased in the presence of negative nitrogen balance (15,16). Likewise, the most efficient use of protein does not necessarily correlate with the net nitrogen balance (16). Many studies have not been able to control for those metabolic variables introduced by dialytic therapy or by uremia itself (4). Few studies have directly measured the quantitative needs of children with varying degrees of renal insufficiency or receiving various forms of renal replacement therapy.

In one attempt to measure the protein and energy requirements for non-dialyzed infants with renal insufficiency, we have used the daily urinary urea content as an estimate of net protein catabolism (16). Infants whose serum creatinine levels varied between 1.4 to 8.4 mg% at entry into the study were fed commercially available modified cow's milk formulae, fortified with varying amounts of polycose, corn oil, medium chain triglycerides and casein to produce a broad range of protein and energy intake. Over the course of the study energy intake varied between 1.8 and 15.4 kcal/cm of length/day (18.6-145 kcal/kg/day), while protein intakes extended from 0.03 to 0.37 gm/cm/day (0.3 to 3.5 gm/kg/day). A gradual decline in urinary urea appearance was noted as protein intake increased from 0.03 to 0.14 gm/cm/day (R = 0.55). However, when protein intake exceeded 0.15 gm/cm/day, urea appearance increased directly with protein intake (R = 0.68). The urea excretion, in fact was almost fourfold higher when the protein intake was above 0.16 gm/cm/day, when compared to a diet that provided under 0.15 gm/cm. Although there was a correlation between protein and energy intake (R = 0.64), there was little relationship between the rate of urea appearance and the energy intake (R = 0.3), suggesting that the absolute amount of protein, rather than a relative deficit of calories, may be crucial. On the other hand, urea appearance also varied directly with the proportion of total energy represented by protein, with the percent of energy contributed by protein significantly higher in those whose protein intake was 0.16 gm/cm or higher. This suggests that the relative amount of protein may be significant, too. The experimental design did not allow a determination of which was the more important.

Urea appearance was maintained below 10 mg/cm/day when daily energy intake was between 6 and 11.4 kcal/cm and protein intake remained below 0.14 gm/cm. (Fig. 1). In this circumstance, the amount of total calories represented by protein ranged from 1.4 to 7.4% ($\bar{x}$4.1%). Below 6 kcal/cm the higher rate of urea appearance suggests inadequate nutrient intake, while at energy intakes above 12 kcal/cm, the protein intake was regularly above 0.15 gm/cm and, as expected, the urea appearance was once more elevated. For each energy intake cluster, increasing the protein intake increased the urea appearance (Fig. 1). At all levels of protein intake, the urea appearance was the lowest at energy intakes between 9 and 11.4 kcal/cm.

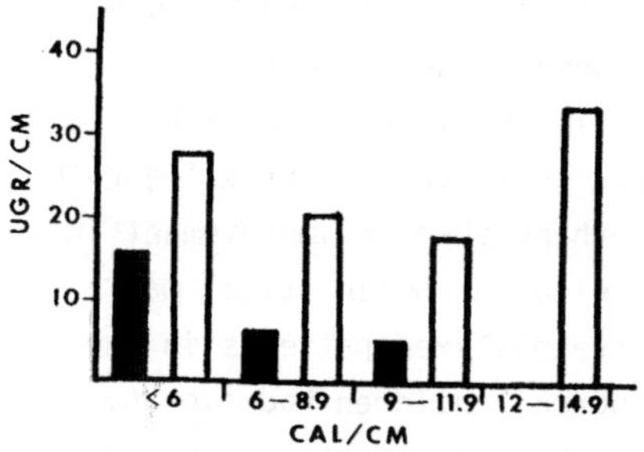

Fig. 1. Relationship between urea appearance (UGR/CM) and energy intake (CAL/CM) in infants whose daily intake of protein was either ⩽ 0.14 gm/cm (closed bars) or > 0.15 gm/cm (open bars).

Growth was maintained in all five infants with accelerated growth in three and a normal growth rate in one. Neither the rate of urea appearance nor the level of blood urea seemed to decide the rate of growth. The patient in the study who had the highest BUN and the highest urea appearance rate grew as well as the patient who had the lowest of each.

These preliminary data suggest that standard dietary sources can stimulate efficient, if not optimal, nitrogen utilization at energy intake between 6 and 11.4 kcal/cm/day provided that protein intake does not exceed 0.15 gm/cm/day. Increasing the protein intake above 0.15 gm/cm/day, or increasing the proportion of total energy represented by protein to more than 7% merely increases the amount of nitrogen appearing as urea.

All values were indexed to statural height rather than the more conventional index of body weight (17). The reasons are several. Height is a more reliable reference for creatinine production and lean body mass. This may be of more value in uremia, since variations in muscle mass correlate well with changes in total body protein. Although basal oxygen consumption in normally proportioned children is accurately predicted by weight, weight is a poor measure of the amount of metabolically active tissue. This is particularly apparent in the chronically ill or malproportioned child where it has been noted that height factored for weight improves the accuracy. Further, the degree of protein repletion or depletion cannot be predicted from weight alone, because of variations in adiposity. Since it is not legitimate to expect a child in renal failure to have the same lean or metabolically active mass as a normal child of the same age or weight, intake referenced for height appears to offer a more easily measured alternative.

The quantitative protein and energy needs of children with renal failure who are receiving renal replacement therapy are only partially known. Conley et al., using N^{15}-lysine enrichment, noticed a decreased protein flux in chronic renal failure which reverted towards normal with the initiation of hemodialysis (18). However, a similar improvement was produced in both the dialyzed and non-dialyzed children by increasing both the energy and nitrogen intake, suggesting perhaps that an improvement in the nutritional status (i.e., the attainment of an anabolic state) may lessen the requirement for dialysis. The three dialyzed patients in their study whose protein flux approached that of normal children had average daily intakes of 48 kcal/kg and 2.2 gm protein/kg, with protein representing an average of 22% of the total energy intake.

In another attempt to measure the protein and energy requirements more directly in children receiving chronic hemodialysis, we used kinetically determined urea appearance to determine the relationship between nutrient intake and protein balance (17,19). We found that neutral protein balance occurred at 10 kcal/cm of height/day and 0.3 gm protein/cm/day. Three mg of nitrogen were retained for each calorie increase in energy, which is a slope similar to that noted in normal adults on marginal protein intakes (15). The net protein catabolic rate diminished as protein balance increased suggesting that the production of positive protein balance, despite increased protein intake, reduced urea generation when protein represented 12% of the total energy intake. Furthermore, for any given protein intake, the net catabolic rate was uniformly lower in those children in positive protein balance (17,20). Thus, these patients did not require additional hemodialysis despite their higher protein intake, which, like Conley's data, suggests that an improvement in nutritional status may reduce the requirement for dialysis. Protein intake appeared to be a better predictor of protein balance than energy intake when both variables were considered simultaneously (20). Of some concern is the suggestion that the amount of energy required to attain neutral balance when protein intake was low could be as much as 20% higher than when protein intake was above 0.3 gm/cm/day (19,20). This apparent requirement for additional energy could conceivably exceed the appetite of many uremic children.

These data argue that the commonly held practice of protein restriction could be counterproductive in advanced renal failure. Children on hemodialysis probably require relatively normal protein to energy ratios and little if any protein restriction when energy levels are maintained (17). Energy intakes above 12 kcal/cm/day and protein intakes approximating 12% of the total energy seem to produce positive protein balance, improve protein flux, and increase lean body mass (17-19).

The nutritional requirements during peritoneal dialysis have been incompletely determined also. Salusky et al. found that children treated with continuous ambulatory peritoneal dialysis had a total energy intake that averaged 68 kcal/kg/day (2,21). Calories acquired by the absorption of glucose from the peritoneal dialysate amounted to 12% of the total. Although the protein intake was reported at 2.4 gm/kg/day, protein losses in the dialysate ranged from 0.12-0.28 gm/kg/day, and protein balance was not determined (2). Net protein intake approximated 13-15% of total energy intake. In a parallel study by Baum et al. total energy intake averaged 60 kcal/kg/day including 7.5 kcal/kg/day from the absorption of dialysate glucose (3). Protein intake averaged 2.0 gm/kg/day from which 0.16 gm/kg/day of protein was lost in the dialysate. Although both of these studies describe only the spontaneous dietary intake of these children, without any measure of actual requirements, positive nitrogen balance has been reported in children undergoing CAPD.

The absorption of carbohydrate from the peritoneal dialysate, combined with significant protein losses through the peritoneal cavity, create the potential for obesity, particularly if the additional energy serves to decrease the spontaneous ingestion of conventional foods and/or a lower protein to energy ratio (3,21-23). High energy relative to protein produces an increase in fat deposition. Whatever lean mass does accumulate appears to be related to the support of the increasing fat mass. Studies in overfed adults show that only 25-37% of the weight gain is lean body mass (24). An increase predominantly in energy intake would be expected to replace only 1/4 of the lean mass lost during periods of undernutrition. Restoration of the major portion of the loss of lean mass, therefore, requires a change in nitrogen intake that is independent of energy. Obesity is a common occurrence in peritoneally dialyzed children and is not an appropriate goal in the management of children with renal failure (23). Even with careful nutritional management, triceps skin fold thickness increases without a significant change in either mid-arm circumference or mid-arm muscle circumference (8). Although it has been suggested that this propensity towards obesity is evidence of an alteration in intermediary metabolism (8), it seems more likely to be the result of relative energy excess similar to that noted in normal man (6,15).

Maintenance of appropriate levels of both energy and protein intake is a formidable challenge in children with chronic renal insufficiency. Supplements may improve nutrition for the undernourished child whose intake is inadequate (1). Unfortunately, when dietary intake is already adequate and the body weight is appropriate for the height, energy supplementation alone may be deleterious; the provision of extra calories can reduce the spontaneous intake of other foods, especially protein (7). Carbohydrate supplements additionally may aggravate hypertriglyceridemia and lead to obesity without an increase in lean body mass or linear growth (1).

Although many authors advocate high quality protein in the diet, the importance of the biologic value has not been established in uremia. For children especially, the palatability of the diet may be at least as important as the content (5,23,25,26).

Why uremic children fail to attain a dietary intake sufficient for compensatory repair or normal growth is not known. Spontaneously, the intake is usually enough to maintain their current body mass and weight for height is often normal (12,14,27). It can be inferred that some internal signal controls hunger in those children with barely enough renal function to sustain life. However, the factors that restrain appetite are ill defined.

An altered taste ability is quite common in uremia. In 1978, we reported that taste acuity for one or more of the four primary tastes was abnormal in 27 of 33 children receiving chronic hemodialysis therapy (28). The ability to taste sweet (sucrose) and sour (HCL) was reduced in half of the children, often when the ability to taste bitter (urea) was intact. It is not hard to imagine how such dysgeusia could significantly alter food preferences, such as the uremic child's inability to accept protein restriction (25). Taste acuity improved immediately post-dialysis accompanied by a subjective increase in hunger and an increased food intake. The improvement was not sustained between dialyses, however. This rapid repetitive and unsustained recovery suggests that the taste abnormality in renal failure is functional and related to the control of uremia. The role of trace metals such as zinc in taste perception is not clear in uremia (28,29). Taste may not be the only important factor for appetite, however. Hospitalizations, altered activity, iatrogenic restraint and psychological factors can be profound adverse influences (5,6).

An increasing number of studies have explored the value of synthetic diets in infants and children whereby nitrogen intake can be reduced without adversely affecting protein metabolism (6, 16, 25-27, 30-32). There are ample data to demonstrate that the child with chronic renal failure can utilize both essential and complete amino acid mixtures. However, no study has documented that these contrived diets offer more than a theoretical advantage over an appropriately designed and consumed conventional diet (6,25,26,31). One study in undialyzed children found significant increases in growth velocity, upper arm circumference, cell mass, serum transferrin, and plasma calcium in children maintained on a protein restricted diet where 20% of the protein was replaced by an amino acid, ketoacid mixture over a 0.4-1 year treatment period (27). The diet seemed well-accepted and well-tolerated by the children. What is not clear is the extent to which the improved growth was a function of the improvement in calcium and phosphorus metabolism and the suppression of hyperparathyroidism related to the calcium content of the ketoacid mixtures. Concern over long-term toxicity, even with new formulations of the synthetic mixtures, demands continued caution in uremic children. With few exceptions, the promise of good results is still dampened by severe metabolic complications and/or poor patient compliance (6,27,32).

It is a major and regular management problem to persuade these children to remain on prescribed intakes, with or without synthetic or nutritional supplements (7,13,25). In general, such diets have been regularly successful only when spontaneous intake has been bypassed by nasogastric, gastrostomy or parenteral feedings (13,30,33,34). Since no study has shown any demonstrated advantage to synthetic diets, for many children those diets using predominantly standard foods and a normal protein to energy ratio seem more palatable and, therefore, more likely to be maintained over the longer term (5,7,11,17,18).

In summary, the protein and energy requirements in chronic renal insufficiency remain poorly defined. Using conventional foods, there are some data to suggest that infants with renal insufficiency who do not yet require dialysis reach efficient utilization of both energy and nitrogen with daily intakes between 6 and 11 kcal/cm and protein intake of 0.15 gm/cm. On hemodialysis, the requirements approximates 12 kcal/cm/day and 0.3 gm/cm/day of protein. Peritoneal dialysis may require 60-70 kcal/kg/day and 2.5 gm protein/day. Of interest is the suggestion that the optimal proportion of total energy represented by protein might be 7% in renal insufficiency, 12% during hemodialysis and 15% during peritoneal dialysis. In all circumstances, however, there is no substitute for a patient supportive team willing to recognize each child's individuality. Simply prescribing a diet, no matter how scientifically based, is rarely successful and is the least effective therapy of all.

REFERENCES:

1. Wassner, S.J. Pediatr. Clin. N. Amer. 29:973-990, 1982.
2. Salusky, I.B., Lucullo, L., Nelson, P., and Fine, R.N. Pediatr. Clin. N. Amer. 29:1005-1012, 1982.
3. Baum, M., Powell, D., Calvin, S., McDaid, T., McHenry, K., Mar, H., and Potter, D. N. Eng. J. Med. 397:1537-1542, 1982.
4. Harmon, W.E., and Ingelfinger, J.R. In: Mendoza, S.A. and Tune, B.M. (eds). Contemporary Issues in Nephrology, Vol. 12, Churchill Livingstone, Inc., New York, 1984, pp.343-379.
5. Spinozzi, N.S. and Grupe, W.E. J. Amer. Diet. Assoc. 70:493-497, 1977.
6. Grupe, W.E. In: Walker, W.A. and Watkins, J.B. Nutrition in Pediatrics. Basic Science and Clinical Application, 1985, Little Brown, Boston, pp. 423-444.
7. Betts, P.R., Magrath, G., and White RHR. Brit. Med. J. 1:416-418, 1977.
8. Wassner, S.J. and Corcoran, M. In: Brodehl, J. and Ehrich, J.H.M. (eds). Pediatric Nephrology, 1984, Springer-Verlag, Berlin, pp. 92-95.
9. Bergstrom, W.H., deLeon, A.S. and vanGemund, J.J. Ped. Clin. N. Amer. 11:563-575, 1964.
10. Stickler, G.B., and Berger, B.J. Pediatr. Res. 7:978-982, 1973.
11. Broyer, M. Pediatr. Clin. N. Amer. 29:991-1003, 1982.
12. Arnold, W.C., Danford, D. and Holliday, M.C. Kidney Intern. 24:205-209, 1983.
13. Chantler, C., El-Bishti, M., and Counahan, R. Am. J. Clin. Nutr. 33:1682-1689, 1980.
14. Grupe, W.E. In: Suskind, R.A. (ed). Textbook of Pediatric Nutrition. Raven Press, New York, 1981, pp. 527-536.
15. Garza, C., Scrimshaw, N.S. and Young, V.R. Br. J. Nutr. 37:403-420, 1977.
16. Wassner, S.J., Abitbol, C., Alexander, S., et al. Am. J. Kid. Dis. In press.
17. Grupe, W.E., Harmon, W.E., and Spinozzi, N.S. Kidney Intern. 24:(suppl 15)6-10, 1983.
18. Conley, S.B., Rose, G.M., Robson, A.M., and Bier, D.M. Kidney Intern. 17:837-846, 1980.
19. Harmon, W.E., and Grupe, W.E. In: Fine, R.N. and Gruskin, A.B. (eds.) End-stage Renal Disease in Children. W.B. Saunders & Co., Philadelphia, 1984, pp. 54-66.
20. Grupe, W.E., Spinozzi, N.S., and Harmon, W.E. Kidney Intern. 23:149, 1983.
21. Salusky, I.B., Kopple, J.D., and Fine, R.N. Kidney Intern. 24:S101-S105, 1983.
22. DeSanto, N.G., Capodicasa, G., Pluvio, M., Gilli, G., Giordano, C. In: Gahl, G.M., Kessel, M., and Nolph, K.D. (eds). Advances in Peritoneal Dialysis, 1981, Excerpta Medica, Amsterdam, pp. 397-404.
23. Grupe, W.E., Spinozzi, N.S., and Harmon, W.E. In: Cummings, N.B. and Klahr, S. (eds). Chronic Renal Disease, Causes, Complications and Treatment, 1985, Plenum, N.Y., pp. 309-320.
24. Keys, A.J., Andersen, J.T., and Brozek, J. Metabolism, 4:427-432, 1955.
25. Jones, R.W.A., Dalton, N., Start, K., El-Bishti, M.M. and Chantler, C. Amer. J. Clin. Nutr. 33:1696-1702, 1980.
26. Counahan, R., El-Bishti, M., and Chantler, C. Clin. Nephrol. 9:11-14, 1978.
27. Jones, R., Dalton, N., Turner, C., Start, K., Haycock, G., and Chantler, C. Kidney Intern. 24:95-103, 1983.

28. Spinozzi, N.S., Murray, C.L., and Grupe, W.E. Pediatr. Res. 12:442, 1978.
29. Arbus, G.S., Wolffe, E., Williams, V., et al. In: Gruskin, A.B. and Norman, M.E. (eds). Pediatric Nephrology, Boston, Martinus Nijhoff Publishers, 1981, pp. 495-496.
30. Abitbol, C.L. and Holliday, M.A. Clin. Nephrol. 5:153-158, 1976.
31. Dalton, R.N., and Chantler, C. Kidney Intern. 24:S11-S15, 1983.
32. Motil, K.J., Harmon, W.E., and Grupe, W.E. J. Parent. and Enteral. Nutr. 4:32, 1980.
33. Holliday, M.A., Wassner, S., and Ramirez, J. Am. J. Clin. Nutr. 31:1854-1860, 1978.
34. Guillot, M., Broyer, M., Cathelineau, L., Boulegue, D., Dartois, A.M., Folio, D., and Guimbaud, P. Arch. Fr. Pediatr. 37:497-505, 1980.

PROGRESSION OF CHRONIC RENAL DISEASE IN CHILDREN: THE UNIVERSITY OF MIAMI EXPERIENCE

Gaston Zilleruelo, M.D., Nuria Dominguez, M.D., Michael Freundlich, M.D., Carolyn Abitbol, M.D. and Jose Strauss, M.D.

Various reports have emphasized the multiplicity of causes leading to chronic renal failure (CRF) in children and the wide variety of clinical presentations of chronic renal disease in this age group (1-3). However, the definition of CRF has varied and the rate of progression of chronic renal disease to end stage renal disease (ESRD) seems to be quite variable (4, 5). Here, we shall review our experience with the different causes of CRF and the outcome of afflicted patients over a period of ten years. A total of 101 patients with CRF followed by the Division of Pediatric Nephrology at the University of Miami/Jackson Memorial Medical Center between 1972 and 1982 were included in this study. Chronic renal failure was defined as a persistent (over two months duration) and progressive decline in renal function to values < 80 ml/min/1.73 or by serum creatinine > 2 SD from the mean for age and sex (6). End stage renal disease was defined by a glomerular filtration rate < 7 ml/min/1.73m^2 or serum creatinine > 8 mg/dl.

According to the original disease, patients were classified into obstructive uropathies, congenital renal malformations, primary glomerulopathies and secondary glomerulopathies. The diagnosis of obstructive uropathies and congenital renal malformations was based on radiological, radionuclide and/or abdominal ultrasound studies. Most children with glomerulopathies were diagnosed through percutaneous renal biopsy. The deterioration rate of renal function was estimated through the time intervals from apparent onset of the renal disease to CRF and from onset of CRF to ESRD.

As in a previous report (3), we have found that the most frequent cause of CRF in children at the University of Miami/Jackson Memorial Medical Center is the group of congenital malformations, combining obstructive uropathies and renal malformations. Reflux nephropathy, posterior urethral valves and ureteral malformations were the most common types of obstructive uropathies (Table I). Among congenital renal malformations, the most frequent type was medullary cystic disease; renal dysplasia was documented in a small number of patients (Table I).

Partially funded under an agreement with the Department of Health and Rehabilitative Services, State of Florida, Children's Medical Services.

TABLE I

MAIN CAUSES OF CRF IN 101 CHILDREN
UNIVERSITY OF MIAMI 1972 - 1982

DIAGNOSIS	(%)
Obstructive Uropathies N=35	
Ureteral malformation	13
Posterior urethral valves	11
Reflux nephropathy	9
Neurogenic bladder	2
Congenital renal malformation N=15	
Cystic diseases	6
Hypoplasia	7
Dysplasia	2
Primary GN N=31	
Chronic GN	11
FSS	7
Crescentic GN	5
MPGN	4
MGN	3
IgA GN	1
Secondary GN N=20	
SLE	10
HUS	3
Sickle Cell GN	3
Vasculitis	3
Diabetes mellitus	1

The mean follow-up in these patients was 5 years with a range from 1-10 years; during this period of time, 60 percent of the patients reached ESRD. The rate of progression of these patients was analyzed according to the type of original disease; a striking difference was found between obstructive uropathies and acquired glomerulopathies. Although age of onset of nephropathy was clearly earlier in the congenital diseases, the rate of deterioration was more rapid in the glomerulopathies. The mean time interval in primary glomerulopathies was 2.5 years to CRF and 1.6 years to ESRD as compared to obstructive uropathies with 3.1 and 5.1 years, respectively (Table II). Congenital renal malformations also had a prolonged time interval to reach ESRD; however, the longest interval involved was from onset of disease to CRF. Once these patients reached CRF, the apparent course was much more rapid than in obstructive uropathies.

TABLE II

RATE OF RENAL FUNCTION DETERIORATION X AGE (RANGE) IN YEARS

DIAGNOSIS	AGE AT APPARENT CLINICAL ONSET	ONSET CRF	CRF ESRD
Obstructive Uropathies	1.1 (0.08-15)	3.1 (0.16-11)	5.5 (0.7-12)
Renal Malformations	3.9 (0.08-16)	7.0 (0.16-16)	1.7 (0.08-4)
Primary Glomerulopathies	10.6 (1-16)	2.5 (0.16-15)	1.6 (0.08-8)
Secondary Glomerulopathies	11.0 (1-18)	1.1 (0.16-5)	1.2 (0.08-4)

Mean time interval to reach ESRD in the patients with obstructive uropathies was about nine years from onset of the nephropathy (considered to be at birth). This result is similar to others reported in the literature (7). It should be emphasized that most of these children were detected in the first year of life and all had some type of corrective surgery, despite which there was progression to ESRD. This clearly suggests that there are various causes of progression of renal disease in children apart from the mechanical factors related to the obstruction.

Table III summarizes factors that may affect recoverability of renal function in patients with obstructive uropathy and CRF (8). In addition, immunological factors, possibly related to the development of autologous immune complex nephritis with antibodies against Tam-Horsfall protein or various other antigens, may affect progression of renal disease (9-10). Among other non-immunological mechanisms, the hypothesis of hyperfiltration with intrarenal hypertension proposed by Brenner et al. (11) has attracted considerable attention. Also, the possibility that hyperparathyroidism and hyperlipidemia may contribute to the progression of chronic renal disease is actively being investigated (12-13).

TABLE III

OBSTRUCTIVE UROPATHY

FACTORS THAT MAY AFFECT RECOVERABILITY OF RENAL FUNCTION

Magnitude of intrapelvic pressure
Degree of obstruction
Duration of obstruction
Stage of renal development
Unilateral or bilateral obstruction
Associated renal disease (dysplasia)
Presence or absence of infection
Extrarenal vs. intrarenal pelvis

When analyzing the factors determining progression of CRF, we found that there were significant differences that could explain the more rapid course in patients with acquired glomerulopathies. Hypertension, heavy proteinuria and hyperlipidemia were significantly more frequent in this group of patients. On the other hand, in the obstructive uropathy group there was a greater incidence of marked renal osteodystrophy, hyperparathyroidism, growth retardation, metabolic acidosis and recurrent urinary tract infections.

Our results suggest that once a patient reaches a level of GFR close to 25 $ml/min/1.73m^2$ or serum creatinine > 3 mg/dl, the patient progresses inexorably to uremia. However, the wide variation in individual results suggests that prolonged follow-up periods are necessary to assess the ultimate outcome of children with CRF. The presence of intact renal function for many years during childhood does not preclude deterioration of renal function later on in life. In addition, corrective surgery performed in cases of obstructive uropathy does not seem to prevent, or even modify, the course of progressive nephron loss in a high proportion of cases. Hypertension, proteinuria and hyperlipidemia seem to be important factors which need to be followed closely and hopefully controlled in children with acquired glomerulopathies if the time interval before reaching ESRD is to be prolonged. Studies comparing various nitrogen to calories ratios in infants also may give further insight into factors that determine progression of renal disease in this age group.

In conclusion, we are still far from understanding what are the mechanisms in the progression to CRF and then to ESRD. More information concerning the causes of CRF in children and rate of deterioration in each entity is needed.

REFERENCES

1. Habib, R., Broyer, M. and Benmaiz, M.: Chronic renal failure in children. Nephron 11:209, 1973.

2. Fine, R.N., Malekzadeh, M.H., Pennisi, A.J. et al.: Long-term results of renal transplantation in children. Pediatrics 6:641, 1978.

3. Zilleruelo, G., Andia, J., Gorman, H.M. et al.: Chronic renal failure in children: analysis of main causes and deterioration rate in 81 children. Int J Pediatr Nephrol 1:30, 1980.

4. Heikki, O., Pasternack, A., Luomala, M. et al.: Progression of chronic renal failure. Nephron 35:31-34, 1983.

5. Adler, S.G. and Kopple, J.D.: Factors influencing the progression of renal insufficiency. Seminars in Nephrology 3:335, 1983.

6. Schwartz, G., Haycock, G., Chir, B. et al.: Plasma creatinine and urea concentration in children: normal values for age and sex. J Pediatr 88:828-830, 1976.

7. Warshaw, B.L., Edelbrock, H.H., Ettenger, R.B. et al.: Progression to end-stage renal disease in children with obstructive uropathy. J Pediatr 100:183, 1982.

8. Walker, R.D., Richard, G.A., Bueschen, A.J. et al.: Pathophysiology and recoverability of function and structure in obstructed kidneys. Urol Clin North Am 7:291, 1980.

9. Torres, V.E., Velosa, J.A., Holley, K.E. et al.: The progression of vesicoureteral reflux nephropathy. Ann Intern Med 92:776, 1980.

10. Pascal, R.R., Sian, C.S., Brensilver, J.M. et al.: Demonstration of an antibody to tubular epithelium in glomerulonephritis associated with obstructive uropathy. Amer J. Med 69:944, 1980.

11. Brenner, B.M., Meyer, T.W. and Hostetter, T.H.: Dietary protein intake and the progressive nature of kidney disease: the role of hemodynamically mediated glomerular injury in the pathogenesis of progressive glomerular sclerosis in aging, renal ablation, and intrinsic renal disease. New Engl J Med 307:652, 1982.

12. Ibels, L.S., Alfrey, A.C., Haut, L. et al.: Preservation of function in experimental renal disease by dietary restriction of phosphate. New Engl J Med 298:122, 1978.

13. Moorhead, J.F., Chan, M.K., El-Nahas, M. et al.: Lipid nephrotoxicity in chronic progressive glomerular and tubulointerstitial disease. Lancet 2:1309, 1982.

MINERAL METABOLISM IN CHILDREN WITH END STAGE RENAL FAILURE

Russell W. Chesney, M.D.

Abnormalities in calcium and phosphate balance which beset children with chronic renal insufficiency have been recognized for over a century (1). The intestinal malabsorption of calcium characteristic of uremic children results in severe secondary hyperparathyroidism and indicates dysfunction of the vitamin D endocrine system (2). The finding that these children are resistant to conventional doses of vitamin D can be explained by the discovery of Kodicek and Lawson, Norman and Haussler and DeLuca's group that the kidney is an essential organ in the biotransformation of vitamin D to more active metabolites (3). This endocrine function of the kidney now excludes vitamin D as "a vitamin" since one of the renal synthesized metabolites - $1,25(OH)_2$ vitamin D ($1,25(OH)_2D$)-acts at target tissues remote from the site of its production such as the intestine and bone (Fig. 1). The hormonally active form of vitamin D appears to be $1,25(OH)_2D$ since it is responsible for active intestinal calcium and phosphate absorption, since it releases calcium from the greatest body depot of minerals - bone - and since it probably contributes to calcium and phosphate conservation by the kidney (4). Again, since many other vitamin D metabolites - among them $24,25(OH)_2$ vitamin D; $25,26(OH)_2$ vitamin D and 25(OH)D - 23,26 - lactone - as well as $1,25(OH)_2D$, are produced by the kidney, it is to be anticipated that the blood levels of these metabolites would be reduced in uremic individuals. Indeed, at least 3 groups have reported that a significant reduction in the circulating values of $1,25(OH)_2D$ occurs in children experiencing renal diseases and whose creatinine clearance is under 50 ml/min/1.73M^2 (5-7) and a significant decline in $24,25(OH)_2D$ has been reported as well (5) with end stage renal disease; the values of $1,25(OH)_2D$ and $24,25(OH)_2D$ fall even farther and many of the findings of vitamin D deficiency develop (8). This chapter is an attempt to outline how changes in the circulating level of $1,25(OH)_2D$ brought about by uremia result in malfunction of the vitamin D - endocrine system and how this influences overall mineral balance in the child with end-stage renal failure.

THE VITAMIN D - ENDOCRINE SYSTEM

Under ordinary circumstances when any vertebrate, including man, becomes hypocalcemic the secretion of parathyroid hormone (PTH) will be stimulated and the kidney will produce more $1,25(OH)_2D$. This metabolite increases local bone resorption, net active calcium and phosphate absorption by the intestine and renal tubular reabsorption of calcium and possibly of phosphate (2, 3). These actions restore the level of calcium in the extracellular fluid and the excessive PTH will promote phosphaturia so that phosphate levels are normal as well. Normalization of serum calcium leads to reduced PTH secretion

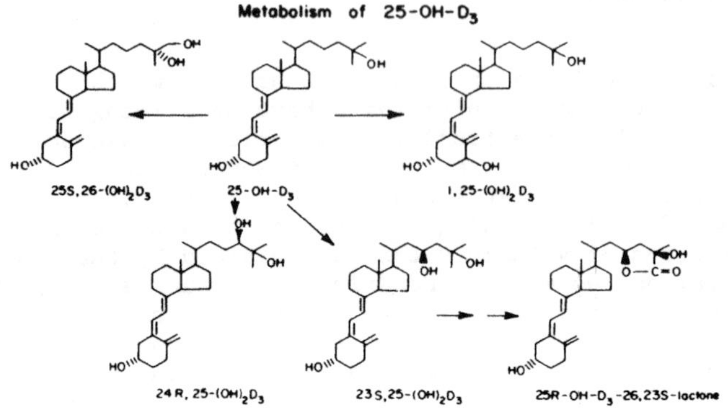

Figure 1. Vitamin D metabolism by the kidney.

with a fall in renal 1α-hydroxylase activity completing the feedback loop.

A second limb of this system is responsive to hypophosphatemia, which of itself stimulates 1α-hydroxylase activity in the absence of PTH secretion. Since PTH levels are normal, bone resorption does not occur and urinary phosphate excretion remains low. However, the increased circulating level of $1,25(OH)_2D$ activates intestinal phosphate resorption (as well as calcium) thereby restoring serum phosphate to normal. In the absence of PTH, the excess calcium is excreted in the urine and the restoration of serum phosphate level dampens 1α-hydroxylase activity in another feedback loop.

On balance both limbs result in normalization of serum (extracellular) calcium and phosphate levels as well; when serum calcium and phosphate are normal, the production of $24,25(OH)_2D$ is stimulated. If this slowly turning over metabolite is important in bone mineralization as has been suggested in previous studies (8), then bone mineral deposition is also favored.

MINERAL IMBALANCE IN UREMIA

In the child with end-stage renal failure, extensive evidence exists that there is impairment in intestinal calcium absorption, both by the finding of hypocalcemia and by direct measurements of intestinal calcium absorption performed over 50 years ago (8). The child with a creatinine clearance of under 20 ml/min/1.73M^2 will usually have hypocalcemia along with hyperphosphatemia for the following reasons. First, the intestine is the major site for the regulation of body calcium stores and $1,25(OH)_2D$ appears to be the hormone regulating this process, except where the patient receives more than 2.5 to 3.0 gm of elemental calcium daily and passive intestinal calcium uptake can assure positive calcium balance. With the reduction in $1,25(OH)_2D$ synthesis found in uremia, ordinary dietary calcium is poorly absorbed. Phosphate, by way of contrast, is not regulated at the intestine, but rather in the kidney. Gut absorption of this mineral is normal and as the GFR falls, the serum value of this anion rises progressively despite the high levels of immunoreactive PTH. Thus on balance, hypocalcemia and hyperphosphatemia are evident along with a very high level of PTH, low levels of $1,25(OH)_2D$ and radiologic evidence of osteopenia.

The nature of the bone defect in end-stage disease is very complex and it involves increased bone resorption - as evidenced by osteitis fibrosa cystica - and decreased bone formation rates - as evidenced by widened osteoid seams and osteomalacia (9). A variety of other factors may contribute to the bone defects found in childhood uremia including aluminum deposition, oxalate deposition and impaired somatomedin activity (8-10). Bone histologic studies in children with uremia are few (11), but the same lesions as found in adults appear to predominate. Nevertheless, bone mineralization in children with renal disease is significantly reduced (12, 13) and this bone does not appear to be a good enough reservoir of mineral to overcome this hypocalcemia. The myopathy of uremia is probably of complex origin and may involve the myopathy

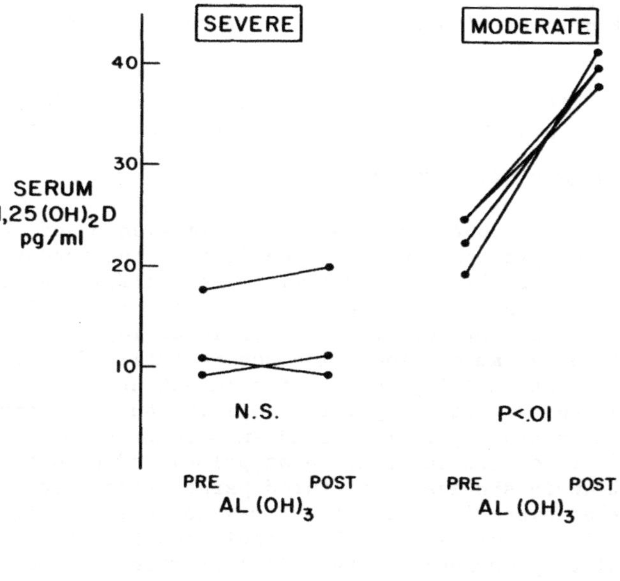

Figure 2. Serum $1,25(OH)_2D$ before and after phosphate restriction and oral $Al(OH)_3$ at 60mg/kg/day. Serum $1,25(OH)_2D$ rises in patients whose creatinine clearance is between 20 and $35ml/min/1.73M^2$.
From Brodehl, J. and Ehrich, J.H.H. (eds.): Paediatric Nephrology. Berlin: Springer-Verlag, 1983, pp 395.

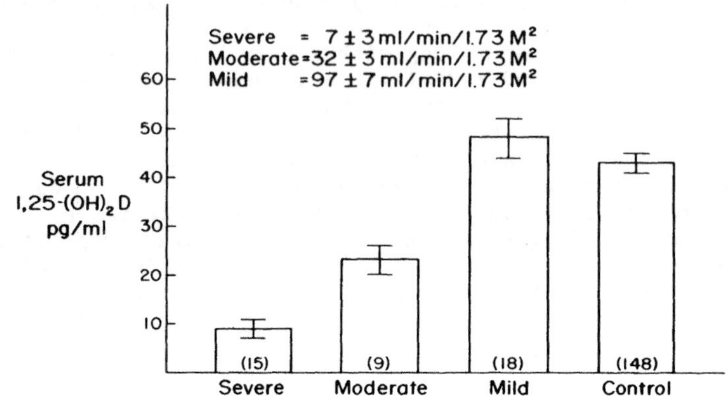

Figure 3. The effect of renal function on the circulating levels of $1,25(OH)_2D$. (Reprinted with permission from reference 8).

characteristic of vitamin D-deficiency, bone pain, bone aluminum deposition, and the poor nutritional status of uremic children.

PATHOGENESIS OF UREMIC OSTEODYSTROPHY

At least 2 factors contribute to mineral imbalance and the development of osteodystrophy in uremic subjects - the retention of phosphate and the abnormalities in vitamin D metabolism. At present it is not established which of these factors is of principal importance, but both factors clearly have an interplay that results in disruption of the vitamin D endocrine scheme outlined above.

Hyperphosphatemia, arising because the intestine is readily permeable to this anion, plays a pivotal role in the development and maintenance of secondary hyperparathyroidism because of a fall in the plasma level of ionized calcium. Slatopolsky and coworkers (14) have recently shown in studies of cultured parathyroid glands from uremic animals that hypocalcemia, per se, may not even be required. Experimental studies in uremic dogs have indicated that the restriction of dietary phosphate intake in proportion to the reduction in GFR prevents the development of secondary hyperparathyroidism (15). Further, in adults at least 2 groups have reported preliminary results indicating that reduction of phosphate intake early in the course of renal failure will be associated with a fall in PTH levels and some amelioration in the development of bone disease (16, 17).

However, it is possible that hyperphosphatemia or phosphate retention may be influencing intestinal calcium absorption and serum ionized calcium values by reducing the rate of conversion of 25(OH)D to $1,25(OH)_2D$. Recent evidence from Portale et al.(18) and from Chesney et al. (19) strongly suggests that if children with a GFR of 30-50 $ml/min/1.73M^2$ undergo phosphate restriction, their serum $1,25(OH)_2D$ values will rise. Chesney et al. (20) examined 6 children with chronic tubulointerstitial disease, but differing levels of renal function In the 3 children whose clearance was less than 15 $ml/min/1.73M^2$ the serum value for $1,25(OH)_2D$ was uninfluenced by a month of the administration of double dose of aluminum hydroxide (60 mg/kg/24h) (Fig. 2). However, in three children with moderate renal insufficiency (clearance between 22 and 38 $ml/min/1.73M^2$) the same manipulation led to a significantly higher level of $1,25(OH)_2D$. In Portale's study, the dietary restriction of phosphate in a much larger group of children with moderate renal insufficiency not only resulted in higher $1,25(OH)_2D$ values but induced a change in the serum concentration of iPTH (18). In other words, phosphate supplementation resulted in higher iPTH levels and restriction in lower iPTH values. As well, supplementation of phosphate resulted in a fall in $1,25(OH)_2D$ values. Taken together, these data indicate that the hypocalcemia of renal insufficiency may be caused by the influence of phosphate on the synthesis of 1,25(OH)D.

These data imply that the synthesis of $1,25(OH)_2D$ and other renal metabolites is influenced by the degree of renal impairment. This is the case and the serum level of $1,25(OH)_2D$ is lowest in children with severe impairment renal function (Fig. 3), despite the fact that the immunoreactive PTH levels are very high (Fig. 4) and that these patients are usually quite hypocalcemic. Thus, despite these signals which ordinarily stimulate the synthesis of $1,25(OH)_2D$, the vitamin D endocrine system is dysfunctional and the levels of the hormone do not rise.

As well, the values of $24,25(OH)_2D$ are reduced in uremic subjects (5). As a consequence, if this metabolite participates in bone mineralization as suggested by some investigators, then uremia is associated with a deficiency of this metabolite. With our present knowledge it is difficult to appreciate the interplay between these two vitamin D metabolites produced in the kidney, but most clinical trials to date have not indicated that the combination of $1,25(OH)_2D$ and $24,25(OH)_2D$ is a more potent form of therapy than $1,25(OH)_2D$ or high dose vitamin D_2 alone (21).

It has recently been reported that the extrarenal sites of $1,25(OH)_2D$ synthesis may account for low, but measurable, levels of $1,25(OH)_2D$ in anephric individuals. Using both a receptor assay after high pressure liquid chromatography and a separate bioassay, Lambert et al. (22) reported serum $1,25(OH)_2D$ values ranging from 3.2 to 23.8 pg/ml. We carefully examined the serum values for $25(OH)D_2$ and D_3 and $1,25(OH)_2D$ in 5 anephric hemodialyzed children (20). As indicated in figure 5, the serum values for $1,25(OH)_2D$ were nondetectable in each of the 5 patients, but 2 patients had a single serum sample with a value of 12 pg/ml. Based on these results and our previous data (5), we do not feel that circulating values of $1,25(OH)_2D$ are found in anephric children.

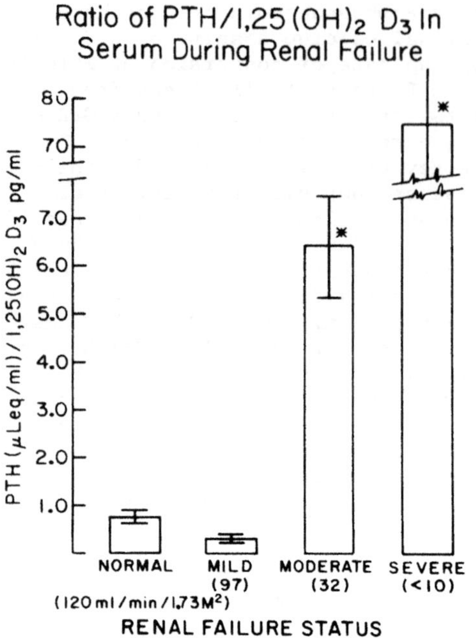

Figure 4. The ratio of immunoreactive PTH to 1,25(OH)$_2$D in the serum of children with various degrees of renal impairment and healthy controls. Note the failure of PTH to simulate the synthesis of 1,25(OH)$_2$D with progressive renal failure.
From Brodehl, J. and Ehrlich, J.H.H. (eds.): Paediatric Nephrology. Berlin:Springer-Verlag, 1983, p 393.

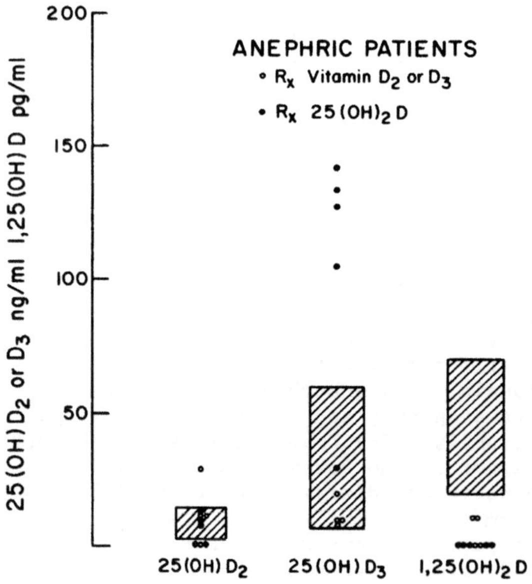

Figure 5. Serum vitamin D metabolite values in five anephric children.
From Brodehl, J. and Ehrich, J.H.H. (eds.): Paediatric Nephrology. Berlin: Springer-Verlag 1983, p 396.

Another factor that may play an important role in the pathogenesis of osteodystrophy, particularly in patients with long term uremia or who have experienced prolonged dialytic therapy, is the potential toxicity of aluminum (23). First recognized as an important factor in dialysis encephalopathy (24, 25), it is now apparent that the bones of patients receiving hemodialysis in centers using high aluminum content water or infants and young children who are administered high levels of oral aluminum hydroxide will contain extensive levels of aluminum (23, 26-28). These latter studies in children who have never undergone dialysis have led to the assumption, as yet unproven, that the gut of young children is perhaps more permeable to aluminum and that these children may be at greater risk for aluminum-induced osteomalacia. It is clear, however, that the portion of dietary aluminum absorbed by the gut is ordinarily excreted by the kidney into the urine and, thus, is retained by patients with renal insufficiency.

The bone lesion associated with high bone aluminum content is osteomalacia, or bone undermineralization (29). When bone turnover studies are carried out in subjects with high bone aluminum levels, they consistently demonstrate low bone turnover rates (23, 29). Despite the appreciation that aluminum is associated with this type of osteomalacia, at present the pathogenesis of this disorder is not known. Regardless of pathogenesis, at least 4 approaches can be taken to prevent aluminum-associated ostemalacia. Reverse osmosis of dialysate is an important first step. Aluminum-containing phosphate sequestering agents should be used with caution. There is a current trend to try to block phosphate absorption by using high doses of calcium carbonate. However, no controlled trial of this agent in children has been published. Unfortunately, the amount of calcium carbonate needed to block intestinal phosphate absorption is so high that hypercalcemia is frequent, particularly if vitamin D analogs are being administered. Finally, aluminum can be removed from bone by the use of the chelating agent desferrioxamine (DFO) (30). Preliminary studies in children indicate that DFO at a dose of 40 mg/kg/24 hours may actually remove aluminum from bound tissue sites and into the dialysate (31).

THERAPY OF MINERAL HOMEOSTATIC DEFECTS

The abnormalities of mineral homeostasis that accompany uremia can, at least in part, be improved by replacement of the vitamin D whose synthesis is impaired and by the avoidance of high doses of aluminum. The first priniciple of therapy is to improve intestinal calcium absorption. This can be accomplished by increasing dietary calcium intake, by reducing phosphate intake and by the use of vitamin D analogs. Several of these analogs - $1,25(OH)_2D$, $1\alpha(OH)D$ and dehydrotachysterol (DHT) - replace the 1α-hydroxy group that is lost with the progressive reduction in renal mass. The use of these analogs has generally improved our capacity to treat renal osteodystrophy since massive amounts of vitamin D_2 or D_3 are required to reverse calcium malabsorption in uremia. Indeed, as much as 50,000 to 100,000 IU of vitamin D may be required to reverse the defects in mineral homeostasis in uremic subjects (32). The provision of only a fraction of a microgram of $1,25(OH)_2D$ to a uremic child will increase serum calcium concentration by augmenting intestinal calcium absorption and will reduce fecal calcium excretion (32). In addition, the therapy of childhood uremic osteodystrophy should be aimed at providing sufficient doses of whatever vitamin D analog is used which can improve bone disease and still be safe. The hypercalcemia, hypercalciuria and the further decline in renal function that occurs in association with hypervitaminosis D are a major concern (13). No analog of vitamin D is completely safe if the potential for hypercalcemia is not anticipated and if serum calcium values are not frequently monitored (33).

As has been shown in studies in uremic adult subjects, the bone lesions in children include osteomalacia, osteitis fibrosa or a combination of the two (34). The 1α hydroxy compounds almost always improve or heal pure osteitis in conjunction with a decline in circulating PTH values and in alkaline phosphatase. Unfortunately osteomalacia is not completely healed (8, 10).

The value of phosphate restriction has been emphasized earlier in this review. However, it is important to realize that reduction of dietary phosphate intake in children with moderate to severe renal impairment has 3 major benefits. First, the influence of phosphate on the development of secondary hyperparathyroidism is so pervasive that dietary restriction has been shown to diminish parathyroid gland hypersecretion (15-17). Second, the newly recognized importance of phosphate restriction in terms of the regulation of $1,25(OH)_2D$ synthesis in children with moderate renal insufficiency (18-20) possibly indicates that phosphate restriction may forestall the decline in $1,25(OH)_2D$ synthesis. This point needs to be shown by human studies. Third, if less phosphate is ingested then lower doses of aluminum hydroxide can be used, potentially avoiding aluminum toxicity (23-30).

Several studies have indicated a dramatic, but unfortunately short lived, augmentation in height velocity which persists for the first year to year and one half of therapy, but other studies have not found this acceleration in growth (8, 10). It is important to recall that growth is the greatest during the first year of life where a child normally increases his length by more than 23-25 cm. Obviously, if a child has severe renal osteodystrophy during this period of rapid growth, his stature may be impaired. However, few studies have examined the role of early intervention in infants born with obstructive uropathy or another congenital disorder (35). The defect in mineral homeostasis brought about by uremia and by disruption of the function of the vitamin D - endocrine system, along with other factors such as acidosis and increased water needs, may be important factors contributing to growth failure during infancy. The impact of renal insufficiency on the young child may be devastating with mineral imbalance playing an important role. Finally, older children who develop osteodystrophy because of acquired disease after the age of 2-3 years may not experience growth failure to the same degree, since growth retardation during the first year of life seems to be a critical event. These older children, nonetheless, may experience serious bone disease and all of the usual manifestations of osteodystrophy.

To conclude, the discovery of the vitamin D - endocrine system and the importance of the kidney in its function has clarified our knowledge of the causes and the extent of childhood uremic osteodystrophy. Since the vitamin D endocrine system is perturbed in uremia, we can now appreciate the factors contributing to hypocalcemia and to hyperphosphatemia and secondary hyperparathyroidism. Therapy should be directed toward restoring the vitamin D hormone that is not produced by the declining kidney. Since phosphate retention may play a role in suppressing $1,25(OH)_2D$ synthesis, particularly in children with moderate renal insufficiency, phosphate intake should be reduced. Because of the potential for hypervitaminosis D and aluminum toxicity, these therapeutic measures must be carefully monitored.

Supported in Part by NIH Grants AM 19489, AM 31682 and by a Research Career Development Award AM 00421 and by Grants from Hoffman La Roche and Miles Laboratories.

REFERENCES

1. Lucas, R.C.: On a form of late rickets associated with albuminuria, rickets of adolescents. Lancet 1:933, 1883.

2. Chesney, R.W.: Metabolic Bone Disease. Pediatr in Review 5:227-237, 1984.

3. DeLuca, H.F.: The vitamin D system in the regulation of calcium and phosphorus metabolism. W.O. Atwater Memorial Lecture. Nutrit Rev 37:161, 1979.

4. DeLuca, H.F. and Schnoes, H.K.: Vitamin D: Recent Advances. Ann Rev Biochem 52, 411-439, 1983.

5. Chesney, R.W., Hamstra, A.J., Phelps, M., DeLuca, H.F.: Vitamin D metabolites in renal insufficiency and other vitamin D disorders of children. Kidney Int 24 (Supp 15):563-569, 1983.

6. Portale, A.A., Booth, B.E., Halloran, B.P., Morris, R.C., Jr.: Effect of dietary phosphorus on circulating concentrations of 1,25-dihydroxyvitamin D and immunoreactive parathyroid hormone in children with moderate renal insufficiency. J. Clin. Invest. 73:1580-1589, 1984.

7. Norman, M.E., Taylor, A.: Interrelationship of serum $25(OH)D_3$ and $1,25(OH)_2D_3$ levels in juvenile renal osteodystrophy during therapy with $25(OH)D_3$. Calc Tissue Int 33:340A, 1981.

8. Dabbagh, S. and Chesney, R.W.: Treatment of renal osteodystrophy during childhood. In Fine, R.N. and Gruskin, A. (eds.): Treatment of End-Stage Renal Disease in Children. W.B. Saunders, 1984, pp 251-270.

9. Mehls, O., Ritz, E., Krempien, B., Gilli, G., Link, K., Willich, E., and Scharer, K.: Slipped epiphyses in renal osteodystrophy. Arch Dis Child 50:545, 1975.

10. Chesney, R.W. and Avioli, L.V.: Childhood Renal Osteodystrophy In Edelmann, C.M., Jr. (ed.) Pediatric Kidney Disease, 2nd Edition. Boston: Little, Brown and Company, in press.

11. Hodson, E.M. Shaw, P.F., Evans, R.A., Dunstan, C.R., Hills, E.E., Wong, S.P., Rosenberg, A.R., Roy, L.P.: Growth retardation and renal osteodystrophy in children with chronic renal failure. J Pediatr 103:735-740, 1983.

12. Chesney, R.W., Mazess, R.B., Rose, P., Jax, D.K.: Bone mineral status measured by direct photon absorptiometry in childhood renal disease. Pediatrics 60:864, 1977.

13. Chesney, R.W.: Treatment of calcium and phosphorus abnormalities in childhood renal osteodystrophy. Dialysis & Transplant 12:270-279, 1983.

14. Lopez, S., Galceran, T., Chan, W., Rapp, N., Martin, K. and Slatopolsky, E.: Hypocalcemia may not be the cause of the development of secondary hyperparathyroidism. The American Society of Nephrology, 17th Annual Meeting, December, 1984.

15. Slatopolsky, E., Caglar, S., Gradowska, L., Canterbury, J.M., Reiss, E., Bricker, N.S.: On the prevention of secondary hyperparathyroidism in experimental chronic renal disease using "proportional reduction" of dietary phosphorus intake. Kidney Int 2:147, 1972.

16. Maschio, G., Tessitore, N., D'Angelo, A., Bonucci, E., Lupo, A., Valvo, E., Loschiavo, C., Fabris, A., Morachiello, P., Previato, G., Fiaschi, E.: Early dietary phosphorus restriction and calcium supplementation in the prevention of renal osteodystrophy. Am J Clin Nutrit 33:1546, 1980.

17. Llach, F., Massry, S.G., Koffler, A., Malluche, H.H., Singer, F.R., Brickman, A.S., Kurokawa, K.: Secondary hyperparathyroidism in early renal failure: Role of phosphate retention. Kidney Int 12:459, 1977.

18. Portale, A.A., Boothe, B.E., Halloran, B.P., Morris, R.C., Jr.: Effect of dietary phosphorus on circulating concentrations of 1,25-dihydroxyvitamin D and immunoreactive parathyroid hormone in children with moderate renal insufficiency. J Clin Invest 73:1580-1589, 1984.

19. Chesney, R.W., Hamstra, A.J., Phelps, M., DeLuca, H.F.: Vitamin D metabolites in renal insufficiency and other vitamin D disorders of children. Kidney Int 24 (Supp 15):563-569, 1983.

20. Chesney, R.W., DeLuca, H.F., Dabbagh, S., Mahan, J. and Kim, Y.K.: Vitamin D metabolism in longstanding nephrotic syndrome and chronic renal insufficiency. In Brodehl, J. and Ehrich, J.H.H. (eds.). Paediatric Nephrology. Berlin: Springer-Verlag, 1983.

21. Evans, R.A., Hills, E., Wong, S.Y.P., Dunstan, C.R., Norman, A.W.: The use of 24,25-dihydroxycholecalciferol alone and in combination with 1,25-dihydroxycholecalciferol in chronic renal failure. In Vitamin D: Chemical, Biochemical and Clinical Endocrinology of Calcium Metabolism. Berlin, Walter de Gruyter & Co., 1982, p. 835.

22. Lambert, P.W., Stern, P.H., Avioli, R.C., Brackett, N.C., Turner, R.T., Greene, A., Fu, I.Y. and Bell, N.H.: Evidence for extrarenal production of 1α,25-dihydroxyvitamin D in man. J Clin Invest 69:722-725, 1982a.

23. Wills, M.R., Savory, J.: Aluminium poisoning: Dialysis encephalopathy, osteomalacia and anaemia. Lancet 1:29-33, 1983.

24. Alfrey, A.C., Le Gendre, G.R., Kaehny, W.D.: The dialysis encephalopathy syndrome: Possible aluminum intoxication. N Engl J Med 294:184, 1976.

25. Baluarte, H.J., Gruskin, A.B., Hiner, L.B., Foley, C.M., Grover, W.D.: Encephalopathy in children with chronic renal failure. Proc Clin Dial Transplant Forum 7:95, 1977.

26. Griswold, W.R., Reznik, V., Mendoza, S.A., Trauner, D., Alfrey, A.C.: Accumulation of aluminum in a nondialyzed uremic child receiving aluminum hydroxide. Pediatr 71:56-58, 1983.

27. Andreoli, S., Bergstein, J.M., Sherrard, D.J.: Aluminum intoxication from aluminum-containing phosphate binders in children with azotemia not undergoing dialysis. N Engl J Med 310:1079-1084, 1984.

28. Sedman, A.B., Miller, N.L., Warady, B.A., Lum, G.M., Alfrey, A.C.: Aluminum loading in children with chronic renal failure. Kidney Int 26:201-204, 1984.

29. Hodsman, A.B., Sherrard, D.J., Alfrey, A.C., Ott, S., Brickman, A.S., Miller, N.L., Maloney, N.A., Coburn, J.W.: Bone aluminum and histomorphometric features of renal osteodystrophy. J Clin Endocrinol Metab 54:539, 1982.

30. Brown, D.J., Ham, K.N., Dawborn, J.K., Xeipell, J.E.: Treatment of dialysis osteomalacia with desferrioxamine. Lancet 1:343-345, 1982.

31. Salusky, I.: Personal communication.

32. Brickman, A.S., Coburn, J.W., Norman, A.W.: Action of 1,25-dihydroxycholecalciferol, a potent, kidney-produced metabolite of vitamin D_3, in uremic man. N Engl J Med 287:891, 1972.

33. Massry SG: Requirements of vitamin D metabolites in patients with renal disease. Am J Clin Nutrit 33:1530, 1980.

34. Baron, R., Norman, M., Mazur, A., Gruskin, A., Rasmussen, H.: Bone histomorphometry in children with early chronic renal failure treated with 25(OH)D_3. In Vitamin D: Basic Research and Its Clinical Application. Berlin: Walter de Gruyter & Co., p. 847, 1979.

35. Chesney, R.W., Dabbagh, S., Uehling, D.T., DeLuca, H.F.: The importance of early treatment of renal bone disease in children. Kidney Int, in press.

THE USE OF CYCLOSPORINE IN PEDIATRIC RECIPIENTS OF RENAL TRANSPLANTS

B.D. Kahan, M.D., Ph.D., C.T. Van Buren, M.D., S.B. Conley, M.D., M.I. Lorber, M.D. and S.M. Flechner, M.D.

The superior results of cyclosporine (CsA) immunosuppression in combination with prednisone (Pred), which was initiated at the University of Texas Medical School at Houston for adult patients in August, 1980, compared to the previous azathioprine-Pred combination, led to application of this regimen to pediatric recipients one year later (1). On the one hand, there were the concerns of carcinogenicity, and particularly in a pediatric population that CsA-induced nephrotoxicity would produce chronic renal dysfunction sufficient to prevent post-transplant growth and development. On the other hand, the possible benefit of improved graft survival and reduced numbers of rejection episodes decreasing the cumulative steroid dose proffered better rehabilitation. The present communication describes our four year experience with the CsA-Pred regimen in 34 children aged 1.5 to 16 years.

MATERIALS AND METHODS

Patients

The 34 pediatric renal transplants were performed between September 1981 and September 1985 at The University of Texas Medical School at Houston in children aged 1.5 to 16 (mean 10.5) years. These patients received only CsA-Pred for immunosuppression. Of the 20 males and 14 females, 26 patients were prepubertal. The etiology of end-stage renal disease (ESRD) included glomerulonephritis (nine), dysplasia with reflux or obstruction (eleven), posterior urethral valves (four), hereditary nephritis (two), Eagle-Barrett syndrome (two), polycystic disease (two), renal hypoplasia (two), congenital nephrotic syndrome (one), and primary oxalosis (one). The donor source was a mismatched cadaver kidney in 17 patients. Seventeen children received haploidentical living related kidneys, 16 from parental and one from a sibling donor.

Pretransplant Preparation

No intentional third-party or donor-specific blood transfusions were administered in preparation for transplantation; however, 11 living related (LRD) and 12 cadaver (CAD) donor recipients had been previously given at least two historical third-party units. Pretransplant nephrectomy was performed in 16 children; one, splenectomy. Seven children underwent pre-emptive transplantation, never having experienced chronic dialysis therapy. Twenty had been treated with hemodialysis, and seven with peritoneal dialysis. CAD kidneys from crossmatch-negative, blood-type compatible donors displayed greater than 2 HLA-A,B matches in six cases; less than 2 HLA-A,B matched kidneys, in 11 instances. None of the CAD kidneys were 2 HLA-DR, nine were 1 DR, and eight were 0 DR matches.

Immunosuppression

Prior to transplantation, CAD kidney recipients were given CsA 14 mg/kg orally. LRD recipients usually received CsA by continuous intravenous infusion for five days at 6 mg/kg/day for children less than 20 kg, and 3 mg/kg/day for larger children. No CsA was given intraoperatively. Postoperatively an intravenous infusion was utilized until resolution of gastrointestinal ileus, which usually occurred by day 3. The 14 mg/kg oral dose was tapered to 12 mg/kg at weeks 2-3, and 10 mg/kg by weeks 4-12. Thereafter the dose was adjusted to maintain serum trough levels between 50-200 ng/ml by radioimmunoassay determinations using the kit available from Sandoz. Drug absorption and elimination were assessed by pharmacokinetic analysis, as previously described in detail (2). Children who displayed a short $t_{1/2}$ were administered CsA on a B.I.D. or T.I.D. dosing schedule. In the few instances that the total CsA dose was increased, there was either documented poor gastrointestinal absorption, or persistently low drug levels attributed to concomitant drug therapy with cytochrome P-450 activating drugs, particularly anti-convulsants. The steroid regimen included 125-250 mg methylprednisolone administered at the time of transplant, followed postoperatively by Pred at 2 mg/kg, rapidly tapered to 0.5 mg/kg the first week, 0.25 mg/kg at one month, and a maintenance dose of 0.10-0.15 mg/kg by three months.

Renal Function

Episodes of renal dysfunction associated with elevated CsA trough levels (greater than 200 ng/ml) were treated by progressive dose reduction by 25-100 mg/day at weekly intervals. The syndrome of progressive renal dysfunction in the presence of low CsA levels (less than 50 ng/ml) demanded renal biopsy. If rejection appeared most likely based upon the biopsy and the clinical picture (3), the patient received one to three intravenous bolus injections of methylprednisolone (15-20 mg/kg) followed by a recycling of oral steroids beginning at 3 mg/kg. Renal function was recorded at intervals post-transplant according to the serum creatinine value (mg/dl). The height of each child in centimeters (cm) was recorded prior to transplantation. Linear growth measurements for those children, whose transplant had functioned more than one year, were plotted on standard curves adapted from National Center for Health Statistics, Hyattsville, Maryland (4).

RESULTS

Patient and Graft Survival

There was no patient mortality during the entire follow-up period of 3-51 months (5). CAD graft survival is 87% at one year and 76% at two years (Fig. 1); LRD graft survival is 82% up to four years post-transplant (Fig. 2).

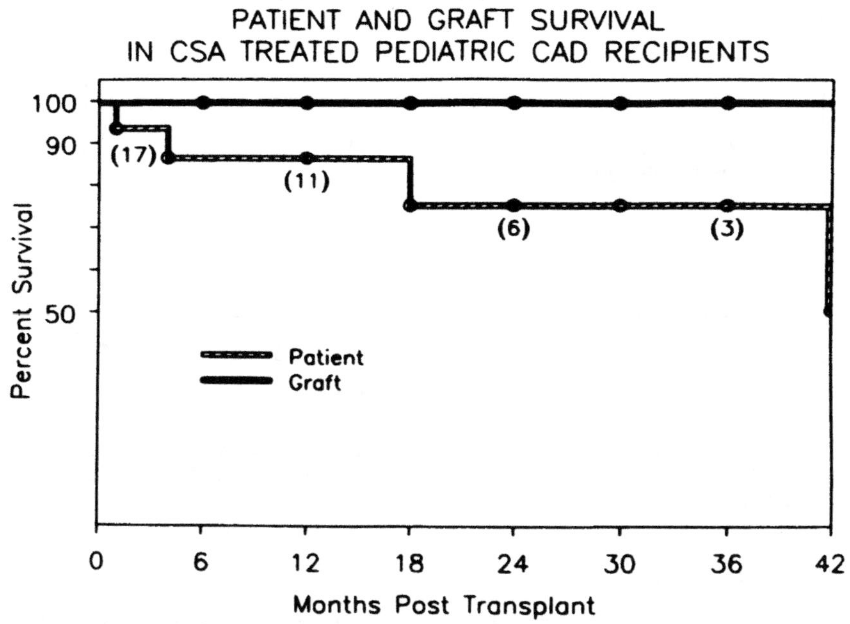

FIGURE 1. CAD graft survival in pediatric recipients using life table methods. Numbers in parentheses represent number of patients at risk.

The three LRD graft losses included two cases of steroid-resistant, accelerated rejection leading to transplant nephrectomy within the first week, and a case of recurrent focal sclerosing glomerulonephritis, who displayed heavy proteinuria (greater than 15 gm per 24 hr) and recurrent disease within one month. The four CAD graft losses included one case of primary nonfunction, probably compounded by ongoing rejection, two instances of chronic rejection at 14 and 40 months, and one graft lost at four months due to recurrent oxalate deposition. Three of the four graft losses occurred in retransplanted patients. The overall graft survival for first CAD grafts was 10/10 of those at risk for at least one year, and 6/7 of those at risk for two years.

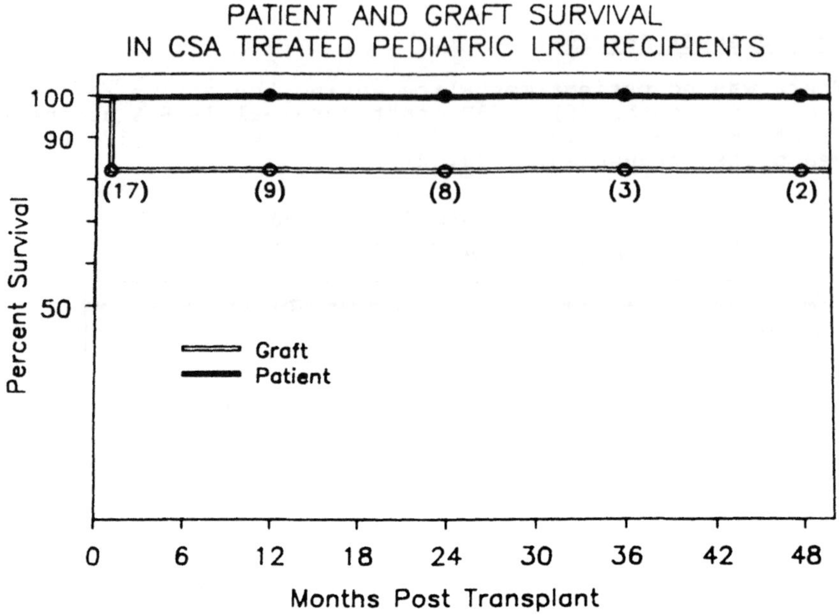

FIGURE 2. LRD graft survival in pediatric recipients using life table methods. Numbers in parentheses represent number of patients at risk.

Allograft Rejection

The incidence of allograft rejection was similar between 7/17 (41%) children receiving LRD and 6/17 (35%) recipients of CAD grafts. While 6/7 LRD rejection episodes occurred during the first post-transplant month, rejection episodes of CAD grafts occurred during the first, second, seventh, twelfth, and eighteenth months.

Quality of Renal Function

The post-transplant renal function and CsA blood levels in CAD and LRD recipients are summarized in Table 1 and Table 2, respectively. The daily administered dose of CsA decreased with time, stabilizing at 5-7 mg/kg per day. These doses were about 40% greater than comparable doses administered to adult renal transplant recipients. The mean serum CsA trough levels at each interval were higher in CAD recipients, even though the mean CsA doses were lower than in the LRD recipient group, suggesting a role of persistent renal injury during the procurement process or of subclinical allograft rejection. The mean serum creatinine values and mean creatinine clearances although elevated at three years compared to six months, remained stable in both CAD and LRD recipients without progressive deterioration.

Table 1. Laboratory Values in CAD Recipients

Post-Transplant (mean ± SE)

	MONTHS					
	6	12	18	24	30	36
n	14	12	9	5	5	4
CsA (mg/kg)	7.8 ±.85	7.7 ±.77	6.9 ±.75	6.3 ±.81	5.8 ±.81	5.3 ±.94
CsA trough (ng/ml)	91 ±10	86 ±11	73 ±12	65 ±16	78 ±25	74 ±18
Creatinine (mg/dl)	1.12 ±.38	1.21 ±.42	1.31 +.20	1.51 +.10	1.50 +.19	1.47 +.22
Creatinine clearance (ml/min)	61 ±8.3	62 ±6.8	63 ±6.7	56 ±6.3	58 ±3.6	60 ±2.1

Table 2. Laboratory Values in LRD Recipients

Post-Transplant (Mean ± SE)

	MONTHS						
	6	12	18	24	30	36	42
n	14	11	8	8	6	3	2
CsA (mg/kg)	9.1 ±.73	7.8 ±.91	7.1 ±(1.1)	6.5 ±1.3	6.5 ±1.3	7.1 ±1.2	5.7 ±2.3
CsA trough (ng/ml)	58 ±11	49 ±10	38 ±8.7	35 ±5.8	33 ±6.7	37 ±8.5	36 ±7.0
Creatinine (mg/dl)	1.01 ±.13	1.14 ±.15	1.30 ±.21	1.13 ±.19	1.24 ±.21	1.60 ±.31	1.4 ±.30
Creatinine clearance (ml/min)	56 ±3.8	61 ±3.6	58 ±3.8	63 ±8.5	74 ±6.9	63 ±6.9	65 ±6.4

Complications

The immunosuppressive complications included 13 bacterial infections, 6 viral infections, and 3 fungal infections requiring in-patient therapy. One 4-year-old LRD recipient suffered initial ureteral necrosis requiring operative repair, followed by four severe bouts of pyelonephritis. Three children suffered severe viral gastroenteritis necessitating intravenous fluid replacement. There have not been any lymphomas or other tumors.

CsA-associated side effects summarized in Table 3 reveal a prevalence of hypertrichosis, which in several female patients required applications of depilatory cream. Five children required seizure medications post-transplant, including two with a previous history of seizure disorders. No localizing neurological findings were identified in the other three children. Hepatotoxicity, which was defined as transaminase elevations twice the normal value and/or a bilirubin greater than 2 mg/dl in the absence of complicating conditions, was uncommon, and uniformly responded to dose reduction. No child required discontinuance of CsA due to an uncontrolled side effect.

Table 3. Side Effects in Pediatric Patients Treated with CsA and Pred Immunosuppression

		CAD	LRD	TOTAL (%)
n		(17)	(17)	(34)
Hepatotoxicity		2	1	3
Hypertrichosis	mild	10	9	19
	severe	2	2	4
Tremor		4	5	9
Seizures		2	3	5
Gum hyperplasia		0	0	0
Hypertension		12	7	19
Osteonecrosis		1	2	3
Tumors		0	0	0

Linear Growth Determinations

Four female and seven male recipients of LRD kidneys, and five female and six male recipients of CAD kidneys demonstrated continued linear growth post-transplant. Some children experienced growth acceleration and catch-up growth. However, the curves of many of the older children continued to be flatter than those predicted for non-ESRD children (6).

PHARMACOKINETIC DATA

Although the number of pharmacokinetic studies available in children are far fewer than the adult data base, they do show significant differences from adults (Table 4). There is a three-fold increased rate of mean drug clearance, namely 39.6 ml/min/kg in children versus 12.3 ml/min/kg in adults, which may explain the almost 50% reduction in area under the plasma concentration versus time curve from 765 in adults to 386 in children. There also appeared to be somewhat better oral absorption of CsA by children, 59%, compared to adults (29%). The major conclusion drawn from this information is that children require shorter dosing intervals and slightly higher total CsA doses than do adults.

Table 4. Comparison of Pharmacokinetic Parameters

in Children and Adults

Parameter+	Adult Value (n)*	Pediatric Value (n)*	"p"†
AUC/dose	765 ± 593 (386)	386 ± 277 (20)	<.01
$t_{1/2}$ (hr)	9.6 ± 5.8 (382)	8.2 ± 5.0 (21)	NS
CL (ml/min/kg)	12.3 ± 8.2 (138)	39.6 ± 30.5 (15)	<.001
F (%)	29 ± 24 (57)	52.1 ± 48.5 (7)	.05

+ Parameters include area under the plasma concentration time curve corrected for the administered dose (AUC/mg), drug half-life in hours ($t_{1/2}$), drug clearance rate (ml/min/kg), and percent oral bioavailability compared to intravenous administration. All parameters defined in (2).

* n in parenthesis refers to the number of patients studied.

† "p" values as determined by unpaired t-test.

DISCUSSION

Renal transplantation has become the optimal management strategy for the child afflicted with ESRD, for it has the potential to return the child to pre-illness levels of growth and development (7), a particularly important factor for small infants. Although successful renal transplantation permits growth, allograft rejection with its concomitant consequences of treatment diminish rehabilitation potential.

Cyclosporine, a fungal endecapeptide of novel chemical structure and potent immunosuppressive properties, has been widely used in renal transplantation in adults. CsA interrupts the generation of lymphokine signals necessary for lymphocyte activation and amplification, while sparing non-specific host resistance by monocytes, macrophages and granulocytes, as well as hematopoiesis of platelets and red blood cells (2). On the other hand, CsA use is associated with nephrotoxic effects resulting in significant, but not progressive, renal impairment. Thus a major concern about the use of the agent in the pediatric population is that the CsA-associated nephrotoxicity would produce chronic renal dysfunction and thereby engender growth impairment.

This report describes the improved allograft survival, diminished incidence of rejection-associated complications, and acceptable levels of renal function permitting growth and development achieved with the use of CsA in pediatric patients. Not only has there been no mortality up to 51 months post-transplant, but also the four year LRD graft survival is 82% and the 3½ year CAD graft survival of 72% are essentially the same as observed in adult recipients (8).

In contradistinction, the 35-40% incidence of rejection episodes has been greater than that observed in adult patients, probably related to the more rapid elimination of CsA in the pediatric age group. Thus pharmacokinetic studies in these patients are necessary to discern patients demonstrating rapid clearance, who require twice or thrice daily, divided CsA doses. This approach avoids the use of excessive CsA doses (<20 mg/kg), which are likely to predispose to toxic or infectious complications.

In accord with the unique pharmacokinetic parameters, nephrotoxicity due to drug intoxication has not been a serious problem in the pediatric age group. First, it has been rare to have to decrease the CsA dose in a child because of impaired renal function. Second, there has not been a trend toward chronic deterioration of renal function up to four years. The mean values for 24 hr creatinine clearances (uncorrected for size) have remained between 50-60 ml/min at each follow-up interval. While it is generally agreed that the ultimate adult height achieved by the pediatric ESRD patient will be depressed (9), nearly all CsA-treated children demonstrate continued linear growth. However, it appears that only the younger children experience "catch-up" growth; postpubertal patients display a flat growth curve.

The experience in pediatric renal transplantation using CsA and Pred at our Center has yielded excellent patient and graft survival with acceptable morbidity. This factor was particularly evident with re-transplanted patients, who were at high risk for graft loss. Attention to tissue matching may be prudent in the re-transplanted patient, in contradistinction to primarily allograft adult or pediatric CsA-treated recipients, wherein tissue typing and prospective blood transfusions do not appear to have a major impact on graft survival.

In conclusion, CsA-Pred represents an efficacious immunosuppressive regimen for pediatric recipients of both CAD and LRD renal allografts up to four years post-transplant. Although CsA-induced nephrotoxicity has not been a serious problem in this population, the incidence of rejection is appreciable due to the rapid clearance of CsA by children with consequent low blood drug levels. These unique pharmacokinetics demand individualization of the drug regimen. No child has required discontinuation of CsA for toxic side effects. To date growth and rehabilitation of these children has been satisfactory.

REFERENCES

1. Kahan, B.D., Van Buren, C., Flechner, S., Payne, W.D., Boileau, M., and Kerman, R.: Cyclosporine immunosuppression mitigates immunologic risk factors in renal allotransplantation. Transplant. Proc. 15(4): 2469-2478, 1983.

2. Kahan, B.D.: Overview: individualization of cyclosporine therapy using pharmacokinetic and pharmacodynamic parameters. Transplantation 40: 457, 1985.

3. Kahan, B.D.: Clinical summation: an algorithm for the management of patients with cyclosporine-induced renal dysfunction. Transplant. Proc. 17: 303, 1985.

4. Hamill, P.V., Drizd, T., Johnson, C., et al.: Am. J. Clin. Nutr. 32: 607, 1979.

5. Conley, S.B., Brewer, E., Flechner, S., Van Buren, C.T., and Kahan, B.D.: Renal transplantation using cyclosporine in pediatric patients 3 to 17 years old. Transplant. Proc. 15(4): 2528, 1983.

6. Flechner, S.M., Conley, S.B., Rose, G., Van Buren, C., Kerman, R., Lorber, M., and Kahan, B.D.: Cyclosporine and prednisone immunosuppression in pediatric recipients of renal allografts. Actua Sandoz, 1986: in press.

7. Fine, R.N.: J. Pediatr. 100: 754, 1982.

8. Kahan, B.D., Van Buren, C.T., Flechner, S., Jarowenko, M., Yasumura, T., Rogers, A.J., Yoshimura, N., LeGrue, S., Drath, D.B., and Kerman, R.H.: Clinical and experimental studies using cyclosporine in renal transplantation. Surgery 97: 125, 1985.

9. Pennisi, A.J., Costin, G., Phillips, L.: Am. J. Dis. Child. 133: 950, 1979.

DISCUSSION: RENAL REPLACEMENT THERAPY
PROGRESSION OF RENAL DISEASE AND TRANSPLANTATION

PANELISTS: Jacques Bourgoignie, M.D., Russell Chesney, M.D., Richard Fine, M.D., Warren Grupe, M.D., Barry Kahan, M.D., George Kyriakides, M.D. and Gaston Zilleruelo, M.D.

MODERATOR: Jose Strauss, M.D.

COMMENT-QUESTION: The Einstein Group in the 1960's had an abstract showing that the rate of increase of GFR in infants after birth was influenced by the level of protein intake. What the study did not do was look at the parallel effect of increases of sodium and other nutrients that go along with the protein. In the human studies, have people controlled sodium intake, mineral content intake, and so on?

RESPONSE: In the acute studies, yes. In the long term studies, I do not know. In the acute studies, which focus on protein and amino acids, yes, sodium is not a factor. In the long term studies, no. That has not been controlled. In the study from Holland, for instance, the last three years' results were recently published; they have not controlled phosphate either. So, there may be other factors intervening there. Prospective studies are badly needed. The NIH is starting a study on modest clinical renal insufficiency to look at these effects.

QUESTION: In that same vein, in the study reported in Lancet, do we know that phosphate increase, PTH, or other related items did not play a role? Obviously, when you restrict proteins you are probably restricting phosphate, among other things. Could that be playing a role?

RESPONSE: It certainly could. In that study, phosphorus was not controlled, as I just mentioned. In animals, however, there are studies where these effects were controlled; clearly, I do not think that it is a phosphate effect or a PTH effect. Several studies have appeared, one from France, one from England, where protein restriction was applied while maintaining phosphates constant in the diet of the two groups, and the same level of GFR decrease and focal sclerosis occurred.

QUESTION: Does control of protein intake have any influence on the blood pressure of rats or of humans?

RESPONSE: Not in the rat. In people, if you malnourish them and deplete their protein tremendously, then yes, you can see a lowering effect on blood pressure. But otherwise, no, there is very little effect on blood pressure as long as they are not malnourished. This was reviewed in the Annals of Internal Medicine recently. That was obviously an issue in these studies.

QUESTION: So, then hypertension could not explain the whole picture.

RESPONSE: In the minds of the researchers, hypertension is not the variable that explains the observations.

QUESTION: I have two problems with the outcome measures. Would you comment on them? One is that in the face of a falling GFR, in the ablation model, the BUN goes down; this to us in Pediatrics is an indication of malnutrition. I wonder if that lower urea generation has anything to do with malnutrition. The second is that the proteinuria goes down as the GFR goes down, which is similar to what we see as a toxic effect of indomethacin in the nephrotic syndrome; the decrease in proteinuria really does not reflect an improvement. It may be that the lower GFR actually lowers the proteinuria. Would you comment on those?

RESPONSE: The decrease in blood urea nitrogen could reflect malnutrition, you are right, if it decreases drastically. But, if you decrease simply protein intake in a normal human being, you will see a change in blood urea nitrogen. The changes are more dramatic here because these animals had a low GFR to start with, so they start with a high blood urea nitrogen. If you decrease their protein intake, they do not need to develop malnutrition to decrease their blood urea nitrogen, at least in the adult population.

QUESTION: But it could be malnutrition. Right?

RESPONSE: It could be.

COMMENT: From what I can see, it has not been excluded that, in fact, what one has done is produce malnutrition and a lowered muscle mass which could account for some of the changes seen. It is certainly not the inulin clearance in the rodent.

RESPONSE: No.

COMMENT: But what about some of the other changes, including the human studies?

RESPONSE: They looked very carefully for malnutrition. That is one of the concerns, of course. In the 1960's, when we were giving a low protein diet to people with advanced renal disease, we were malnourishing them when we were giving them 20 grams protein/day. Clearly, malnutrition was developing. At the level of 0.6 g/kg, there was no evidence of malnutrition. There is little evidence of malnutrition in these subjects, at least for those in the Dutch study. That also is the level while I think the NIH is going to recommend in terms of their study for follow-up of patients with modest chronic renal insufficiency.

COMMENT: The MIT people though have found that a 0.5-0.6 g/kg in the adult as the limit is too low. You cannot maintain muscle mass.

RESPONSE: It is the limit, you are right. The proteinuria may decrease because GFR decreases, that is correct.

QUESTION: So, it need not be a beneficial effect. As an outcome measure, it need not be a beneficial outcome. Right?

RESPONSE: Except that these animals survived--the ones that had a higher GFR to start with. Pathologically, morphologically, their kidneys looked better and those that started with a higher GFR, survived.

COMMENT: What I am getting to is that maybe there is, indeed, an increased survival in the rodents. We are not sure about other animals. It is not clear to me from the studies, what rent is being paid to gain that survival. And, from a pediatric point of view, if that rent is decreased muscle mass and malnutrition, we are in deep trouble.

RESPONSE: You are absolutely right. That is a concern, obviously, and for children you have an even bigger problem than for adults. One cannot jump on these conclusions from rodents and extrapolate them to man; one needs additional data. If these conclusions, so far, are correct, how are we going to implement them? That is going to be another question especially in the pediatric group. You are absolutely correct.

COMMENT-QUESTION: In your summary here, you mentioned that with high protein restriction, endurance training exercise can also retard progression of renal disease. I am a little concerned. I would like to hear you comment on this since with exercise you naturally have an increase in proteinuria.

COMMENT: I do not know how the proteinuria occurs with exercise. I am not sure that it is related at all to this. Here proteinuria has been demonstrated to result from a change in permeability at the glomerular basement membrane level as a result of hyperfiltration or hypertension. With exercise does the same occur in the kidney? I do not know.

QUESTION: Does hydrostatic pressure come up during exercise?

RESPONSE: I am not sure we can assume that. Because, during non-isovolumetric exercise, pressure tends to go down. I do not know how to extrapolate there.

QUESTION: Since local production of prostaglandins as vasodilators has been implicated in hyperfiltration, and we know that fatty acid composition in the diet could influence prostaglandin synthesis, do you have any thoughts on the role of fatty acid composition in the progression of renal failure?

RESPONSE: Yes, I talked mainly of proteins but there are other dietary factors. In a recent abstract published from St. Louis, it was stated that the main factors which affect progression of renal disease are not different protein but different lipid intakes especially diets rich in linoleic acid; a diet poor in linoleic acid was desirable and they demonstrated also that lipids can influence the rate of decrease in GFR of rats with remnant kidney. So, clearly, diet can have an influence; the lipid composition of diets should be taken into consideration as well.

COMMENT: There seem to be differences in some of the studies, whether you use creatinine clearance or inulin clearance, at least in some animals. Knowing that at least in children, at low levels of GFR there seems to be up to a 40 to 60% over-estimation when using creatinine clearances; I see some real problems with that. On the other hand, since there is probably a concomitant decrease in muscle mass, serum creatinine should be lower; that could be another factor that affects creatinine clearance. This is even truer for the estimation of GFR from body height and serum creatinine. Perhaps some of the studies could be done better if GFR was measured with inulin clearance rather than creatinine clearance.

COMMENT: That is absolutely correct. GFR really has been looked at carefully in adults at Stanford. It was found that the GFR of about 80 ml/min creatinine overestimated GFR by 20 percent. But other GFRs of about 30 ml/min creatinine clearance overestimate true inulin clearance by 90 percent. So that could be a variable. Although cumbersome, I think that certainly some long-term studies should be done with inulin clearances. Iodothalamate clearance may be easier than inulin clearance.

MODERATOR: The important assessment, the important problem with the excessive protein intake is,is itthe protein that reaches the glomerulus or is it the protein that appears in the urine? I want to tie this question in with some suggestions for clinical applications. There are pediatric nephrologists who are restricting the protein intake of nephrotics in an attempt to reduce proteinuria, I guess in the belief that proteinuria is what damages the glomeruli. Do you have any thoughts on that?

RESPONSE: No, I do not. I do not think it is the proteinuria that damages the glomeruli. The proteinuria is a consequence of the damage rather than producing the damage itself. And, in regard to restricting proteins in nephrotics, I do not do it in adults because I am afraid of malnutrition in these patients. The data are in. By restricting protein in patients with chronic renal insufficiency who are not proteinuric, I think the damage of malnutrition may probably be greater than the saving which at most, in patients with progressive renal disease, may be a few months extension of the period away from hemodialysis. In patients with normal GFR who are proteinuric, I do not restrict protein intake at the present time. Should we? I am not sure, because then they need their protein for survival. And really, restricting protein intake is not going to decrease that much their level of proteinuria. There are some studies in which non-steroidal anti-inflammatory agents are used to reduce proteinuria; it is assumed that proteinuria is mediated by prostaglandins. I know of one group that has used non-steroidal anti-inflammatory agents for many years in the treatment of nephrotic syndrome; it seems that they decrease proteinuria, but have no effect on improving GFR.

QUESTION: Do you administer blood transfusions to patients receiving a live-related kidney transplant?

COMMENT: With an azathioprine (Imuran) protocol whereby the day before they get the transfusion, the day of the transfusion and the day following the transfusion, the patients receive Imuran, the sensitization rate has been reduced to less than ten percent. With live-related protocols and donor specific blood transfusions, the one year survival rate has been 100 percent. Really not 100 percent because there were two with technical problems. But from the standpoint of immunologic phenomena, we had no immunologic losses with the live-related donors during the first year with the donor specific transfusion protocols.

QUESTION: This is not a topic that was discussed, but I would like to ask for the panelists' opinion about iron in the pediatric population. In children who require frequent transfusions and continuously run ferritins that are over 1,000, is anyone prophylactically treating these patients for the development of iron overload?

RESPONSE: Well, I can tell you that if you transplant them, you frequently find that the ferritin levels will come down following transplantation. But, in addition, if you do autopsies on children who have been on dialysis for prolonged periods of time and required multiple transfusions, you will find that they have considerable hemosiderosis. In the pediatric population I have not seen any patient who has gone on to cirrhosis or has developed hemochromatosis with regard to involvement of the pancreas or the heart from the iron overload. I think it has been described in adult patients and it is a concern. One of the things that I would really advise against is the use of oral iron supplementation or certainly intravenous iron without following the serum ferritin; that is probably the best indicator for iron status in the patient. I am not aware of anyone, at least in the pediatric age group, who is using Desferoxamine to remove iron but I suspect that if the patients were symptomatic with their iron overload, that might be a reasonable alternative.

COMMENT: Last year at the Pediatric Meetings we submitted an abstract of a single patient in whom we had used DFO for precisely what you are talking about—very high ferritin levels. By using DFO in association with hemodialysis, we were able to reduce the ferritin level. This patient was subsequently switched to CCPD and actually has gone 14 months without requiring a transfusion. We have continued to use DFO in his dialysate and the ferritin levels have come down. This was a child who had been on dialysis for ten years. I have to tell you that his myocardium is very stiff; I think if we were to do a biopsy we would find evidence of iron, because he has not had other causes of cardiomyopathy.

COMMENT: I would like to extend the discussion on iron supplementation for these children and point out the large number we find who have had the uremic anemia treated with iron before we have seen them. I confess to you that there are times when we have not looked into the history carefully, and therefore have missed finding the children with prolonged uremia who are still getting iron at home. They should not be started on iron but if they have been started on it, we should stop it.

COMMENT: There is another facet of iron toxicity in chronic renal failure patients to which we have not given much attention. I believe last year in the ASN Meeting, there was an abstract from the Mayo Clinic describing bone disease that for all practical matters looked like aluminum bone disease ; they found iron deposits in the bone rather than aluminum. If I may, a comment and two questions. I have not heard in four days anything about essential amino acids. We used to hear a lot about it—two or three years ago. I saw in one of your slides that the effect of their administration is not sustained. I wonder if you could make some comment on that. Is there any role, indeed, of oral or parenteral essential amino acids in the treatment of acute or chronic renal failure in children?

RESPONSE: We have not used very much of them. We have used, in terms of chronic, the sorts that you saw presented relative to the child before dialysis. The levels that we have been able to attain on dialysis can maintain a reasonable amount of nutrition. Our aim is not to make these children fat. I do not think there is any demonstration that there is any specific advantage to essential amino acids or complete amino acids in this group of children. There is one report stating that children who received essential amino acids grew much better while they were taking them; it turns out that those children were on a calcium and essential amino acids supplementation and that their PTHs fell. It may be that they grew not because they were getting the amino acids but because their bone disease was being better treated. The control was not done on an equal group of children on standard meat and potatoes who got the calcium supplement. The other concern I have is that we have tended to use the essential amino acids when we are forced to use a parenteral form of nutrition. That usually comes up in the child with acute renal failure. I would caution that essential amino acids in the small child, at levels that will produce positive nitrogen balance, also produce hepatotoxicity and these children get hyperammonemia. That hyperammonemia is avoided if one turns to a complete amino acid mixture probably because of the histidine and the arginine that is in the complete mixture.

COMMENT: I want to say a few additional things about essential amino acids. Important work has shown that in the uremic state there are amino acid imbalances of a very different degree, both within the muscle and in the plasma. One may need to tailor to each patient an essential amino acid mixture to facilitate this. The observation about the calcium salts, I think, is an important one. Finally, there are some data from Madison on uremic rats and the fact that when their diet is supplemented with leucine (one percent leucine), these rats rapidly develop anorexia and refuse to eat. In addition, it seems that using essential amino acids when giving leucine may result in additional fractures. That is in rats; it is not in man. We have to think about some of these things critically before we embark on the use of essential amino acids. Obviously, I think the time to prescribe these essential amino acids is not with us yet. We need a lot more baseline data.

COMMENT: There have been some suggestions that one would want to replace glucose in the dialysate solution with an amino acid as an osmotic agent. It is worth cautioning everyone that if one is going to do that, one cannot (or should not) use the commercially available amino acid formulas. In the commercially available formulas the amino acid composition is really inappropriate for someone with uremia; one can get into significant difficulty with some of the amino acids. Specifically I am referring to methionine and trionine, where one can get very high and toxic levels in the blood. I think we do not, as yet, have any amino acid formulation that takes into consideration the perturbations in the amino acid pattern that exists in uremia.

COMMENT: Let me come back to what both of these comments really mean, at least to me. That work, in fact, not only showed that unusual things happen when one gives essential amino acids to the uremic patient. If one carries that information into the cell a little bit further, it looks more as if the cell is in trouble because of inability to synthesize, not from breakdown or storage difficulties. Thus, if one continues to give these amino acids, one is bound to get backups in the serum and backups in a variety of other places because the cells cannot use them. My concern is that if we then change the formulation to reduce these abnormally high levels in the plasma back to normal, we should not necessarily conclude that we have changed the intracellular status because there still may be intracellular amino acid abnormalities.

COMMENT: I would clearly agree with that. I mean, in other words, until we find ways of improving synthesis in uremia, recommendations on essential amino acid administration are far too preliminary.

COMMENT: I want to address just what was said about amino acids. We did some studies in San Francisco in which we gave acutely uremic-anuric patients essential amino acid solutions. Even though the data looked "good" in terms of nitrogen retention, obviously there was a deficiency in protein accumulation of body mass. In fact, in one patient, I feel sure that it was the cause of her ultimate demise. Some have said for a long time, relative to supplementation with essential amino acids, that we cannot forget that there is a requirement for non-essential nitrogen. You cannot go on the premise that if you give essential nitrogen, it will be converted to non-essential nitrogen; that is incorrect. We have to give adequate non-essential nitrogen. The same thing goes when studying amino acid patterns in premature infants. Any time you give any one of these intravenous solutions, they cause tremendous aberrations in the aminograms even when given through the dialysate. So, again, I echo the caution just stated and that is: do not use what is on the market; it is inappropriate. We do not know what is appropriate. One little point about iron supplementation in end stage disease or chronic renal insufficiency: there is a little hooker in the whole thing. There is not enough substantiation at this point for what I am saying, but there is evidence that high doses of vitamin C given concurrently with iron, and perhaps with any iron load to anyone, can cause abnormalities in the binding of that iron and, therefore, may make it more available for deposition in tissues; in other words, the development of hemosiderosis. So, at this point, I think we ought to be very cautious about giving to all of our dialysis patients these vitamin supplements which contain 500 mg of vitamin C.

COMMENT: Concerning what was mentioned about the use of calcium carbonate, I think we agree that we have to be very cautious. We have not collected our data yet, but anecdotally we have a fair number of patients currently on calcium carbonate. I do not think we have encountered prominent hypercalcemia and we are using up to four, five, sometimes six grams of calcium carbonate a day. We have to be extremely cautious in the hypoalbuminemic patient and the patient who has the nephrotic syndrome also as part of the chronic renal failure. There we probably ought to measure ionized calcium because we certainly can have a total calcium of 8 and have an ionized calcium of 2.8 or 3 mEq/L leading into a state of ionized hypercalcemia with normal total calcium. I think that is a very important aspect to consider.

COMMENT: One of the things I indicated was that uremia is a malfeasance of the vitamin D endocrine system and one does not produce calcitriol [1,25$(OH)_2$D], but if one gives calcitriol exogenously, one is also inducing a state of malfeasance. This is a very, very potent compound. In a young child, even 0.25 mcg a day, if there is a lot of available calcium, will result in hypercalcemia which fortunately may last only for a few hours. These studies need to be done; if you have data on this you should look into it and publish this. The point that I was making before, and I hope I made it clearly, was that in good hands it is fine to use it because I think that a calcium of 11.5 is probably not all that harmful to the child on dialysis. But if you are worried about the progression to renal failure, you may find problems. That was my basic point. We have used calcium carbonate, we have not gotten into trouble with it in general (we have in one or two specific instances). We have not switched completely away from aluminum hydroxide but it has certainly allowed us to lower our dose of aluminum hydroxide.

COMMENT: I would agree with you. But very young children may be a bit more susceptible and, of course, these are the patients about whom we are much more concerned when giving aluminum; therefore, we would like to avoid aluminum and only give calcium carbonate. I am sure you would agree with that. What we have tried to do is to initiate calcium carbonate therapy independent of 1,25D; only after they are on a stable dose of calcium carbonate and their calcium and phosphorus levels are stable, do we then add the 1,25D. We have found that even in doing it this way we have gotten into difficulty with calcium levels in the range that we would not like to have them, and we have had to back off with either the calcium carbonate or the vitamin D. So your point is well taken that it is not something one should rush into and do immediately. One needs to have very close surveillance if one is going to use these drugs especially in very young children.

QUESTION: In some of your patients you restricted phosphorus and there was not any increase in 1,25D levels. You did not show if there was a change in serum phosphorus; as you mentioned, others did not show any change in serum phosphorus either. As you know, it has been stated that it is the phosphorus load in the remaining nephrons which modulates the synthesis of 1,25D. Do you have any thoughts about what determines the change in those 1,25D levels, if not a change in serum phosphorus?

RESPONSE: This is a very complicated issue. What we would agree on is that if a patient has moderate renal insufficiency, if you can reduce phosphate, you can stimulate the synthesis of 1,25D or allow the 1,25D to return to a more normal level. In other words, with moderate renal failure, you have a significant suppression of 1,25D synthesis. What we also agree on is if you have severe renal failure, reducing the phosphate intake or reducing it by binding with aluminum hydroxide does not appear to change 1,25D synthesis. Now, what I did not do, I did not phosphate deplete those patients with severe renal failure. That is what you would almost need to do. Another study is much more elegant than mine. What they did was to give phosphate back and to show that the production of 1,25D could be suppressed. So, there is reasonable evidence that phosphate is an important factor in this. The problem with these types of studies is that they are looking at one factor of this considerable number of factors that actually contribute to the synthesis of 1,25D. If you look at this in the individual patient, it is probably a combination of the reduction in nephron mass and of the hyperphosphatemia that is going to change the levels of 1,25D. I really do not know how to interpret the data. I do not think that from the available data we can have the answer. What I was trying to show with my studies was that if you limit phosphate intake, you will probably have a slightly higher 1,25D value, and that that may be of benefit. Although I did show it, it was a short term study; I would not advocate leaving people on higher doses of aluminum hydroxide for long periods of time. If we have ways to limit phosphate intake, then this whole question of calcium carbonate, aluminum hydroxide and all of those things does not become as important. I do hope that all of us who are treating young infants who have chronic renal failure are using a formula somewhat similar to the one that was shown here, similar to PM 60-40, with a low phosphate content.

QUESTION: Along those lines, when do you start using phosphate binders? At what level of renal function do you start using vitamin D analogs and phosphate binders? Do you individualize it, or do you think that it should be used in mild, moderate, or just severe?

RESPONSE: This is a very difficult question. Obviously, when you are interested in a subject, you start doing it very early and you start looking at your data. In general, I think you have to be aware of the potential for bone disease in the young child who has renal failure. Certainly, we saw children with GFRs of 50 $ml/min/1.73m^2$ who had elevated PTHs and who had evidence of a decline in 1,25D levels. If you look at their bone histology you can see changes. In the young child who has that, we could certainly begin phosphate binders and usually at a level of 35 $ml/min/1.73^2$. We use the Schwartz' formula, as most of us do. We would go ahead and start a vitamin D analog cautiously. In the older child, in the child who has a focal sclerosis and comes to you with a creatinine of 5 or 6, often the period of time until he can be transplanted is so short, that we tend to treat hypocalcemia when it occurs. In other words, we obviously restrict phosphate, but if they become hypocalcemic, we treat that with a vitamin D analog. Very often it seems to me spinning the wheel to be treating a child, say a 15 year old girl with membranoproliferative G.N., for two months with a D analog when you know that she has a good match for a transplant.

COMMENT: I do not have a specific interest in this area but we still start earlier with treatment Part of the reason is that when we looked at what happened at the kidney level, looking at nephrogenous cyclic Amp as a measure of the biologic effect, we saw it very early. In children whose creatinines are 2 mg/dl whose function is at the level of 30-$35/m^2$, which is actually a little higher than what you have, we have become very aware of this. I think it is a lot easier to stay ahead of these children than to play catch-up further down the line.

QUESTION: At least in the adult population, cyclosporine seems to change the ratio of cadaveric versus living related donor transplants. Just hearing the discussion regarding transplantation over the last several days, I just wondered if that is true in the pediatric population or is there still aggressive use of living related transplants.

RESPONSE: The list of cadaveric recipients that we have at the University of Miami is quite small in pediatric renal failure patients who are potential transplant recipients. However, overall in the country as a whole there is an increase of cadaveric transplants being performed in pediatric patients. The truth, however, is that when you are presented with a pediatric patient that has a potential related donor, it is very hard to turn the donor down and put the patient on the cadaver list. My response is that whenever there is an available donor, we use the donor.

COMMENT: I think it depends on what section of the country you live in. There are some areas of the country that do predominantly live-related donor transplants with cyclosporine; there are other sections of the country that shy away from live-related donor transplants. They think it is unethical. If you look at the data and at what the transplant surgeons say, they talk with a "forked tongue". On the one hand they say cyclosporine is God's gift to humanity and we are getting 90 percent survival rate with cyclosporine; on the other hand, they are using cyclosporine for HLA identical sibling transplants, for live-related donor transplants. To me, those two concepts are incompatible. If cyclosporine is so good, we should stop doing live-related donor transplants and just do cadaver donor transplants if the results are what everybody says they are (90 percent or so). I believe that we need a little bit more time before we can really evaluate all the data that are available and find out what are the long-term effects of cyclosporine. We really do not know. As a matter of fact, the data in the literature with regard to the outcome of transplantation in pediatric patients with the use of cyclosporine with cadaver donor transplantation are not so good. If you look at results from one of this country's largest programs (which have not been published but were presented at the ASN meeting last year), one year's results were between 50 and 60 percent. In a couple of short reports from Europe, results with cadaver donor transplants have not been that outstanding. Some people have tried to intimate that maybe children do not handle cyclosporine as adults do. Others have tried to say that the reason their results with cyclosporine were not as good even as the results with azathioprine or prednisone reported from adults, was because there was a learning period, that it took a year or two of using cyclosporine before you really knew how to use the drug and then you could get the good results that everybody else has. I think that there really are minuscule data on the use of cyclosporine in the pediatric age group to really discuss it intelligently at the moment.

COMMENT: I basically agree that cyclosporine definitely is not the miracle drug that everybody was hoping for. Hopefully in the future, an analog of cyclosporine will be both more effective and less toxic than the present preparation. In those centers that traditionally had good results with conventional immunosuppression, cyclosporine did not prove to be very advantageous. I can mention several such centers as a matter of fact that have published their results. In our center here, we had always fairly good results with conventional immunosuppression; we have not really improved our graft survival with cyclosporine. Maybe we have seen less infections--opportunistic infections mainly--with the use of cyclosporine, but even that I am not really sure about. The only centers that have shown improvement of transplantation success rates with cyclosporine seem to be those centers which had very poor survival with conventional drugs; with the use of cyclosporine it became easier for them to achieve results comparable to the good centers.

QUESTION: In relation to the progression of chronic renal failure, when you have a reflux nephropathy in a child with not very severe renal failure, do you ever correct the reflux?

RESPONSE: The question is, if you have a child that has reflux but also has renal failure, do you correct the reflux? You could presumably want to correct the reflux for two or three reasons: 1) because you think that the course is going to change, and that he may not progress to renal failure; 2) because you hope that the number of infections that he may or may not have will change; 3) because you think that if the patient has persistent reflux, when he goes on to renal failure the transplant surgeon, will not want to transplant him without taking out his kidneys. I do not think that there is any reason to correct the reflux because I do not think that there is any evidence that correcting the reflux in any way changes the course to chronic renal failure. The group from the Mayo Clinic studied patients with a creatinine between 1.5 and 2.0, they fixed the reflux in some patients but not in others with the same degree of renal insufficiency. The progression rate to chronic renal insufficiency was exactly the same. So, once you have a patient who has reflux nephropathy and progressive renal insufficiency, the fact that he has reflux does not in any way affect the subsequent course. I do not think that there is a reason to do it. There are no data that I am aware of in the literature to indicate that correcting reflux has anything to do with subsequent infections. The incidence of infections, pre- or post-correction of reflux, whether the patient has renal failure or not, is essentially the same in almost every study that I have read. There might be some justification when you have a patient who has a creatinine of 1.7-2, a GFR of 30-40, reflux nephropathy, and you know that he is going to go on to renal insufficiency, but he has grade IV reflux (V reflux, or maybe III). Maybe it will be a good idea at that time (with a creatinine of 1.7-2) to correct the reflux so that when the patient comes to end stage disease you do not have to get into an argument with the transplant surgeon about whether or not they should transplant the patient with reflux. My bias would be that there is no problem in transplanting the patient with reflux; we do it all the time. There are some transplant surgeons who are reluctant to do that, so you can avoid that whole issue by reimplanting the patient. But, if you are reimplanting because you think that you are benefiting the patient, I think that there is no reason to do it.

COMMENT: I fully agree with what was just said. I would like to add a qualitative statement. In some occasional patients that have presented with reflux nephropathy, severe proteinuria, and focal segmental glomerulosclerosis, there have been some hypotheses on the effect of reflux immune complex nephropathy due to Tamm-Horsfall protein In fact, there was a recent publication in the American Journal of Medicine on this subject; but I think it is going to happen only in very occasional instances. I would like to comment on another aspect somebody raised: if these patients are going to go anyway to renal failure, are we not just delaying the time when they are going to come to dialysis? I agree and that is supported by our experience. I want to add a word of caution in terms of not being too optimistic that if you correct, even early in life, something from the mechanical aspect, that you have solved the problem. You probably have not taken care of what is going on in the kidney itself and that is going to lead that child to renal failure later on in life.

COMMENT: We do transplant patients with reflux. The only indication to remove those kidneys and ureters is if they have a persistent infection. If they do not have infection, then we feel comfortable in transplanting them.

QUESTION: Are you feeling more pressure to transplant smaller children, like below the age of two years now that CAPD keeps them going? We are getting a lot of developmental problems. Does transplant improve developmental aspects? We will not find out, I guess, unless we transplant the small ones. Are you feeling that pressure?

RESPONSE: In our particular group we are transplant-oriented, and we will transplant anybody who is available for transplantation. Especially in these little children that you mentioned, if there is a donor, a living-related donor, then we will not hesitate. I do not consider that as pressure, though. We currently have one little baby whom we are following; he is about 11 months, nine kg, and he has not been doing well on CAPD. He has not been growing very well, and has had multiple problems--infections, GI bleedings and so forth. I think that that is a definite indication for a transplant.

QUESTION: Are you using loading doses when starting out treatment for a routine peritonitis? When using Vancomycin if you give it too fast as a loading dose, you can get hives. The other question is, how long do you treat a routine peritonitis? Three days? A week?

RESPONSE: Our peritonitis protocol is as follows. We use a cephalosporine without any oral or parenteral supplementation. If, after 48 hours, there is no significant improvement--by that I mean the bags are still cloudy or the patient is symptomatic--we automatically add an amino glycoside at the same dose (6-8 mg/L) because that is the level we want to maintain. We treat patients with uncomplicated peritonitis by a gram positive organism; just with a cephalosporine for 10 days. It is actually 12 days because at 10 days we take a culture and two days later, if the culture is negative, then we stop the treatment. If the patient has a gram negative organism, then he is treated for two to three weeks. In addition, if the patient has a staph aureus, because of the problems that we have seen with this organism, he is given intravenous antibiotics initially and then orally for five to seven days; no loading dose is necessary.

QUESTION: Even though you do not find out about the staph aureus peritonitis for a day or two, you have them come into the hospital to get the parenteral medication?

RESPONSE: If we find out and the patients are home, then we would put them on oral antibiotics. Depending on how the patients are doing, we may just give them oral supplementation at home. But usually patients with staph aureus peritonitis are in the hospital because they often present with significant symptomatology and fever; they do not clear up the fluid in 48 hours, etc.

QUESTION: I wanted to raise the question about candida albicans in the peritoneum in children on CAPD, and actually throw this open to whoever has had any experience with it. We have found this to be extremely difficult to get rid of. I wonder what the panelists think.

RESPONSE: We have had two cases and in both instances we have lost the peritoneum. I think that we contributed to the loss of the peritoneum because we tried to eradicate the infection with amphotericin which I think may be toxic. I do not know, but that is the feeling that I have. Our modus operandi at the moment, if we get candida in the peritoneum, is to immediately pull the catheter. I think that anybody who tries to treat it intraperitoneally leaving the catheter in runs the significant risk of loss of peritoneum. Once we pull the catheter, depending on the clinical symptoms, we either treat them with parenteral amphotericin or try to use one of the other antifungal agents systemically. After two to three weeks, if things are stable, we put another catheter in.

RESPONSE: We do exactly the same. Our first thought is to get the catheter out of there. We will then keep the child off dialysis for as long as we physiologically can because we have found that moving right back in through a different route, i.e. putting a cannula in a subclavian or femoral vessel for hemodialysis, also gets infected. We try and wait about five or six days, then go to hemodialysis, and finally back to the peritoneum.

COMMENT: It sounds like we are doing the right thing.

COMMENT-QUESTION: I would like to have some discussion on the point that was made, that pediatric patients tolerate higher doses of immunosuppression. Personally, I do not like the concept because I think that pediatric patients may tolerate it but I looked at your list of infections; they did not tolerate it so well. I think that it depends on what you mean by tolerating it. Do you mean that they do not die from overwhelming infection or do you mean that they are growing as well as they could grow if we did not give them such high doses of immunosuppression? I think the whole concept of children tolerating more immunosuppression is reflective upon the fact that in an adult patient, similar doses of immunosuppression may cause overwhelming infection. An overwhelming infection in a 55 year old is going to cause demise much more readily than it will in a younger patient. But, I do not think that that justifies us giving inordinate doses of immunosuppression to a young patient.

COMMENT: I want to clarify that I am not advocating higher doses of immunosuppression in children. We had only two children of 33 patients who were admitted to the hospital because of severe high fever, and we found that they had CMV or other opportunistic infection. So, the incidence of infection in our pediatric patients was really quite low. The incidence of sepsis of 10 percent is from another center and not from ours. What we are saying by the concept "increased tolerance to immunosuppression" is that it is much easier with the same per kg dose of Medrol, let us say, to kill an adult without opportunistic infection than it is to cause the opportunistic infection in children and, therefore, their demise as a result. What I am saying is that we are not worried about treating a rejection in children or a second rejection or even a third rejection with high doses of steroids as long as we are following the T_4/T_8 ratios and we know that they are not already immunosuppressed. When the ratio starts decreasing and becomes inverted, then it does not matter whether it is a child or an adult;if there is evidence that the person is already immunosuppressed, the danger for opportunistic infection is very real.

QUESTION: Isn't the more relevant question whether or not children require more immunosuppression to maintain their grafts?

RESPONSE: Our immunosuppressive protocol is that we start off with 0.5 mg/kg body weight. When we compared our current data to our data from when we were using 3 mg/kg to start with, our one year survival rates were the same. What the patients looked like was considerably different. Children can tolerate a lot, but I am not sure that justifies the fact that we do it or that it means that they really need it. I think the tendency is to give less and less immunosuppression; that would be my pitch.

COMMENT: I definitely agree with that. There are many centers now where they are starting out with a maintenance dose of Medrol and they do not load their patients at the beginning. Unquestionably, it is a controversial topic. We do feel comfortable, and again that is based on our experience, that it is safe to start out with a large dose because most of the rejections and loss of kidney happens initially, as everybody knows. Therefore, we feel comfortable in starting out at large doses. However, most of our patients, if we look at them a year after transplant, are taking a minimal dose of Medrol; they are down to 0.2 mg/kg or sometimes even less, depending on their immune responsiveness, their incidence of infections, rejections, and so forth.

COMMENT: We share your concern about the possibility of over immuno-suppressing our patients and, as was mentioned, our incidence of infection is very low. On the other hand, although your number of patients is huge compared to other pediatric areas, your two year survival is around 50 percent, while in this area it is close to 100 percent. So, that also must be considered.

COMMENT: To add to that, it is the discriminate use of immunosuppression that is important, and not the dose. What we have found out retrospectively is that you can give high doses (if you have to) to children without harming them as much as you harm the adults. But, definitely we are not advocating that children should be on higher doses. As I already mentioned, at one year they are taking very, very little immunosuppression with cyclosporine as well as with conventional therapy.

COMMENT: That is difficult. In the 33 patients that you have done, 29 of them have been live-related donor. You have treated the majority of the live-related donor transplants with ATG, Medrol and "relatively high dose steroids". With the protocol with donor specific transfusions (DST) and with live-related donors, one could possibly not need any ATG and have a considerably less dose of prednisone. You did not show what your growth data were during the first year or two and how much adverse effect the high dose steroid had. It is not a cut and dried issue. It is difficult to extrapolate what is one's experience and make generalized statements. Certainly the results that you have obtained are superb. The question is, is there a similar way you can get those results without the risks that maybe you are taking. That is the only point I wanted to make.

COMMENT: There is no question that DST with immunosuppression could be in the future the way to treat all transplant patients who receive a kidney transplant from a living donor. I agree with you. We have not initiated that because we are happy with our present results. As far as growth is concerned, maybe one of my pediatric colleagues can comment on that. One of our small children has shown evidence of quite a bit of growth but I do not have any data; my impressions are anecdotal.

COMMENT: Our data also are anecdotal. We have to go over all carefully. We do not have data on the growth rate accurately charted.

QUESTION: To clarify this in my mind, are you doing DSTs on all living-related donors or only those with high mixed lymphocytes?

COMMENTS: With regard to living-related donors, I do not think it makes much difference whether they are high or low responders. Most people now are just doing the high responders; we are doing both the low and high responders. Any one haplotype.

COMMENT: I want to go back to one of the talks we heard today. I appreciate the emphasis on the relationship between protein and calories. My ideas and maybe yours have been changed about calorie supplements; the emphasis is that it is important to give adequate nutrition. If we give calorie supplements, especially at a time when growth velocity is not high normally--children who are greater than three years of age and who are in the adolescent pre-pubertal stage--that we might end up making them fat. That is not a good thing. I was giving high calorie supplements to that group of patients. I think now that those high supplements caused one patient to rapidly progress in his pubertal development, and he never achieved any increase in growth velocity. Calorie supplements may be detrimental, stimulate production of hormones, and limit the patient's ultimate height. Since the height is not going to be great to start with, we do not want to make it worse. We might still be in the hieroglyphic phases of our knowledge of nutrition and uremia, but our data and that presented are similar. It is a fact that nitrogen retention is increased at a greater rate when you are in negative nitrogen balance and the cost of that retention in terms of energy is greater and it levels off as you improve your nitrogen balance . It is good that that is true in uremia, but the lingering question is, is it different in the uremic as opposed to the normal? Is the calorie cost of nitrogen retention greater or is the nitrogen cost of nitrogen retention greater in the uremic?

COMMENT: If you correct for the status of the child at the moment, I have yet to find very much difference between the uremic child and the normal child. Their rates of change, in a post-surgical stage, are very similar to what was found in normal adults post-surgically. The efficiency of utilization at different stages seems to be the same as in some of the studies done in adults. I have not found them to be that inefficient even though I expected that we would. They really are very close to normal provided that we do not overwhelm them.

QUESTION: To go back to problems with cyclosporine therapy, what is the name of the unique amino acid at the 1 position?

RESPONSE: I do not know. It should be called paralamine. It is called "C-9 ene" meaning athalene bonding, but it does not have a specific name.

QUESTION: Do you feel that children who have had the hemolytic uremic syndrome and are getting a transplant should not be treated with CSA?

RESPONSE: I definitely do. We just had a child come to us with hemolytic uremia for living-related donor transplant and we elected to give the child azathioprine and specific transfusions. I do not think these children should received cyclosporine.

QUESTION: May I ask why?

RESPONSE: There have been several reports of recurrent hemolytic uremic syndrome in cyclosporine treated patients apparently related to the capacity of cyclosporine to decrease the production of prostacyclin stimulating factor. The first report was from Vienna, but this has been confirmed by a number of people. Now someone is sure to stand up and tell me, "But there was one report which said that they did a hemolytic uremic patient and did not have recurrent disease". Unfortunately, in my transplant practice, I cannot afford to take that kind of chance; namely, 10 positive reports and one negative. So I would not recommend it.

COMMENT-QUESTION: I know of at least five reports. You did not address questions about hypertension and CYA. all of us who have used CYA are curious about your thoughts on hypertension and the mechanism leading to it.

RESPONSE: It is said to be low renin hypertension. Our problem in analyzing the hypertension is that we have such a high incidence of hypertension in our azathioprine-prednisone treated children that we could not clearly see any increase in hypertension in the cyclosporine treated group. When we looked in the adults, however, we did see a difference in that the adults treated with cyclosporine had a much higher requirement for blood pressure medications. Their mean blood pressures were not higher, but they required more medications in higher doses of beta blocker, vasodilators and diuretics. Interestingly enough, when we examined the adults over the course of several years, by two years post transplant the azathioprine group and the cyclosporine group were comparable. The initial hypertension seems to be more of a problem early after transplant in adults. In children we cannot see a difference between the conventional and the cyclosporine groups. In children we do have a big problem with hypertension; I think some of that is related to fluid and salt problems in addition to the drug therapy.

COMMENT-QUESTION: I am delighted to see a surgeon come to the rescue of our pediatric patients in the sense that you are trying to explain elevated serum creatinine on a basis other than poor compliance on the part of pediatric patients. For some pediatric patients it seems to be, indeed, an inherent problem with bioavailability. We have been facing that problem since we also use cyclosporine in some of our patients. One explanation which has been given is the children do not take the medications, thus let's not transplant them again. I am sure you know that with corticosteroids some people have found that children seem to tolerate higher doses proportional to weight; higher doses are required to invert the H/S ratio as compared to adults. Have you found something similar with cyclosporine? Is the child's tolerance to cyclosporine higher than that of adults?

RESPONSE: Basically, that is what we are saying. You have made a good point: our results in pediatric transplantation have been excellent with azathioprine and prednisone. Most of you have very good results in pediatric transplantation, and the reason is what was just said: children tolerate a lot more corticosteroids than adults do. Therefore, you can really blast them for rejection, and do other things which in adults would not be possible. The only reason for wanting to get away from that strategy is to see if we can improve growth in these children by reducing the amount of corticosteroids they take. That is the reason for looking at cyclosporine. Regarding your question, "Will children tolerate more cyclosporine", that is inherent in what I am saying. We are giving much more cyclosporine to children than we are to adults. We are using prolonged intravenous infusions of 4 mg/kg for usually three weeks; this is much more than we are giving to adults. When we measure half-lives, a child's half-life is much shorter so children are getting higher doses; there is no question about it. The only thing I caution you about is that it is better to make the total dose intravenously, not to give them an enormous dose by mouth. It would be a tragedy if we got back to the days of giving 20 or 25 mg/kg by mouth to a child. They will tolerate more cyclosporine, maybe more than the 14 mg/kg that I am giving them, but I would not go to very high doses because I would be afraid of complications.

QUESTION: I may have heard wrong, and it may be that you made a Freudian slip. Let me ask you to please clarify that. You mentioned that growth was different in the population getting cyclosporine. You did not imply or think that it was the cyclosporine inducing the growth, did you? It was that they were taking less corticosteroid, so there is no question about it having no effect on growth results.

RESPONSE: There are no questions from our data that the cyclosporine treated children are receiving half or less than half the corticosteroid than the children previously treated with azathioprine. Yes, that is right. In a letter in Lancet about a month ago acceleration of growth was observed in a very small series (I think only five pediatric patients were treated) but a marked acceleration of growth upon transplantation was noticed. Some raised the possibility that cyclosporine exerted a pro-androgen effect which actually increased growth. There are some effects of cyclosporine at the level of the CNS; they are not well documented but there are changes in CSF, in prolactin and other hormones, suggesting that cyclosporine has some central effects. So I should not say absolutely that cyclosporine has no growth promotion; it is possible. The steroid sparing is a fact. It is possible that there is a pro-androgen effect and this should be looked at particularly in pediatric patients. I think serial hormone levels would be worth doing (prolactin levels and androgen levels).

QUESTION: Do you think that a patient who has been on a donor specific transfusion (DST) protocol is at any special risk by receiving cyclosporine after transplantation?

RESPONSE: You mean for living-related donor? My interpretation of that strategy is that you are taking the risks of DST and the risks of cyclosporine and getting the benefits of neither. The benefit of giving DST is that you do not have to give cyclosporine. The benefit of giving cyclosporine is that you do not have to give DST and take a chance of sensitizing a patient. If I did a DST protocol for a child (I am very much against them because they tend to sensitize patients), I would just treat that child with azathioprine post-transplant even if he were not sensitized. I do not think that there is any risk in cyclosporine therapy but it is a hazard the child does not need if he has already been protected or conditioned by DST.

QUESTION: Even in a high risk patient? Is that what you would do? If you keep him on a DST protocol you would not put him post-transplant on cyclosporine A therapy?

RESPONSE: No. If I have treated a patient with DST and he has a negative cross-match after three transfusions, I would use azathioprine because the results are very good with azathioprine once the patient has been conditioned by DST. On the other hand, I am totally against DST except for cases of hemolytic uremic syndrome. I never use DST, and I think you are much better off to proceed immediately with the transplant and just use cyclosporine without any transfusion.

QUESTIONS: Do you suggest doing a pharmacokinetic study in all children whether they are getting live or cadaveric transplants?

RESPONSE: Yes, I do.

QUESTION: Is it the same group that has absorptive problems that has elimination problems?

RESPONSE: No, it is not. They are overlapping groups but one does not define the other group. I mean one does not necessarily mean the other.

QUESTION: Can you make any comments on whether any of the children you reported have been on chronic anticonvulsant therapy?

RESPONSE: I did not discuss that in detail because it was not necessary for them to have had anticonvulsant therapy to have rapid elimination times. However, it is clear that children treated chronically with dilantin or phenobarbital will have rapid elimination times by activation of P450. I think it is more significant to know that many of the children who had rapid elimination times were never treated with anti-seizure medications, never received any P450 activators such as isoniazide or rifampin or any other drugs that are known to be P450 activators.

QUESTION: Would you comment on measurements of cyclosporine levels by the radioimmune assay versus the HPLC method? Which method do you personally use?

RESPONSE: This question really is two questions: the first is HPLC versus RIA, and the second is whole blood versus serum. In terms of HPLC versus RIA, our preference is for the radioimmune assay. Our very simple problem is that we have a thousand blood levels to do a week at our center and we just have not been able to hire 16 chimpanzees with HPLC machines working all day round. As you know, the HPLC takes about 25 minutes to do by the time you wash the column, prepare it, and do it each time, and we just cannot do HPLC tests on all of our patients. Column switching techniques have been introduced to cut this time down but it is still way out of the range for a thousand samples a week.

Regarding the question of whole blood versus serum, we prefer serum. As you know, the majority of cyclosporine in the blood, after it has been absorbed, is associated with erythrocytes. As the hematocrit changes (which happens in end-stage renal disease patients), obviously the amount of cyclosporine in the total blood changes rapidly. In addition, what we are really interested in is a trough value--in other words, what is not on cytoplasmic receptors. The way in which we constructed the value of 100 ng/ml was, we looked at the concentration of cyclosporine that we had to add to a mixed lymphocyte culture reaction to cause 50 percent inhibition. We reasoned that since this is not a cidal drug, it is a static drug, we wanted to achieve that concentration as a baseline, as a trough. We think we can measure the trough best if we look at plasma or what you might call the free, not cell associated cyclosporine. So, our recommendation has been to look at serum radioimmune assay levels. Each center develops its own strategy; after you see enough of these values, you learn how to use them. I can tell you that they are not 100 percent reliable. You will see a patient with high trough values who has unequivocal rejection because he has poor pharmacodynamic handling of cyclosporine, and you will see some patients with low levels who do very well and never have a rejection episode. Levels are just a useful guide; they are just another parameter in the clinical picture. But those are my preferences.

QUESTION: I would like to focus on your last comments. In your slides you recommended that we keep the blood levels between one and two hundred. You have recommended that for a long time, as have other people. Yet in the paper that you published with your pediatric experience, almost every patient long-term had blood levels around 50. That seems to me to mean that either we do not need the high levels which everyone is recommending initially, cyclosporine is inducing some kind of a tolerance effect, or cyclosporine is accumulating and has its immunosuppressive effect as it accumulates, with time. If the latter is true, then possibly the toxicity will also accumulate with time. It is difficult for me to understand why a patient needs a blood level of one to two hundred at one point post-transplant but at another point post-transplant he can tolerate a blood level of 200--if the drug is doing the same thing.

RESPONSE: We do need to clarify this. We have advocated only that you keep a level of 100 to 250 for roughly the first two months. After that we generally let the levels drift. The children who were reported who had low levels, generally were much further out. In other words, we are talking about where they were at the time of reporting. Most of them were about 50. At the time that paper was written they were 18 months out; now they are over two years out. We believe in a very high level initially, this 100-200 range, and then we tend to back off from there as we follow the taper. You have pointed out a very important aspect of this which deserved more detail or some explanation. Cyclosporine has some important metabolites which are not detected by the HPLC and by the radioimmune assay. In time, cyclosporine metabolism changes such that these metabolites are generalized and parent compound is eliminated even more rapidly. That is the reason the levels tend to drift down. If you measure these metabolites, you can see them appearing in higher concentration than you had before. It is these metabolites that have strong immunosuppressive action. What could be happening in some of the pediatric patients who have very low levels initially and have not rejected is that they are already keyed in and metabolizing in the proper direction generating those immunosuppressive metabolites and, therefore, not rejecting. On the other hand, a large number of the patients are not metabolizing in the right direction because the low levels are associated with a high incidence of rejection, presumably, because they are not generating the proper metabolites.

QUESTION: Some transplant centers are now using cyclosporine in combination with both corticosteroids and azathioprine. The reason given is that they can use lower doses of both azathioprine and Cyclo A. Would you comment on this approach.

RESPONSE: That strategy emanates primarily from the desire to minimize nephrotoxicity. It was started in England, basically with one mg/kg of azathioprine, 6 mg/kg of cyclosporine and the normal prednisone regimen dealt with before. What was found was that there was the same allograft survival (in one year it was 70%), but a much lower incidence of nephrotoxicity. The problem that I see in applying that regimen in children is first, that even on full dose, cyclosporine does not have very good drug absorption or drug levels. Secondly, nephrotoxicity has not been a major problem; our major problem has been getting immunosuppression, getting adequate amounts of cyclosporine in. While that strategy may be promising in the adult, it does not seem to be useful in children. Our problem is the opposite.

COMMENT-QUESTION: I am amazed by the fact that you do not see hypertension.

RESPONSE: I did not say that. I said I saw hypertension but it was exactly the same incidence and severity as it was in the azathioprine-prednisone treated children.

COMMENT-QUESTION: We have six children, all under 10, who have been treated with cyclosporine; all but one had been hypertensive. We have switched three of these children over to azathioprine; two of them came off three antihypertensives and one of them came off two. That was during the switch-over at six months.

RESPONSE: There is no any question that if you switch patients from cyclosporine to azathioprine you will improve their renal function and improve their hypertension. On the other hand, there is no question that that group in graft survival will now return to the azathioprine line, and the mean survival of the graft is about a year. I can show you the curve in which you can see that these grafts are being lost at six months, nine months post transplant in the azathioprine treated child. As another speaker pointed out, this has been the reason for triple drug regimens. My own recommendation is, if you feel that the hypertension is so limiting, then reduce the cyclosporine to 5 mg/kg; if the patient still has continued hypertension and renal dysfunction, start azathioprine at 1 mg/kg, and continue to reduce the cyclosporine down to 3 mg/kg progressively. At 3 mg/kg, we find that most of the hypertension problems will go away and some of the renal dysfunction will improve. There we are using azathioprine as a kind umbrella yet we still have some cyclosporine effect. But I would not encourage you to totally convert patients; I think this is dangerous. I have very sobering life tables which I can dig out if someone wants to see them. I admit to you that the initial result is great, but when you follow these patients further out, they lose their grafts; you know it is a tragedy to lose a graft.

MODERATOR: We must end now. Thank you.

VII

WORKSHOP

WORKSHOP: FOUR CASES

Jose Strauss, M.D., Moderator

MODERATOR: The first case will be presented by Dr. Norman Siegel.

DR. SIEGEL: This was the first hospital admission for a 12 year old black female for evaluation of proteinuria and edema. The patient had been previously well and the past medical history and family history were non-contributory. Four months prior to admission, the patient noted some headaches and ankle swelling while visiting in Pennsylvania, was seen there, diagnosed as having a urinary tract infection and treated with sulfamethoxazole. During the next two months she felt relatively well, although noticing continued weight gain from her "usual weight of 110 to 115 pounds". One month prior to admission the patient saw a physician because of puffiness. Her weight was 130 pounds, blood pressure 128/80 mmHg, and mild periorbital and ankle edema were noted. Urinalysis revealed a few red cells/HPF, many white cells/HPF, and 3+ albumin. She was given sulfamethoxazole and sent home. Ten days later the patient was seen again because of increasing periorbital and ankle edema. Her weight was 140 pounds, blood pressure 140/94 mmHg, urinalysis with 5-10 red cells/HPF, and 4+ albumin; BUN 17 mg/dl and creatinine 1.1 mg/dl, Hgb 13 g/dl, WBC 6,500/mm^3. Approximately one week later, her weight was 142 pounds, blood pressure 142/94 mmHg, urinalysis with 8-10 red cells/HPF, and 4+ albumin.

Physical examination on admission: Weight 65.3 kg (143.6 lbs), height 160 cm, blood pressure 156/100 mmHg, pulse 76/min, respirations 20/min. General: An edematous black female in no distress. HEENT: Slight A-V nicking in the right fundus and some carious teeth. CHEST: Pubertal breast development without masses. LUNGS: Decreased excursion on inspiration and expiration with bilaterally decreased breath sounds in the bases. HEART: Normal sinus rhythm without murmur, second sound with a physiologic split; pulses 2+ and symmetrical. ABDOMEN: Markedly protuberant with fluid wave, soft, no masses felt, liver and spleen were not palpable. GENITALIA: Normal, pubertal female; Tanner Stage II. EXTREMITIES: Four plus pitting edema from ankle to knees, bilaterally; 3+ edema of the sacrum to the thoracic vertebrae. NEUROMUSCULAR: Within normal limits.

LABORATORY DATA: Chest x-ray: bilateral pleural effusions, right greater than left. Lung fields with normal pulmonary vascularity without evidence of congestion. Serum: BUN 52 mg/dl, creatinine 3.5 mg/dl, electrolytes within normal limits, total protein 4.4 gm/dl, albumin 1.3 gm/dl, globulin 3.1 gm/dl, cholesterol 369 mg/dl, liver function tests within normal limits. Urine: 24 hour urine collection with 6.8 g protein, vol. 400 ml. Urinalysis with 3+ protein, moderate occult blood, specific gravity 1028, sediment 25-30 white cells/HPF, 8-12 red cells/HPF, multiple hyaline, granular and cellular casts, and multiple maltese crosses. Serological data: ASLO 50 units, AHT 128 units, ANA negative, serum complement 130 mg/dl (control 109 ± 31). Cultures: Throat and urine, negative. Hematology: Hemoglobin 13.4 g/dl, hematocrit 40.5%, WBC 6,100/mm^3, differential within normal limits, platelets 290,000/mm^3, PT and PTT within normal limits, fibrinogen 1035 mg/dl. I would be happy to entertain any suggestions as to what her problem might be.

COMMENT: In looking at her CBC, given the fact that she has a normal hematocrit, I would guess that she has acute rather than chronic renal failure, but the latter goes along with her relatively prolonged course of a couple of months. I guess in the old days this would have been called a nephritic- nephrotic. Given the fact that her complements are normal and her ANA is normal, she presumably does not have a collagen vascular disease. My suggestion, besides giving her some reasonable dietary restriction, as far as her renal failure is concerned, would be to biopsy her.

DR. SIEGEL: Any other questions or suggestions in terms of her problem? Any other tests you might want?

COMMENT: I would not call her a nephritic-nephrotic. One thing I would worry about would be a nephrotic who develops massive edema; he then could develop edematous kidneys which could be a cause of renal failure but usually this would be reversible by getting off some of the edema with i.v. albumin.

COMMENT: Any other suggestions.

QUESTION: It would be interesting to know her erythrosedimentation rate.

RESPONSE: Her sedimentation rate was elevated.

COMMENT: The reason I asked this was because of the possibility of Wegener's Granulomatosis.

RESPONSE: She had no evidence of naso-pharyngeal lesions and her chest x-ray was normal except for the pleural effusions. There were no intrapulmonary lesions present.

QUESTION-COMMENT: Since our pathologist requires a clinical impression, how many people think this patient might have had minimal change disease? How many think that she probably had a proliferative disorder and acute glomerulonephritis? How many think she might have had a rapidly progressive or crescentic glomerulonephritis? The proportion here is about what the renal group thought; nobody knew what she had and everybody was willing to guess. So, we did perform a biopsy after her blood pressure was controlled. Bowman's capsule was perfectly normal and she definitely did not have a crescentic glomerulonephritis. The capillary loops were widely patent; they were not thickened in a diffuse manner and the nuclei were randomly distributed; there was a little bit of widening of the mesangium. The tubules appeared normal. This patient had Minimal Change Nephrotic Syndrome. I presented this case because patients with Minimal Change Disease have been reported in the last few years as presenting in Acute Renal Failure or with acutely compromised renal function. The mechanism of that is not well known or understood; it is felt that they have swelling of the kidney usually associated with massive anasarca, as was present in this girl. She responded beautifully to a course of corticosteroids; she began to have a diuresis on about day five; she did not require treatment with albumin. As of today, she has had about six relapses of her disease but has absolutely normal renal function and continues to respond to steroid therapy about once every two years when she has a relapse.

MODERATOR: Talking about "the old days", I worked with Dr. Conrad Riley at Babies' Hospital in New York; he was a great believer in the erythrosedimentation rate in terms of diagnosing a relapse or remission. If you follow the sed rate, you are going to find that most times it is elevated, even in Minimal Change Disease and for unknown reasons, probably for the same non-specific reasons that alpha 2 macroglobulin is elevated.

QUESTION: When this girl had her recurrences, did she get the same azotemia each time?

RESPONSE: No, she did not. We treated her for the first relapse after only a couple of days of proteinuria, although that has not been our policy in most cases. We did not allow her to get massively edematous. She has had a full blown relapse, including edema, on a couple of occasions over the past several years and has not developed a renal insufficiency component. Regarding disease progression, we have to be very cautious about the use of a non-steroidal, anti-inflammatory drug. There is no question that renal insufficiency can be induced in the nephrotic patient with the use of a non-steroidal anti-inflammatory agent. We have seen, in the adult population, two elderly ladies who presented with Acute Renal Failure of unknown etiology and on biopsy did not have substantial interstitial inflammation but they had been on a non-steroidal anti-inflammatory drug. And, after the drug was withdrawn, they regained their renal function only to show us a Nephrotic Syndrome. We have to be very cautious also about drugs like indomethacin which have actually been used to treat the Nephrotic Syndrome, because they can induce a rapid loss of renal function in the nephrotic patient.

QUESTION: The heart size on x-ray I think is critical: if it is normal, is that strongly against it being a nephritic process with real fluid retention as opposed to the nephrotic edema?

RESPONSE: She certainly had some nephritic components. The relative oliguria and the hypertension had us thinking that we could not differentiate, certainly it was not a pure nephrotic syndrome. The reports on this end of the "impure" nephrotic syndrome suggest that it is due to massive swelling of the kidney which causes the compromised renal function and all these other problems secondarily, and they can be made to go away just by getting rid of the edema.

COMMENT: I know that has been the proposed scenario. I am not sure how carefully it has been proven but it certainly is well described.

QUESTION: You thought it was Minimal Change, that was your clinical diagnosis. Did you feel comfortable enough with that diagnosis to have treated the patient with prednisone without biopsing her?

RESPONSE: I would biopsy the patient. There were two things that came together in the patient to make me think that it was Minimal Lesion. I wonder if the group here can challenge them? Acute Renal Failure or renal failure with a specific gravity of 1028 and an ASO titer of 50, which is less than normal for that age child, to me means Minimal Lesion. I am wondering if anybody has seen that with a specific gravity that high and an ASO titer that low?

MODERATOR: But the specific gravity with so much protein, do you pay any attention to it?

RESPONSE: If you got a lot of protein, that protein would add 0.002/g%; it is not going to add all that much.

COMMENT: I think you could see that in the very early stages of a Post Streptococcal GN, but the ASO was low; tubular function is relatively well preserved in those patients.

COMMENTS: It is the combination of those two things. It is not even a normal ASO titer; or it is much lower than you would expect for a child of 12.

COMMENT: I said that this was Minimal Change Nephrotic Syndrome only because a month ago I took care of a child who did the same trick after a year and a half of recurrent course of what I thought was Minimal Change Nephrotic Syndrome. Without a biopsy and after some kind of non-specific gastrointestinal infection with some vomiting, she came to the hospital very, very edematous, in relapse, being on every other day prednisone, and under our eyes, over a two and a half day period, her BUN went to 57 mg/dl, the creatinine was almost 3 mg/dl. At this point, obviously, I got nervous because I really did not have a histologic diagnosis of Minimal Change. We gave her albumin and we gave her steroids, and in three days she diuresed and the creatinine came down over maybe 10 days to 0.6 mg/dl. I did biopsy her, at this point just to see, because we also discussed what it could be in addition to her Nephrotic Syndrome. She did have some tubular changes, very focal, some atrophic changes, very little degenerative changes in the proximal tubules. Several years ago, I had a similar case, a child with peritonitis and nephrosis who also developed severe renal failure. At that time, I found a paper stating that radionuclide studies with hippuran could differentiate acute reversible failure from chronic nephritis. I wonder if anybody knows about it?

RESPONSE: I am not aware of that paper. In the type of patient that you just described, one would have to be very careful in because that patient may have had classical ATN. It seems to me that the children who are edematous and have low serum albumins are very sensitive to other sources of intravascular fluid loss, especially diarrhea, and can become hypotensive with considerably less vomiting or diarrhea than the average patient. We have had two children who were in relapse of their disease and developed a common gastroenteritis; by the time they got to the Emergency Room, they were hypotensive because with low albumin, they really cannot mobilize peripheral edema into their intravascular space. Some of the cases that have been reported as swelling of the kidney may have been cases that have a superimposed ATN due to something else going on. And some of them are also cases where the patients have gotten a prostaglandin inhibitor and have an underlying Nephrotic Syndrome. I think all three of those things happen--the classical swelling of kidneys, ATN induced by what we think would be less of an injury or less a stress than usual, and taking prostaglandin inhibitor.

MODERATOR: You described hypertension in about 20% of children with Nephrotic Syndrome. How do you explain it?

RESPONSE: I do not know exactly how to explain the hypertension that you see in the nephrotic patient. I wish there was a good way to be able to study intravascular volume. As you know, the studies that have been done have shown about a third with an increased intravascular volume, a third normal, and a third with low intravascular volume. It does not seem to have a correlation with the blood pressure, particularly. I am not sure of the pathophysiologic mechanisms by which the patients become hypertensive. Certainly, with a massive degree of anasarca, one would have to assume that the patient was volume overloaded.

MODERATOR: Can you say that just because of the anasarca?

RESPONSE: No, I am not saying that I can. I am saying that I would have made that assumption initially.

MODERATOR: The Cornell group found high renins in some of these patients; that is consistent with the assumption that most nephrotics are volume contracted. But, they also found normal and even low renins in other patients; I believe they concluded that their blood volumes were normal or even increased.

RESPONSE: I think you can find anything you would like in terms of renins and aldosterones, and you can find anything you would like in terms of plasma volumes. The true pathophysiology of the syndrome is not well worked out. Part of our problem is being able to study these patients in a steady state. One of the problems that we have is being able to have a nephrotic patient in a relatively steady state so that we can measure the variables that have to be measured and interpreted to make sense out of renins and aldosterones. The other problem is that there is no adequate measure of intravascular volume that is applicable in these patients.

QUESTION: What about the possibility of it being lupus?

RESPONSE: I do not think that it would be likely to be lupus because the antinuclear antibody was negative and the serum complement was normal. I would have expected at least one of those to be abnormal if it were a case of lupus with severe renal failure.

MODERATOR: The next case (#2) will be presented by Dr. Carolyn Abitbol.

DR. ABITBOL: The patient is a 14 year old girl who was referred from Bogota, Colombia with a two month history of fever to 39.5° C. requiring hospitalization in Colombia for evaluation. At that time laboratory data included a urinalysis which showed blood and pus cells and the diagnosis of urinary tract infection was entertained. Urine culture, however, was subsequently negative. She was treated with antibiotics, initially, on the assumption that she did have a urinary tract infection. She did not seem to improve symptomatically after the antibiotic therapy. After 10 days, the fever recurred and she was readmitted to the hospital in Bogota, where she was treated with IM Chloramphenicol for 8 days. She continued to have fevers and an active urinary sediment. Throughout the two month period her symptoms continued to include undulating fevers, as well as night sweats, associated anorexia, and a 4 to 5 kg weight loss.

A summary of her laboratory data obtained in Colombia during her hospitalizations is as follows: C reactive protein positive, C3 complement 95 mg/dl with a normal range of 60-120, VDRL negative, ANA negative, LE prep negative, Toxoplasma titers negative, febrile agglutinins negative, mono spot test negative, bleeding profile normal, IVP normal, CT scan of the abdomen negative. Serial sed rates and hemograms were as follows: in June 1984, ESR 38 mm/hr; on July 4, 1984, ESR 33 mm/hr; on July 16, 1984, ESR 45 mm/hr; hemoglobin 35.6 g/dl, WBC 9,300/mm^3 with 3% eosinophiles. On June 26, 1984, serum creatinine was 2.2 mg/dl with a BUN of 43 mg/dl and a urinalysis which showed too numerous to count red cells and one to three mixed cellular and hyaline casts. The most recent laboratory exam prior to referral showed a serum creatinine of 1.2 mg/dl, with urinalysis showing persistent cellular casts.

Upon her arrival in the U.S., the patient began experiencing some pain in the left leg which began in the hips and radiated down the posterior thigh. The pain had become so severe in the few days prior to her initial visit to our Medical Center that she was unable to walk and required the assistance of a wheel chair.

Past medical history: Birth weight was 5 pounds. She was the product of an uncomplicated pregnancy of a gravida 1, para 0, aborta 0 mother who was Rh negative and required RHOGAM after the pregnancy. Her childhood illnesses have been minimal and she has not had varicella. She has previously required no hospitalizations for major illnesses, other than the current illness. She began her menses this year at the age of 14 and during the past two months had menstruation more frequently than monthly.

Family history: The mother is 33 years old, the father is 40 years, and there is one male sibling who is well and 11 years of age.

On physical examination the patient was a very cachetic, ill-appearing, pale, young female. She was afebrile. Blood pressure was 100/60 mmHg. Weight was 93 7/8 pounds or 43 kg. Height was 60 3/4 inches. HEENT examination was normal. Chest was clear to auscultation. Breasts were small without masses. Cardiac exam: Grade 2/6 systolic ejection flow murmur at the left lower sternal border; no gallops were audible. Abdomen was slightly rotund, although no fluid wave was demonstrated; spleen was not palpable; liver was palpable four cms below the right costal margin and was non-tender. GU exam: Tanner Stage IV. Extremities showed trace edema. Neurological examination was difficult to perform although she seemed oriented and was appropriate in terms of her response to the situation. Cranial nerves were intact. Gait and station were not performed due to the patient's inability to stand. Sensory examination was intact to a pin prick and light touch. The muscles were wasted in all extremities. Reflexes were 2-3+ and equal bilaterally. There seemed to be two to three beats of clonus at the ankles.

Laboratory examination: Urinalysis - pH 6, specific gravity 1.015, protein 2+, glucose negative, blood large, RBC's too numerous to count, WBC's 25-30/HPF, casts 0-1/HPF (mixed cellular and red cell); hemoglobin electrophoresis was normal. BUN 17 mg/dl, creatinine 1.2 mg/dl, calcium 9.3 mg/dl, phosphorus 4.5 mg/dl, uric acid 4.7 mg/dl, sodium 139 mEq/L, potassium 4.6 mEq/L, chloride 106 mEq/L, CO_2 22 mEq/L, triglycerides 80 mg/dl, total protein 7.3 g/dl, albumin 3.4 g/dl, total bili 0.2 mg/dl, SGOT 14 U/L, SGPT 10 U/L, rheumatoid factor negative, ESR 54 mm/hr. Coombs test was negative. Cholesterol 114 mg/dl, serum iron 17 mg/dl (normal range 30-160), alk-phos. 138 units (normal range 30-115), serum globulins 3.9 g/dl (normal range 2-3.5). Urine protein:creatinine ratio 2.3 (nephrotic range > 1.2). C3 complement 227 mg/dl (normal range 90-230), C4 complement 44 mg/dl (normal range 11-35), ANA negative, Anti-DNA negative, Circulating Immune Complexes (C1Q) 55.5 mcg/dl (normal < 30), Anti GBM negative; Circulating Immune Complexes (Raji cells) < 6.25 mg/dl (normal < 12.5).

The patient underwent percutaneous right renal biopsy on July 26, 1984.

QUESTION: Do you have a chest x-ray and a TB test?

RESPONSE: TB was negative; chest x-ray just showed the asthenic character to the chest with a normal or even small-sized heart.

QUESTION: You do not describe and I am sure that you are not hiding a rash from us. Is that true?

RESPONSE: I searched this child for a rash and asked the parents and there was no history.

QUESTION: No spots?

RESPONSE: No. There was only a little discoloration around the ankles and over the feet. I think this was due to her rapid weight loss and relative malnutrition. Also, pulses were good throughout.

COMMENT: I think that the triad of fever, hepatomegaly and weight loss in this patient meets or is very suggestive of the diagnosis of malaria. Also, considering the area from where the patient comes, that is a very strong possibility that I think needs to be considered. It is well known that patients with malaria can present with the nephrotic syndrome. Also, these patients with chronic antigenemia can develop circulating immune complexes. In some of these cases, the circulating immune complexes can be trapped in the glomeruli; these patients can develop glomerulonephritis with nephrotic syndrome. So far, after reading the clinical history, I think that the possibility of secondary nephrotic syndrome due to malaria is one diagnosis to consider.

RESPONSE: I appreciate that suggestion. I think it is an excellent observation, one that we did not have to follow up but it certainly shows our limitations.

MODERATOR: We expect that the laboratory people, when they get a blood smear for white count and CBC, will look for malaria. And they have made that diagnosis for an American patient who went to Haiti. We do not see malaria, but that is a very good point.

COMMENT: Being an internist, I am not really well versed in the glycogen storage diseases or similar problems, but the pain that this patient had brings me to think of Faber's Disease.

COMMENT: I did not consider that at all. We did have a neurologist examine her and it seems that there probably was a psychological component to her inability to walk. After her biopsy, she had a miraculous recovery from this inability.

MODERATOR: But she did look in distress.

COMMENT: Yes. This was a very sick, chronically ill child.

MODERATOR: Immediately the thought of something systemic was entertained. Any other thoughts?

QUESTION: This patient had fever, hepatomegaly and hematuria. The other diagnostic possibility is schistosomiasis. The patient lived in South America. The problem of schistosomiasis with a glomerulonephritis and even with the nephrotic syndrome is more frequent in Brazil. Another possibility is that of a nephritic-nephrotic syndrome.

MODERATOR: We are not accustomed to thinking about those disorders. For that reason, among others, it is good to have people here from different countries.

COMMENT: Do you want to vote on some possibilities? How many think she had nephritic-nephrotic syndrome? A rapidly progressive glomerulonephritis, or membranoproliferative glomerulonephritis, or a vasculitic picture with possibly a polyarteritis?

COMMENT: This was our thought, but in our minds, she was presenting with a systemic vasculitic picture. We felt that this was totally consistent clinically and we did biopsy her although I have to say that our minds were pretty well settled on this particular diagnosis, having had some experience with other such cases and thinking that she was really quite consistent clinically. Her biopsy showed focal areas of proliferation, and most remarkably, there were areas of cariorrhexis, necrotizing lesions which would be consistent with a vasculitic process. We gave her the "Big Guns", sent her home, and hope that she is doing well.

MODERATOR: We heard from our friend in Colombia who is taking care of her, and apparently she is well controlled. The diagnosis of polyarteritis nodosa was made. It was such a severe disease with systemic involvement that we opted for the "Big Guns"--Prednisone and Cyclophosphamide.

COMMENT: Prednisone and Cyclophosphamide. We might, if anyone wants to, discuss those choices. It would be good to hear other people's opinion about the choice of drugs.

RESPONSE: I did not think that renal biopsy was the way to diagnose polyarteritis.

COMMENT: Well, in my old time in adult medicine, it was not but it seems helpful even if this is not a polyarteritis nodosa specifically. Although, certainly, that is a major diagnosis. It is in my mind a vasculitis and the biopsy is consistent with a vasculitis. The classical polyarteritis nodosa with lesions in the liver and lesions diagnosed by arteriography in the kidney, certainly is of the major vessel type and is found in adults. We do see the small vessel disease with which this biopsy was consistent.

COMMENT: I think that unless you really saw a medium-sized vessel with perivascular infiltrate, you could not call her polyarteritis nodosa. So the renal biopsy is not the way to make that diagnosis unless you like to have post biopsy bleeding. The size of the vessel you need to make the diagnosis is much larger than any of us want to stick a needle into and remove a piece of, at least, percutaneously. What you described was a necrotizing glomerulonephritis which certainly fits this clinical pattern. Hopefully the patient's underlying vasculitis will get better but it is a small vessel vasculitis unless you can prove that you have a medium-sized vessel--just a technical comment, in terms of the nomenclature.

MODERATOR: Thank you. We now go to Case number three which will be presented by Dr. Michael Freundlich.

DR. FREUNDLICH: This is not a diagnostic problem. It is an anecdotal experience which we would like to share with you and welcome any comments. It is really more an ethical problem, maybe a logistic problem, maybe a problem of attitude. This 3,300 g full-term baby girl was delivered by Caesarian section; a prenatal ultrasound had revealed an alive fetus with bilateral enlarged kidneys. The latter was confirmed after birth. The abdominal ultrasound and renal scan demonstrated a right obstructed hydronephrotic kidney and a left multicystic kidney, both with poor function. Despite right nephrostomy, the patient's clinical condition deteriorated; blood chemistries showed BUN 20 mg/dl, creatinine 6.5 mg/dl, calcium 7.8 mg/dl, phosphorus 7.4 mg/dl, sodium 139 mEq/L, potassium 4.5 mEq/L, total CO_2 18 mEq/L, PTH 150 ulEq/ml (normal 10-100).

A peritoneal Tenckhoff catheter was placed during the second week of life and continuous peritoneal dialysis (CPD) was initiated. The peritoneum was sutured around a single dacron felt cuff in a pursestring fashion and a 5 cm segment of catheter was buried in a subcutaneous tunnel. Following a brief break-in period during which small volumes of dialysate were instilled, 100 ml cycles eventually were employed. To deliver accurately this volume out of a 1,000 ml bag, a Y system was implemented. This design allowed changing the dialysate bag only once-a-day. Daily ultrafiltration averaged 260 ml using 8 daily three-hour cycles of the 4.25 g/dl dextrose dialysate. Hyponatremia (serum sodium 123 mEq/L) was corrected and subsequently prevented by supplemental sodium in amounts matching daily peritoneal losses ($\bar{x}$ 34 mEq/day). After two months of CPD, serum calcium and phosphorus remained normal and the PTH concentration was 145 μlEq/ml, without the administration of phosphate binders or calcium supplements. This is the summary of a rather stormy course. Several other problems developed; we could discuss them if the questions arise.

COMMENT: This is a very interesting problem which we are going to have to deal with more and more. In the past, when we were confronted with neonates with ESRD, very few people were willing to take them on because they required intermittent hemodialysis. Also, up until quite recently, the data on transplanting children under a year of age have been dismal. As a matter of fact, if one looks in the literature up until 1982 to 1983, there were reported approximately 15 to 20 children under a year of age who had been transplanted, and 80 percent of them, at the time of the reports, were dead. Now there is a recent paper or abstract from the people in Minnesota reporting nine children under a year of age, and the outcome was relatively good. But that is an isolated experience, and almost all their results were from live-related donor grafts. So, the issue that one is being confronted with is: if one assumes responsibility for the care of a one-week-old, two-week-old, one-month-old with ESRD, what are the end points? When should one propose that the patient be transplanted? And more importantly, when one sits down and discusses the options with the parents, what should one tell them with regard to the ultimate outcome? This is very difficult because there are very few data on what the long-term outcome is in children of this age who have been subjected to ESRD. My personal attitude would have been to do essentially what you have done, with the following exception: you did not indicate what the interaction was with the parents which precipitated your desire to proceed. I would take my cues from what the parents want. I would try to sit down with them and paint about as dismal a picture as I could paint. My experience has been that it does not make any differences; you can tell them that the chances are one in a million and the only thing they hear is that there is a good chance that their child will be the one who is going to do well. They forget about the million that are not going to do well. That is, many parents selectively hear what you tell them. But, if they want to proceed, I personally see nothing wrong with proceeding. The other factor you mentioned is that if you are dialyzing a young child, you have to worry about the sodium. The amount of sodium that you lose in the dialysate is proportionate to the amount of ultrafiltrate you have. As you want to give them more and more calories, you are going to give them more and more fluids, and if they are oliguric, you are going to have to ultrafiltrate a lot. The more ultrafiltering you do, the more sodium the patient loses and the more he has to be supplemented. You pointed that out in your talk, but I think it is worthwhile emphasizing because the first time it happens to you, you are not quite sure why this child is so hyponatremic. And you really have to supplement him quite a bit. You can decide exactly how much you want to supplement by just calculating the difference between the sodium in the spent dialysate and that which he actually loses.

RESPONSE: I think your point about the rapport with the family and interaction is crucial. This was a couple who was 100 percent committed to the care of their child. They knew exactly what they were dealing with because they had a prenatal evaluation. They decided to continue that pregnancy at all cost and once the diagnosis was confirmed, they were 100 percent committed to the entire care of this child. They were completely engaged in all types of prospective planning for that child.

COMMENT: I just want to say two things now. First, I respect the previous commentator, and his frank opinions about the approach to these parents and patients very much because he obviously has a tremendous amount of experience and understands how these parents are thinking. Second, I want to talk about sodium from a nutritional point of view. In basic nutritional thought, if you are going to retain nitrogen, you have to retain it in set proportions to other nutrients. If you do not have those nutrients available--specifically phosphorus, potassium and sodium--then you will not attain growth; if those nutrients are deficient, which frequently they are in these long term diets and patients who are depleted, then the patient will not grow. We have to give them adequate minerals including sodium and potassium.

COMMENT: I also respect what you said but I am sure there are people in the audience who will have a different view about how to approach the ethical problem presented by this baby. I wonder what establishes a healthier balance at home and effective interrelationships among the parents and child, knowing that the prognosis is abysmal or hoping that maybe something good might be at the end.

MODERATOR: Do you have the answers to those questions?

RESPONSE: The problem is not the reality of the situation, at least in my experience. No matter what you say to parents, and no matter how dismal the outlook you provide, they hear what they want to hear. Once they have made the decision, they are like any other parents. They are up and down, depending on how the child does. If the child is doing well, then they are up; if there are a lot of problems, then they are depressed. I do not think that they look to the future in their everyday activities or concern themselves about what is going to happen a year, two or three from that moment, once they have made the decision. My point is that in most instances, no matter how honest we try to be, parents still will ask: "Well, what else can you do?" And, if there is nothing else, then, "Do whatever you can". We have certain abilities and we need to be honest with patients and their families, and let them know what is available. I personally feel that it is dishonest to say that for a two-week-old infant there is nothing available, there is nothing to do. But it is also important when you are telling the parents what is available, to paint the picture as the picture is. According to the literature, taking on a two-week-old is an awesome responsibility because what you can offer these parents long-term, even five years, is a huge question mark. There are so little data as to what the outlook is for a two-week-old once you start end stage care. I think that is what you need to tell them. You also need to tell them all the other potential problems that they are going to get involved with along the line, including the fact that there may be severe growth retardation and bone disease despite everything we do, and so on. Even after you tell them all that, they only hear one thing--that is, yes, you have something you can do and if you do nothing, their child is going to die.

COMMENT: I would like to obliquely address part of the same issue. I am very concerned about maternal/child and paternal/child interactions and the effect these have on the new addition to a family and existing siblings. Could you comment, or anyone else who has dialyzed newborns chronically, on how this has impacted on a family in a very important period of its life?

RESPONSE: That is a critical issue, a critical point. I can tell you the experience we have with three infants. In one instance, prior to delivery there was full commitment of both parents. Following delivery of the baby, there was full commitment of the mother, much less support on the part of the father; there was some distancing among the father and mother throughout the period. Progressively, the mother took a predominant role in the care and the father a much more observant role, not very supportive. In the second infant, the beginning was very similar. The mother was probably the best nurse you can imagine for CAPD and there was an exquisitely strong bonding between child and mother. Again, the father was not playing a very supportive role. In the third infant, my personal feeling is that neither mother nor father are playing a very important role in the establishment of a healthy bond; in addition, I think that the mother is progressively withdrawing in the care of this child. It is a very complex issue. The impact on the family is tremendous, and the situation is very tough even for the strongest parents imaginable.

COMMENT: I give you four anecdotal bits of information about three children under a year of age whom we dialyzed, two of them for over 18 months. Both of those mothers (they were the ones who took almost all responsibility for the care), became pregnant during this period of time. So, obviously, the family relationship was relatively good. In one family, there was an older sibling and the mother was about seven or eight months pregnant. In the second family, there were some teenage siblings from a previous marriage and this baby with the renal failure, and the mother got pregnant. In the third one, the child had oxalosis and the family could not decide what to do. The impact is there. One can sit down and begin to contemplate about all the problems ahead and I think we have seen them all. But there is also the possibility that despite this, families will go on and have a relatively normal existence.

COMMENT: To continue in the anecdotal train, we have had this problem in our unit. We have been very realistic in presenting the data to the parents. Specifically, we had a pair of 1,100 gram premature twins with bilateral cortical necrosis in each of them and we presented the data to the parents with the uncertainties noted here. In this instance and nearly all others, the parents have chosen not to continue. There are two aspects of this which I think are critical. My prediction would be for your three families, where the parents are withdrawn and the parent-child interaction is very poor, that child will not develop either psychosocially or in terms of body length, etc. You are going to find that this is a very important and crucial aspect. This is something we need to think about a great deal—that parent-child interaction in early infancy is going to be very, very important. The second point I want to share with you is some papers that I have been asked to review. It has come to my attention that some infant formulas have a lot of aluminum in them. It is critical to realize that some of the formulas you are using may have a fair amount of aluminum in the preparation. It is not very much and, obviously, in a normal newborn this is going to be excreted by the kidneys fairly rapidly. But in these infants where the removal of aluminum is impaired (these children are not making urine), there are going to be problems. This is another piece you need to add to the formula--not to the feeding formula, but to the overall picture. Hopefully, as more information comes out about the effects from aluminum in formula, formula manufacturers will see that the aluminum is removed.

QUESTION: May I ask one related question? How do the people here feel about putting on dialysis a fairly significantly retarded child, 10 years old, who goes into end stage?

MODERATOR: We have two. One right now and we had one around Christmas time.

RESPONSE: That is a question for a one day seminar--a really tough one. There are many answers: a legal answer, an ethical answer, a medical answer. It depends upon your approach, where you practice medicine, what your ethical, religious, moral beliefs are. That is such a complicated issue, I really do not have an answer to the question.

RESPONSE: I have had several experiences in two different places--one was when I was in another institution and had very little to say about a patient who was significantly retarded and hyperactive but was definitely the love object and very cohesive force in the family. When I presented the child for dialysis, she was refused treatment and that was that. To tell you the truth, in that situation perhaps all was in the presentation to the family because it ended all right. The verdict was accepted and the child's course was a natural course. On the other hand, my more recent association is not dissimilar from the approach mentioned earlier. It is the most fair to the physicians, the nurses, the family and the patient to be very frank about the situation, to let the parents be participants in the decision, to not render verdicts, so to speak, but to allow everyone to realize what it means to offer treatment to a child who probably will not be a candidate for transplantation and who ultimately is not rehabilitatible.

MODERATOR: It is very important to realize that what is needed is a team effort. I was impressed by the strength of the parents in the case of this child whom we allowed to die, how the nurses on the floor knew the mechanics of how to facilitate all the family's interaction and reduce their suffering as much as possible. The nurses were very effectively respectful and helpful to all who were suffering in that complicated situation.

COMMENT-QUESTION: I think that we have two obligations in dealing with families like this one. The first is that we should tell them the truth, that in fact it is feasible to embark on a therapeutic program. The second is what was alluded to a little bit earlier: to tell the parents that this is not a conventional form of therapy. From our perspective, dialysis therapy for the newborn is still experimental and the parents have to recognize that it is not easy to get them to listen to what you say. We should not regard it as a conventional form of therapy and should make parents recognize the fact that it is heroic therapy, outside the norm, because technology outstrips viability in this situation. Until we know that viability can match the technology of being able to do something, we have to worry about the situation we are getting the family into.

MODERATOR: Would you go as far as considering this a research project and asking the Committee for the Protection of Human Subjects for approval?

RESPONSE: We have had a lot of experience at our institution with both the Committee for Human Investigation and the Ethics Committee, appointed because of our notorious problems in taking care of newborns and handicapped individuals. My own experience is that neither committee will be of much help to you. It is your personal relationship with the family, your ability to relate to them on a one-to-one basis, and understanding of that family interaction which is not easy if you have not seen them. Most often, our Ethics Committee meets at least two or three times and by then the child is either too sick to be treated or the decision has been made.

COMMENT: There is one other issue that has to be dealt with. That is the parent who says: "I have a child who is slightly retarded and I do not want him to be dialyzed because he is never going to be perfect and I will accept nothing less than a perfect child". Do you accept the parents' decision in that case? Despite the fact that there is therapy available, they do not want to take advantage of it because they are going to be saddled with imperfection?

MODERATOR: In the State of Florida in particular and the United States as a whole, it is illegal to withhold proven therapies for mild (or even severe) mental retardation.

COMMENT: We had a nine-year old boy who had an I.Q. of 70 or 80, and the father said he did not want to have the child dialyzed; of course, the child mimicked everything the father said. The court said it is okay, whatever the father wants is acceptable.

RESPONSE: We as physicians and pediatric nephrologists taking care of those problems have to define our limitations and I very strongly believe that there are problems in terms of psychological bonding, etc., social problems, that we cannot handle. A very rude truth is that we do not have the time to deal with these problems. We need the help of paramedical personnel to be effective in assisting those families. We cannot do it alone.

MODERATOR: Thank you. We go now to the final patient, our fourth case, who will be presented by Dr. Warren Grupe.

DR. GRUPE: M.D. was born after 33 weeks gestation, delivered by Caesarian section following the spontaneous initiation of premature labor. Oligohydramnios was noted in the third trimester by ultrasonography performed because of small maternal size. Apgar score was 8 at one minute and 9 at five minutes. She had mild respiratory distress treated with two days of supplemental O_2. Her urine output was noted to be low and unresponsive to furosemide. Serum creatinine was 3.2 mg/dl on day three and 8 mg/dl on day 11 at a time when BUN was 54 mg/dl, potassium 9.0 mEq/L; phosphorus 7.6 mg/dl and calcium 8 mg/dl.

She was transferred for further care on her 11th day of life. Weight was 2,200 gm, length was 41 cm, pulse - 120/min, blood pressure 64 mmHg/palp. Both kidneys were palpable and firm; bladder was not palpable. Admission laboratory in serum: BUN - 47 mg/dl, creatinine - 8.4 mg/dl, sodium 129 mEq/L, potassium 4.8 mEq/L, chloride 98 mEq/L, bicarbonate 11.7 mEq/L, calcium 9.3 mg/dl, and phosphorus 7.2 mg/dl. Abdominal ultrasonography demonstrated bilaterally small and echogenic kidneys without hydronephrosis. Voiding cystourethrogram failed to demonstrate vesicoureteral reflux; the bladder and its outlet appeared normal. Kidneys failed to visualize by radionuclide scan.

By discharge, without dialytic therapy, her BUN was 12 mg/dl and her serum creatinine was 6.8 mg/dl. How is this possible? What should be her management and clinical course following discharge? The family was in a dilemma. The mother was faced with the circumstances of one set of in-laws praying and saying everything would be fine; the other set of in-laws saying, "Don't you dare buy a crib. This is not a keeper, throw it back and go fishing again". The child, in fact, looked fine. Potassium was brought under control very quickly with Kayexalate; bicarbonate was brought under control very quickly with Bicarbonate; phosphorus, it seems, was brought under some control by decreasing intake. Please notice several things about her: first of all, we put her on a formula. This formula was designed to increase her protein and caloric intake; protein intake was increased to create an anabolic phase for this infant. Our hope at that point was that by creating an anabolic state we would decrease the urea load by creating a positive nitrogen balance. The other circumstance is that this was an infant with horrible renal function. If it were taken on a per kilo basis, a serum creatinine of 8 mg/dl for this child is about a 40 for me. The idea was that if we could create this positive balance, we also could create circumstances that would allow compensatory hypertrophy to take place. The only thing that has been known to interfere with compensatory hypertrophy of the kidney is actually a protein restricted state. This was a circumstance that we have had on several occasions with infants, certainly not one with a creatinine of 8 mg/dl. But by creating anabolic conditions, we have been able to enhance their compensatory hypertrophy and see a course very similar to what happened in this child. The fact that her BUN fell from 47 to 12 mg/dl, despite her being on a formula (#1) which was basically a PM 60-40 formula, was gratifying to us. The hope was that if we put her in an anabolic state, despite the fact that she had such a high intake of protein, her BUN would fall; since it fell, that was evidence of her anabolism. At the same time that she became anabolic, her phosphorus fell from 7.2 to 2.8 mg/dl. We have seen this happen on several other occasions, including one child who became hypophosphatemic and phosphorus supplements had to be started. Nobody had remembered to take the child off the aluminum hydroxide. If you ever want to see pharmacologic ping-pong, see aluminum hydroxide given with phosphorus. The aluminum really works; it holds to even phosphorus supplement! She also, as she became anabolic, got out of her acidosis because she was away from her nitrogen breakdown. Her bicarbonate was stopped and she was continued on that formula for a period of time. As her BUN fell, her serum creatinine continued to fall; she remained in some degree of balance. As her formula intake increased, her caloric intake increased and suddenly by the end of two and half months, we saw the BUN take a jump at the same time that her serum creatinine had fallen; it still is continuing to fall. At that point, we put her on formula #2 which removed the protein supplement she was on. Formula #1 was PM 60-40 plus Polycose plus corn oil plus a casein hydrolysate supplement. We took the protein out; her BUN came back down and we noticed that by three and a half months of age, she had a BUN of 9 mg/dl and a serum creatinine of 3.9 mg/dl. It is usually around four to six months of age that we have seen the maximum compensatory hypertrophy. Serum creatinine will level off at whatever level it is and then, at a period of time later, begin to have an increase as renal function continues to deteriorate. We saw that with her, at about four and half months of age; her creatinine had bottomed, out and then begun to turn around. Some of that may be from an increase in muscle mass; but I can tell you from following the child a little bit longer that the creatinine has continued to climb and she is going to be ready for some form of therapy. The fact is that this works. By four months we started her on vitamin D. Later on she was started later on calcium carbonate. Formula #3 was made by just reducing the amount of carbohydrate supplement that she was receiving. This works under severe circumstances, very severe renal insufficiency. We saw a pattern of catch-up growth in terms of weight, length, and weight for height. We were able to maintain her intake to balance her weight for height; that was of concern to us. For a period of time, her head circumference increased rapidly. We have seen this in several children including some with congenital nephrotic syndrome who have been very well managed: that, I think, is brain growth. We were worried for a while with that rate of growth; we were afraid we were doing something else. She is at the 90th percentile for head circumference, which makes me a little bit concerned. She eventually will need some form of therapy. My guess is that whatever form of dialytic therapy she will need, it will be by about 10 months of age. By that time maternal and paternal bonding to this child will have taken place. The mother and father are both very clear in their commitment to the child; one set of grandparents is still praying and the other set is still saying throw it back, you have to go fishing again.

COMMENT: These two cases provide a very interesting contrast. One of the infants was dialyzed and the other not. Strictly, by biochemical parameters, it would be difficult to say that patient number one had worse renal failure at the time dialysis was initiated than the case just presented. The second case, managed very carefully, did remarkably well. What should be the indications for initiating dialysis in a newborn infant or a very young infant?

RESPONSE: I am for holding off on dialysis as long as the urine volume is good. We can do a tremendous amount nutritionally and at least we ought to be given the opportunity. So, my bias is to go for nutritional supplementation, then see what we can do as long as urine volume is not a problem. A lot of time in these babies, it is not a problem. In the other baby that was presented, urine volume was a problem; she was effectively anuric and, therefore, there was little choice. If they do not have a good urine volume, it is hard to feed them. The last baby exemplifies what I call fantastic treatment; you were giving high amounts of protein, but low percent protein calories. Again, this reinforces the inviolate fact that the protein:energy ratio is essential in the treatment of uremic patients. The key question is something that has kept me worried for a long time. When we talk about the hyperfiltration theory, all the studies that have been done thus far, to substantiate or not the noxious effect of protein intake, have looked at the absolute protein intake as opposed to the aberrations in protein:energy ratios in rats and patients with protein loads. Every time the question has been studied, it has been studied outside the issue of protein:energy ratio.

QUESTION: Along those lines, of course, this is the opposite of the Giovanetti diet and similar diets. A lot of people feel that that diet has worked because as they reduce protein calories, they increase other calories. Do you think they have been looking at the wrong thing all along?

RESPONSE: Yes, I do. It says that what we need to do is reduce protein intake in order to get a low urea or low nitrogen balance. I do not know of any data that show that that does anything for anybody. The most common secondary reason for dying on dialysis in the European Dialysis and Transplant Society Study has been malnutrition. The criterion I would use for starting dialysis in a child like this, would be if we had tried to do something like this and it did not work, if we had tried to increase her protein intake, tried to create a positive nitrogen balance and, for some reason, were unable to attain it. Then, we would have seen a climbing urea and inability to control serum phosphorus, potassium, and bicarbonate. The fact that we were able to create the anabolic state, I think, is what brought this child out of that. We use the urea to monitor how much protein we ought to give. We aim at a protein as a percent of kilo calories which is very close to what we would give in a normal formula for a child of this age. What we were doing really was giving this child something that was beefed up, and, then, monitoring what we were doing, in terms of both growth and weight for height. I do not want to advocate that children with creatinines of 8 mg/dl ought to be treated by dietary means. That was because of the circumstance of this particular infant. I would point out to you, though, that this experience is not unique and I would refer you also to about eight or nine patients that were reported at the ASN about two years ago by the group at Cornell and subsequently published; they showed exactly the same sort of thing. Some of these infants who look as if they are at the end of the earth when they are first born, if one relies on compensatory hypertrophy and does something to enhance it, these children can go on for a surprisingly long period of time. That was what prompted my comment, "when you get one of these kids that are blowing out their lungs, if you can, in fact, maintain their oxygenation, do not give up on them". In a fair number of these infants one can maintain some balances like this, not only for survival, but to get the kind of growth that has occurred here.

MODERATOR: On that optimistic note, we will call it a day. Thank you.

PARTICIPANTS

and

INDEXES

PARTICIPANTS

Program Chairman

Jose Strauss, M.D., Professor of Pediatrics; Director, Division of Pediatric Nephrology, University of Miami School of Medicine, Miami, Florida.

Guest Faculty

Sidney Blumenthal, M.D., Former Director of the Division of Heart and Vascular Diseases of the National Heart, Lung and Blood Institute, National Institutes of Health, Bethesda, Maryland; New York, New York.

Joan P. Chesney, M.D., Associate Professor of Pediatrics; Head, Pediatric Infectious Diseases, University of Wisconsin, Madison, Wisconsin.

Russell Chesney, M.D., Professor of Pediatrics; Director, Division of Pediatric Nephrology, University of Wisconsin Hospital, Madison, Wisconsin.

Richard N. Fine, M.D., Professor of Pediatrics; Head, Division of Pediatric Nephrology, UCLA Center for the Health Sciences, Los Angeles, California.

Warren Grupe, M.D., Associate Professor of Pediatrics; Director, Division of Pediatric Nephrology, Harvard Medical School, The Children's Hospital, Boston, Massachusetts.

Alan Gruskin, M.D., Professor and Chairman, Department of Pediatrics, Wayne State University School of Medicine; Pediatrician-in-Chief, Children's Hospital of Michigan, Detroit, Michigan.

Julie R. Ingelfinger, M.D., Assistant Professor of Pediatrics; Director, Hypertension Clinic, Division of Pediatric Nephrology, Harvard Medical School, The Children's Hospital, Boston, Massachusetts.

Abdollah Iravani, M.D., Associate Professor of Pediatrics, University of Florida College of Medicine, Gainesville, Florida.

Barry D. Kahan, M.D., Ph.D., Professor of Surgery; Director, Division of Immunology and Organ Transplantation, University of Texas Medical School, Houston, Texas.

Peter O. Kwiterovich, M.D., Professor of Pediatrics and Medicine, Lipid Research-Atherosclerosis Division, Department of Pediatrics, The Johns Hopkins University School of Medicine, Baltimore, Maryland.

Norman J. Siegel, M.D., Professor of Pediatrics and Medicine; Director, Section of Pediatric Nephrology; Vice Chairman, Department of Pediatrics, Yale University School of Medicine, New Haven, Connecticut.

Kirsti Thodenius, M.D. Department of Pediatrics, University of Umea, Sweden.

Local Faculty

Carolyn Abitbol, M.D., Assistant Professor of Pediatrics, Division of Pediatric Nephrology, University of Miami School of Medicine, Miami, Florida.

Jacques J. Bourgoignie, M.D. Professor of Medicine; Chief, Division of Nephrology, University of Miami School of Medicine, Miami, Florida.

Cherry Charlton, R.N., Head Nurse, Pediatric Dialysis Unit, Division of Pediatric Nephrology, Jackson Memorial Hospital, Miami, Florida.

Rosa Diaz, R.N., CAPD Charge Nurse, Pediatric Dialysis Unit, Division of Pediatric Nephrology, Jackson Memorial Hospital, Miami, Florida.

Michael Freundlich, M.D., Assistant Professor of Pediatrics, Division of Pediatric Nephrology, University of Miami School of Medicine, Miami, Florida. (As of August 1985, in private practice in Miami, Florida.)

George K. Kyriakides, M.D., Associate Professor of Surgery, Division of Transplantation, University of Miami School of Medicine, Miami, Florida.

Jorge Lockhart, M.D., Associate Professor of Urology, University of Miami School of Medicine, Miami, Florida.

Joshua Miller, M.D., Professor of Surgery and Microbiology; Director, Division of Transplantation, University of Miami School of Medicine, Miami, Florida.

Victoriano Pardo, M.D., Professor of Pathology; Director, Renal Laboratory, Veterans Administration Medical Center, Miami, Florida.

Victor A. Politano, M.D., Professor and Chairman, Department of Urology, University of Miami School of Medicine, Miami, Florida.

Catherine A. Poole, M.D., Professor and Chairman, Department of Radiology, University of Miami School of Medicine, Miami, Florida.

Gwendolyn B. Scott, M.D., Associate Professor of Pediatrics; Head, Infectious Diseases, Division of Pediatric Immunology, Allergy and Infectious Diseases, University of Miami School of Medicine, Miami, Florida.

George N. Sfakianakis, M.D., Associate Professor of Radiology, Division of Nuclear Medicine, Department of Radiology, University of Miami School of Medicine, Miami, Florida.

Jose Strauss, M.D., Professor of Pediatrics; Director, Division of Pediatric Nephrology, University of Miami School of Medicine, Miami, Florida.

Carlos A. Vaamonde, M.D., Professor of Medicine; Chief, Renal Section, Veterans Administration Medical Center, Miami, Florida.

Gaston Zilleruelo, M.D., Associate Professor of Pediatrics, Division of Pediatric Nephrology, University of Miami School of Medicine, Miami, Florida.

Other Contributors *

Susan B. Conley, M.D., Associate Professor of Pediatrics, Department of Pediatrics, University of Texas Health and Science Center, Medical School, Houston, Texas.

Nuria Dominguez, M.D., Visiting Fellow, Division of Pediatric Nephrology, Department of Pediatrics, University of Miami School of Medicine, Miami, Florida.

Larry E. Fleischmann, M.D., Director of Nephrology, Children's Hospital of Michigan, Detroit, Michigan.

Stuart M. Flechner, M.D., Associate Professor of Surgery, Division of Immunology and Organ Transplantation, University of Texas Health and Science Center , Medical School, Houston, Texas.

Marianne Fordyce, M.D., Associate Professor, Division of Nutrition, Department of Epidemiology and Public Health, University of Miami School of Medicine, Miami, Florida.

Karen M. Gaudio, M.D., Assistant Professor of Pediatrics; Director, End-Stage Renal Disease Program, Division of Pediatric Nephrology, Department of Pediatrics, Yale University School of Medicine, New Haven, Connecticut.

William E. Harmon, M.D., Director, Dialysis Unit, The Children's Hospital, Division of Pediatric Nephology, Department of Pediatrics, Harvard Medical School, Boston, Massachusetts.

S. L. Hsia, Ph.D., Professor, Department of Dermatology and Cutaneous Surgery, University of Miami School of Medicine, Miami, Florida.

Heinz E. Leichter, M.D., Head Fellow, Division of Pediatric Nephrology, Department of Pediatrics, UCLA Center for the Health Sciences, Los Angeles, California.

Gary Lerner, M.D., Assistant Professor of Pediatrics, Children's Hospital of Michigan, Detroit, Michigan.

Mark I. Lorber, M.D., Assistant Professor of Surgery, Division of Immunology and Organ Transplantation, University of Texas Health and Science Center, Medical School, Houston, Texas.

Milan Novak, Ph.D., Associate Professor of Pediatrics, Department of Pediatrics, University of Miami School of Medicine, Miami, Florida.

Antonia C. Novello, M.D., M.P.H, Deputy Director, National Institute of Child Health and Human Development, National Institutes of Health, Bethesda, Maryland.

Isidro B. Salusky, M.D., Assistant Professor of Pediatrics, Division of Pediatric Nephrology, Department of Pediatrics, UCLA Center for the Health Sciences, Los Angeles, California.

Nancy Spinozzi, Renal Dietitian, Dialysis Unit, The Children's Hospital, Boston, Massachusetts.

Charles T. Van Buren, M.D., Associate Professor in Surgery, Division of Immunology and Organ Transplantation, University of Texas Health and Science Center, Medical School, Houston, Texas.

* Co-authors

AUTHOR INDEX

SUBJECT INDEX

GPSR Compliance

The European Union's (EU) General Product Safety Regulation (GPSR) is a set of rules that requires consumer products to be safe and our obligations to ensure this.

If you have any concerns about our products, you can contact us on ProductSafety@springernature.com

In case Publisher is established outside the EU, the EU authorized representative is:

Springer Nature Customer Service Center GmbH
Europaplatz 3
69115 Heidelberg, Germany

Batch number: 10755284

Printed by Printforce, the Netherlands